CARING FOR
HEALTH: HISTORY AND
DIVERSITY

Edited by Charles Webster

PUBLISHED BY
IN ASSOCIATION   UNIVERSITY

 OPEN UNIVERSITY PRESS

 Health and Disease Series, Book 6

The U205 Health and Disease Course Team

The following members of the Open University teaching staff have collaborated with the authors in writing this book, or have commented extensively on it during its production. We accept collective responsibility for its overall academic and teaching content.

Basiro Davey (Course Team Chair, Lecturer in Health Studies, Biology)

David Boswell (Senior Lecturer in Sociology)

Gerald Elliott (Professor of Bio-physics)

Kevin McConway (Senior Lecturer in Statistics)

Perry Morley (Senior Editor, Science)

Clive Seale (Lecturer in Sociology, Goldsmiths' College, University of London, U205 Tutor)

Steven Swithenby (Senior Lecturer in Physics)

The following have contributed to the development of particular parts or aspects of this book.

Sylvia Abbey (course secretary)

Steve Best (graphic artist)

Lucille Eveleigh (course co-ordinator)

John Greenwood (librarian)

Pam Higgins (designer)

Jean MacQueen (indexer)

Eleanor Morris (BBC producer)

Rissa de la Paz (BBC producer)

Liz Sugden (BBC production assistant)

Doreen Tucker (text processing compositor)

Authors

The following are principal authors for the chapters listed below, or have contributed material on certain historical periods or geographical areas as indicated, and have also contributed extensively to the structure and philosophy of the book as a whole.

Chapters 1 and 10, the structure of the National Health Service in Chapters 6 and 7, and Academic Editor for the book

Charles Webster, Fellow of All Souls College, Oxford.

16th–19th-century health care in Britain, in Chapters 2-4; co-ordinator for Chapters 2-4

Margaret Pelling, Deputy Director, Wellcome Unit for the History of Medicine, Oxford.

16th–mid-20th-century health care in continental Europe, in Chapters 3-5

Paul Weindling, Senior Research Officer, Wellcome Unit for the History of Medicine, Oxford.

16th–mid-20th-century health care in the European colonies, in Chapters 2-5

Mark Harrison, Research Fellow, Wellcome Institute for the History of Medicine, London.

20th-century health care in Britain, in Chapters 4-7; co-ordinator for Chapters 5-7

Virginia Berridge, Senior Lecturer in History, Health Policy Unit, Department of Public Health and Policy, London School of Hygiene and Tropical Medicine.

Chapter 8, and 20th-century health care in the Third World in Chapter 6

Gill Walt, Senior Lecturer in Health Policy, Health Policy Unit, Department of Public Health and Policy, London School of Hygiene and Tropical Medicine.

Chapter 9

Alastair Gray, Research Associate, Centre for Socio-Legal Studies, Wolfson College, Oxford.

Co-ordinator, Chapters 8 and 9

Basiro Davey, Lecturer in Health Studies, Department of Biology, Open University.

External Assessors

Course assessor

Professor James McEwen, Henry Mechan Chair of Public Health and Head of Department of Public Health, University of Glasgow.

Book 6 assessors

Professor David Arnold, Head of Department of History, School of Oriental and African Studies, University of London.

Dr Carol Barker, Senior Lecturer in Health Planning, The Nuffield Institute for Health Service Studies, University of Leeds.

Dr Anne Crowther, Reader in Economic History, Department of Economic History, University of Glasgow.

Professor Jane Lewis, Professor of Social Policy, Department of Social Science and Administration, The London School of Economics and Political Science.

Dr David Parkin, Senior Lecturer in Health Economics, Department of Epidemiology and Public Health, The Medical School, University of Newcastle-upon-Tyne.

Acknowledgements

The Course Team and the authors wish to thank the following who, as contributors to the first edition of this book, made a lasting impact on the present volume.

Nick Black, Robert Dingwall, Jennie Popay, Steven Rose, Phil Strong.

We also wish to thank the following for their advice and assistance in preparing the present volume.

Dr A. Batty Shaw
Professor David Hunter
Deborah McGovern
Emilie Savage-Smith

The Open University Press, Celtic Court, 22 Ballmoor, Buckingham, MK18 1XW.

First published 1985. This completely revised edition first published 1993. Reprinted 1995.

A catalogue record of the book is available from the British Library.

Library of Congress Cataloging-in-Publication Data

Caring for health: history and diversity/edited by Charles Webster.
— Rev. ed.

   p. cm. — (Health and disease series; book 6)

Includes bibliographical references and index.

ISBN 0–335–19118–5 (pb): £12.99

1. Social medicine. 2. Medical care—History. 3. Medical care—Great Britain—History. 4. Medical care—Europe—History. 5. Medical care—America—History. 6. Public health—History. I. Webster, Charles, 1936– . II. Series.

RA418.C34 1993

362.1'09—dc20   92–45734

                                                          CIP

Edited, designed and typeset by the Open University.

Printed in the United Kingdom by Page Bros, Norwich.

ISBN 0 335 19118 5

This text forms part of an Open University Second Level Course. If you would like a copy of *Studying with the Open University*, please write to the Central Enquiry Service, PO Box 200, The Open University, Walton Hall, Milton Keynes, MK7 2YZ.

2.2

5705C/u205b6i2.1

Grateful acknowledgement is made to the following sources for permission to reproduce material in this book:

Figures

Figure 1.1 Käthe Kollwitz Museum, Berlin; *Figure 1.2 a, b, d, f, g* Dr A. Batty Shaw; *Figure 1.2c* Norfolk Museums Service/Norwich Castle Museum; *Figure 1.3* Deutscher Archaeologischer Institut, Rome; *Figures 1.4, 1.6* Morley, D., Rohde, J. and Williams, G. (1983), *Practising Health For All*, Oxford University Press; *Figure 1.5* Lithograph by A. F. Tait/British Railways Board. From *Charles Dickens: An Exhibition To Commemorate The Centenary Of His Death*, June–September 1970, exhibition catalogue, Victoria and Albert Museum; *Figure 2.1* Bibliothèque Nationale, Paris; *Figures 2.2, 2.3, 2.6, 2.9* Reproduced from *Medicine and the Artist (Ars Medica)* by permission of the Philadelphia Museum of Art; *Figure 2.4* Herzog August Bibliothek, Wolfenbüttel; *Figure 2.5* Bayerische Staatsgemäldesammlungen; *Figures 2.7, 2.8, 3.6* Wellcome Institute Library, London; *Figures 2.10, 3.2, 4.14, 5.7, 6.5* Hulton/Deutsch Picture Collection; *Figure 2.11* Peabody Museum, Harvard University; *Figure 2.12* Wilberforce House Museum/Hull City Museums and Art Gallery; *Figure 2.13* British Museum; *Figures 3.1a, 4.9, 4.15* Punch; *Figures 3.1b, 3.8* Mary Evans Picture Library; *Figures 3.3a, 5.1* Mackintosh, J. (1944), *The Nation's Health*, The Pilot Press; *Figure 3.3b* University College Library; *Figure 3.4* illustration from Fabre, A. F. H. (1840), *Némésis Médicale Illustrée*, revised ed.; *Figure 3.10* British Library, London; *Figures 4.3, 4.5* Royal Pharmaceutical Society of Great Britain; *Figure 4.4* Royal Holloway and Bedford New College, University of London; *Figure 4.6* Gwynedd Archives Service; *Figure 4.7* Llewellyn Davies, M. (1978), *Maternity*, Virago Press Ltd; *Figure 4.8* Illustrated London News; *Figure 4.10* Shellard P. (1970), *Factory Life 1774–1885*, HarperCollins Publishers; *Figure 4.13* Greater London Photograph Library; *Figure 4.17* Church Missionary Society; *Figure 4.18* Medical Missionary, Vol. 8, No. 9, Bodleian Library, Oxford; *Figures 5.2, 5.3, 5.9* Age Exchange/Alec Schweitzer; *Figure 5.4* The Boots Company plc, Nottingham; *Figure 5.5* Loudon, I. (1991), On maternal and infant mortality 1900–1960, *Social History of Medicine*, **4**(1), © Society for Social History of Medicine; *Figure 5.6* M'Gonigle, G. and Kirby, J. (1936), *Poverty and Public Health*, Victor Gollancz; *Figure 5.8* Greater London Photograph Library; *Figure 5.10* Dorien Leigh/The Pilot Press; *Figure 5.11* Sport and General/The Pilot Press; *Figure 5.12* Indian Medical Gazette, June 1923; *Figure 5.13* Courtesy of the Rockefeller Archive Centre; *Figures 6.1, 6.3* Central Office of Information & Ministry of Health (1948), *The New National Health Service*, reproduced with the permission of the Controller of Her Majesty's Stationery Office; *Figure 6.2* Courtesy of Mrs Carol Ann Danes, c/o Needham & Grant, London; *Figure 6.4* Jean Mohr; *Figure 6.6* Brook Advisory Centre; *Figure 6.7* Saatchi & Saatchi; *Figure 6.8a* WHO/photo by P. N. Sharma; *Figure 6.8b* WHO/photo by Eric Schwab; *Figure 6.9* Diesfield, H. J. and Hecklau, H. K. (1978), *Kenya: A Geomedical Monograph*, Springer–Verlag; *Figure 7.2* Bradford Telegraph & Argus; *Figure 7.5* Vicki White/Photo Co-Op; *Figure 7.7* Times Newspapers Ltd; *Figures 8.1, 8.2, 8.3, 8.6, 8.8, 8.10a* Panos Pictures; *Figure 8.4* Tom Learmonth/Christian Aid; *Figure 8.5* Photograph courtesy of Teaching Aids at Low Cost (TALC), P. O. Box 49, St Albans; *Figure 8.9* Health Division of Ghana Armed Forces; *Figure 8.10b* Tom Learmonth; *Figures 9.10, 9.11* OXFAM.

Tables

Tables 3.1, 3.2 Flinn, M. W. (1965), *Report On The Sanitary Condition of the Labouring Population of Great Britain 1842*, by Edwin Chadwick, Edinburgh University Press; *Table 4.1* Maggs, C. J. (1983), *The Origins of General Nursing*, Croom Helm; *Table 4.2* Lewis, J. (1980), *The Politics of Motherhood*, Croom Helm; *Table 4.3* Scull, A. (1979), *Museums of Madness: The Social Organisation of Insanity in 19th Century England*, Reprinted by permission of the Peters, Fraser and Dunlop Group Ltd; *Table 5.1* Eckstein, H. (1958), *The English Health Service*, Oxford University Press; *Table 7.2* data from the British Medical Association, based on Department of Health (1992), Statistics for general medical practitioners in England and Wales 1980–1990, *Statistical Bulletin*, **4**(2); *Table 7.3* Stacey, M. (1988), *The Sociology of Health & Healing*, Unwin Hyman; *Table 8.1* Heggenhougen, K. *et al.* (1987), *Community Health Workers: The Tanzanian Experience*, Oxford University Press.

Cover photograph

Child in Mali: Panos Pictures.

Contents

About this book

A note for the general reader

Caring for Health: History and Diversity takes a critical look at health care, tracing the historical development of health-care systems in Europe (with particular emphasis on Britain) and in the colonies controlled by European states, from 1500 to the early 1990s. The authors also examine the diversity of health-care systems and the political policies and economic circumstances which have shaped the patterns we see today.

The book contains ten chapters, all of which address the following five main themes to some degree (the prominence given to each theme varies between chapters):

- the contribution of lay health care and boundary movements between lay and formal sectors;

- environmental health problems and the public health movement;

- the professionalisation of health-care occupations;

- the health-care system within the emerging structure of state involvement in social welfare, with particular reference to institutions, the hospital and high technology medicine;

- the impact of European models of health care on the rest of the world, with examples of reciprocal influences.

After the substantial introduction to the scope of the book in Chapter 1, Chapters 2 to 6 follow an historical sequence from 1550 to 1974, arriving in modern times in Chapters 7 to 9, which deal with three different portraits of contemporary health care: British health care in Chapter 7; Third World health care in Chapter 8; and international health care in Chapter 9. The book concludes in Chapter 10 with general comments about main themes in the book as a whole.

The text is fully indexed and the reference list ends with a guide to further reading. A number of abbreviations used in this book are listed at the end of the book for easy reference.

Caring for Health: History and Diversity is the sixth in a series of eight books on the subject of health and disease. The book is designed so that it can be read on its own, like any other textbook, or studied as part of U205 *Health and Disease*, a second level course for Open University students. General readers do not need to make use of the study comments, learning objectives and other material inserted for OU students, although they may find these helpful. The text also contains references to an anthology of previously published material[1] prepared in association with the OU course: it is quite possible to follow the text without reading the articles referred to, although doing so will enhance your understanding of the contents of *Caring for Health: History and Diversity*.

A guide for OU students

Caring for Health: History and Diversity introduces the subject of health care, using a historical and comparative approach to demonstrate the widest possible definition of what constitutes 'caring for health'. The structure of the book (in brief) is set out in the 'Note for the general reader' above, and is developed extensively in Chapter 1.

Study comments are given in a box, where appropriate, at the start of chapters. These primarily direct you to other books in the course series where connections should be made, or to other course components (articles in the Reader and a television programme on health care in Zimbabwe). Major learning objectives are listed at the end of each chapter, along with self-assessment questions (SAQs) that will enable you to check that you are able to achieve those objectives. The index includes key words in bold type (also printed in bold in the text) which can be looked up easily as an aid to revision as the course proceeds, and abbreviations are listed at the end of the book.

The time allowed for studying *Caring for Health: History and Diversity* is four weeks, or about 40–48 hours. The following table gives a more detailed breakdown to help you to pace your study. You need not follow it slavishly, but try not to let yourself fall behind. If you find a section of the work difficult, do what you can at this stage, and then return to the material when you reach the end of the book.

There is a tutor-marked assignment (TMA) associated with this book; about three hours have been allowed for completing it, *in addition to* the time spent studying the material it assesses.

Study Guide for Book 6   (total 40-48 hours, including time for the TMA, spread over 4 weeks).

1st week

Chapter 1	**History and diversity**; revise *Reader* article by Engels (1845)
Chapter 2	**Pre-industrial health care, 1500 to 1750**
Chapter 3	**The Industrial Revolution, 1750 to 1848**; revise *Reader* articles by McKeown (1976) and Szreter (1988)

2nd week

Chapter 4	**The era of public health, 1848 to 1918**; *Reader* article by Stevens (1976)
Chapter 5	**The impact of war and depression, 1918 to 1948**
Chapter 6	**Mobilisation for total welfare, 1948 to 1974**

3rd week

Chapter 7	**The crisis of welfare, 1974 to the 1990s**; *Reader* article by Day and Klein (1991); *Reader* article by Bowling and Cartwright (1982)
Chapter 8	**Health care in the Third World, 1974 to the 1990s**; *Reader* article by Warner (1978) and TV programme on health care in Zimbabwe

4th week

Chapter 9	**International patterns of health care, 1960 to the 1990s**; *Reader* article by Ramesh and Hyma (1981); the TV programme referred to in Chapter 8 is also relevant
Chapter 10	**Conclusions**
TMA completion	

Cover photographs

Electron micrograph of brain cells. (Photo: Tony King)

Illustration from a poem, 'Le triomphe de haute et puissante dame Vérole [pox]', 1539, showing the 'Queen of Love' in procession with her victims. (Source: Claude Quétel, *History of Syphilis*, translated 1990, Polity Press, Cambridge)

A high-speed vaccination 'gun' being used on a child in Mali in one of the mass immunisation programmes organised by international charities in the 1980s. (Source: Panos Pictures)

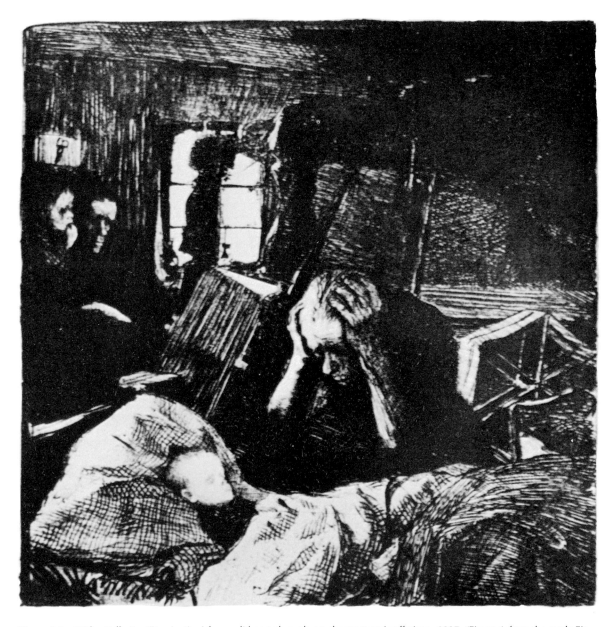

Figure 1.1 *Käthe Kollwitz, 'Deprivation' from a lithograph cycle on the weavers' sufferings, 1897. (Figure 1 from the cycle* Ein Weberaufstand, *Käthe Kollwitz Museum, Berlin)*

1 *History and diversity*

This book builds on the discussion of the growth of medical knowledge and medical technology in an earlier book in this series, **Medical Knowledge: Doubt and Certainty,**[1] which also introduced the concepts of lay care, traditional or folk systems of health care and alternative or complementary therapies—subjects to which we return in this book.

Introduction

This first chapter serves as an introduction to *Caring for Health: History and Diversity.* It performs a set of general but essential functions. We start by explaining the grounds for an historical approach to health care and providing some basic orientation. Then we set out general guidelines for the scope and organisation of the subsequent chapters. And finally we explain some social science concepts that will be used at various points in the book.

Caring for Health: History and Diversity takes a critical look at our health-care system. Health is, of course, one of the great preoccupations of modern civilisation. Indeed, the ability to maintain its population in a condition of relative immunity from pain and with much reduced risk of premature death can be regarded as one of the defining characteristics of modern Western society. This task has involved the creation of a multiplicity of formal and informal agencies devoted to health maintenance.

Most visible among these is the elaborate and expensive mechanism designed for this purpose, involving hospitals, health centres, ambulances, doctors, nurses and a whole host of supporting staff, which is collectively called the **formal health-care system.** The formal system of health care is complemented by an *informal health-care system* drawing on family and community, and also by a variety of alternative healers. Health is also affected by a whole range of factors ranging from the state of the environment to the quality of education. All of these factors must of course be borne in mind when assessing the causes of ill-health and the effectiveness of health care. In modern industrialised countries about ten per cent of the resources of the economy are applied to formal health care. This visible health-care system is therefore a significant and growing burden on the economy, comparable in scale with education or social security, and now surpassing military expenditure in its economic importance. Modern systems of formal health care represent a vast undertaking and a significant civilised achievement. It is therefore tempting to dwell on the successes which have contributed to this record.

However, as we are forcefully reminded by Figure 1.1, ill-health is a source of perpetual anxiety, and in the experience of the great majority of the world's population, past and present, the resources of welfare and health care have proved inadequate to meet essential or even minimal needs.

> ☐ In Figure 1.1, what failures has the artist emphasised as contributing to the ill-health of this working-class family?
>
> ■ Käthe Kollwitz has drawn attention to the lack of ventilation or sunlight and the cramped living conditions, suggesting that the family live and work in a single room, in which the weaving machinery is the dominant element. She powerfully suggests that the struggle for subsistence has drained the health and energies of the family.

Caring for Health: History and Diversity is therefore faced with a difficult task of assessment. It aims to reflect the genuine achievements of biomedical science and health care, without underestimating the magnitude of the failings of the health-care system. This first chapter provides some general guidelines and basic explanation concerning the contents of later chapters. It is useful to begin by explaining briefly the reason for selecting history and diversity as the twin themes for this book.

[1]*Medical Knowledge: Doubt and Certainty* (Open University Press, revised edition 1994).

Why history and diversity?

When considered in all of its dimensions, the modern health-care system is notoriously complex and difficult to understand. This difficulty is in part due to a constant process of change, as the mechanism is adapted to meet rising expectations, the altering pattern of disease, the new capacities of medicine, or shifts in political and social policy. Of course, all of these influences have been exacting their effect over a long period. Present systems of health care are therefore the end-product of a long process of accretion and modification. *Caring for Health: History and Diversity* will examine the process of change in the health-care system in the light of the economic and political determinants that have fashioned the institutions of advanced capitalism as a whole. You will see that present arrangements for health care are the product and to some extent the captive of a long history.

The process of historical change has brought about the dominance of the Western industrial economies and associated value-systems, within which Western bio-medical science is an important component. Western medicine has therefore gradually become predominant, even in regions where traditional medicine preserves some form of co-existence. Consequently, history shows the emergence of increasing uniformity. This process is termed *convergence*.

☐ What features of health care provide evidence for convergence?

■ Many forms of treatment are universal, indicating that the knowledge base of medicine and therefore the training of medical personnel are everywhere largely similar.

Because history shows the progressive dominance of Western biomedical science, it is tempting to regard this trend as the main organising principle. Yet this ideal model constitutes only one strand of a complex situation. It is evident that the application of technical expertise is affected by a wide range of political and economic factors, which collectively have produced wide diversity in the expression of health care. This is the reason for equal emphasis on 'history' and 'diversity' in the title of this book.

As holiday-makers in continental Europe quickly discover, there are stark differences in arrangements for health care even between European Community neighbours. These distinctions reflect deep-rooted differences among social and political institutions. And within Western industrialised countries, evident distinctions in health-care provision between the rich and the poor remind us of the even greater diversity between the affluent advanced nations and the impoverished economies of the Third World. The burden of malnutrition, of preventable disease and premature death borne by the peoples of the Third World, provides the most potent indicator of the selectivity with which the benefits of welfare are made available. The intractable difficulties standing in the way of effective health care in the Third World, discussed in detail later in this book, warn us against believing that improvements in health care naturally and automatically follow from advances in scientific knowledge.

Relentless progress?

The greater realism of recent decades has caused us to revise the once dominant idea of the seemingly relentless advance of health care.

This older view of medical progress is aptly illustrated by quotations from the writings of Sir George Newman, who was the dominant figure in the field of public health in Britain before World War II.

> Men now alive in England have witnessed…the emancipation and enfranchisement of the people, an enormous development of local government, the transformation of the mind of a whole nation by education, and the emergence of a consciousness of natural science and its application to human well-being undreamt-of three generations ago…One illustration of man's increasing knowledge and control of natural forces may be found in the steady advance of the science and art of Medicine, in the prevention and healing of disease, in the increase of health and human capacity, and in their collective application to the whole community…The historical fact is that the four great ideas of Vaccination, Anaesthesia, Antiseptic Surgery and the Causation of Infective Disease swept through Western Europe, relatively speaking, like a whirlwind…as usual, science and humanism won, truth prevailed, and in the event these four ideas extended for men, of every nation and race, the frontiers of life.
> (Newman, 1939, pp. 1–2, 35)

The above extract exemplifies the 'triumphalist' approach to history. Undoubtedly, Newman genuinely identified advances in medical science and health care. What is entirely misleading is the impression given that progress in health care is inevitable and guaranteed by the existing social and political order. Newman reflected the prevailing idea that Western civilisation in general, and Britain in particular, was witnessing a 'silent social revolution', under which all sections of society were benefiting of necessity from the relentless advance of the institutions of liberal democracy. This confidence in the beneficence of the system was communicated to the wider public through the mass media.

☐ What was the consequence of the triumphalist fallacy?

■ It resulted in elevating expectations about health care and other social provision to a level which in practice has proved impossible for even the richer Western economies to realise.

In recent years any false optimism and complacency concerning the advance of Western medicine has been overtaken by a growing sense of realism.

☐ From earlier books in this series and from your knowledge of current world events, can you identify expressions of scepticism about modern biomedicine which have contributed to this realism?

■ You may have thought of the work of Ivan Illich and Thomas McKeown,[2] the anti-psychiatry movement, and the many manifestations of alternative medicine. Also relevant are negative attitudes towards the state and collective provision emanating from both the political left and right.

An indicator of the changing mood was provided in 1977, when the prestigious American general academic journal *Daedalus* devoted a special issue to the crisis of confidence in Western health care, under the heading 'Doing better and feeling worse'.

This title alluded to the perplexing dilemma of modern Western medicine: a profusion of achievement,

resulting in an unparalleled technical capacity to conquer disease, yet even in the richest and most advanced societies an inability to evolve medical services capable of commanding the confidence of the public, or dispelling anxiety concerning ill-health. Developments since 1977 have done nothing to resolve this dilemma. Technical advance has continued unchecked, but confidence in health-care systems has steadily deteriorated, while the gap between rich and poor has if anything widened. Consequently the prospect of progress held out by Newman (and quoted earlier) is only tenable in the most limited sense.

Examples from history

To a greater extent than perhaps we realise, our everyday experience involves exposure to the historical record of health care. Either explicitly or implicitly, we are invited to evaluate the present practice of care in the light of past precedents. As already indicated by the example of the Newman quotation and the critique of his point of view, we are often faced with constructions about the past which are difficult to reconcile or even patently incompatible.

☐ For a further example, can you construct two opposing mythologies about the Victorian period?

■ Traditionally social reformers portrayed the Victorian period as a 'Bleak Age' from which the nation finally emerged into a more civilised and humane society with the post-World War II welfare state. Then during the 1980s we were encouraged to adopt a more positive attitude to 'Victorian values': the welfare state was represented as an extravagance which irrevocably damaged the economy, artificially extended the life of a paternalistic state and eroded the will of individuals to 'stand on their own two feet'.

The controversy concerning Victorian values and the welfare reforms which led to the setting up of the National Health Service (NHS) in the United Kingdom, indicates the sensitivity and contemporary relevance of historical evaluations. The future shape of health care is being determined in the light of judgements about the past. It is therefore essential that our assessment about the past should be based on the firmest foundations.

The extent to which all of us are in possession of much relevant historical data is often not fully appreciated. Such experience can be utilised to develop insights about the sources of present-day arrangements.

[2]Articles by Illich and McKeown appear in *Health and Disease: A Reader* (Open University Press, revised edition 1995), and are set reading for earlier books in this series.

Figure 1.2 (referred to on p.10)
Map showing the distribution of the main hospital buildings of Norwich, with the city wall (dashed line) marking the boundary of the medieval town.

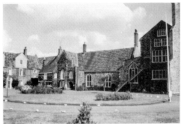

(a) **The Great Hospital** was founded in 1249 by Walter de Suffield, Bishop of Norwich, and was originally part of a monastic institution providing hostels for pilgrims, care for the poor and treatment for the sick. The original buildings were remarkably large, the infirmary hall being 200 feet long. The hospital was divided into men's and women's wards. By 1500 the Great Hospital had ceased to function as a hospital for the sick.
(Source: Dr A. Batty Shaw)

(b) **The Lazar House** was founded in 1119 by Herbert de Losinga, Bishop of Norwich. Lazar houses were hostels for lepers and others with diseases perceived as infectious. The surviving portion on Sprowston Road is the chapel, which you will notice is built on a substantial scale. Such lazar houses were distributed around the city perimeter, safely outside the city walls.
(Source: Dr A. Batty Shaw)

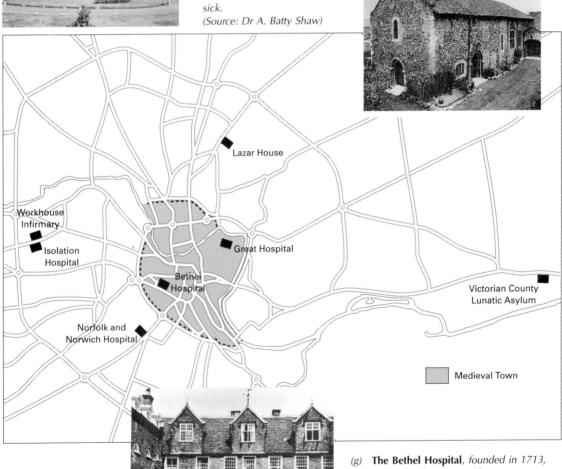

(g) **The Bethel Hospital**, founded in 1713, with a bequest from Mary Chapman, was the first hospital for patients with mental disorders established outside London. This was superseded by the Victorian County Lunatic Asylum built outside the town at the village of Thorpe St Andrew.
(Source: Dr A. Batty Shaw)

(c) **The Norfolk and Norwich Hospital** *was completed in 1775. It was representative of the hospitals which were established in most county towns in the mid-eighteenth century, funded by subscriptions from the prosperous members of the community, and supported by the various religious denominations. This 'voluntary' hospital catered for the sick poor, largely reviving the functions of the Great Hospital.*
(Source: Norfolk Museums Service (Norwich Castle Museum))

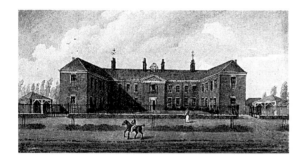

(d) **The Norfolk and Norwich Hospital**
was completely rebuilt in 1879. The spacious site of the original voluntary hospital was big enough to house the grandiose, Tudor-style Victorian voluntary hospital, and the bleak extensions added under the NHS. This site has therefore accommodated the acute hospital services for Norwich and a large surrounding area for more than two centuries.
(Source: Dr A. Batty Shaw)

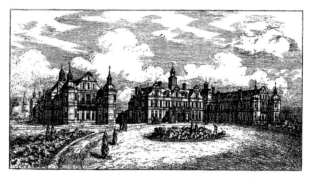

(e) **The Norwich Isolation Hospital** *was built by the County Borough Council in 1893 on a site opposite to the workhouse. Under the NHS this hospital was used also for the treatment of chest diseases.*
(Source: Mike Levers)

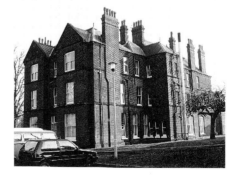

(f) **The Workhouse Infirmary,** *Bowthorpe Road, was developed for sick patients from the workhouse established by the Poor Law authorities in 1859, to replace the old workhouse which had been housed in the converted Blackfriars monastic buildings in the centre of the town. This Infirmary was damaged by bombing during World War II and demolished in 1959. Often such hospitals have continued on as geriatric departments.*
(Source: Standley, P.J. (1989) Norwich: A Second Portrait in Old Picture Postcards, S.B. Publications, Market Drayton, Shropshire)

For instance in any historic population centre it is possible that 'almshouses', often called 'hospitals', are descendants of medieval charities. In town centres there are many former voluntary hospitals or dispensaries, often located in classical buildings dating from the late eighteenth century. They were part of a comprehensive system of philanthropy, religious in origin, but in health (unlike education) inter-denominational. These institutions are dwarfed by dingy workhouses or lunatic asylums bequeathed by the Victorians; they are now located in the outer suburbs, but were well outside population centres when they were built. The sites of old hospitals are frequently used for modern district general hospitals, the product of the hospital building plan which began in the 1960s. Smaller settlements frequently contain examples of the rash of cottage hospitals built by local subscription at the turn of the century. Location and physical character tell us much about the original purposes of the miscellaneous collection of institutions absorbed by modern health authorities. Proposals for closure of hospitals and residential homes for the elderly, or more recently for opting-out from health authority control, expose the deep-rooted feeling of local communities for their local hospitals. Any such change is likely to be resented and resisted, as desecration of a fundamental part of the local heritage.

Figure 1.2 shows the location of the main hospitals of Norwich, a representative larger county town.

☐ Can you suggest why the workhouse and the lunatic asylum are situated at a distance from the town?

■ You may have guessed correctly that the inmates were perceived as a danger to themselves or a bad example to their community. Therefore they were subject to strict regimes of discipline in large prison-like institutions, which were necessarily located outside the town. Also these forbidding institutions served as a deterrent, and they suitably eliminated stigmatised groups of perceived deviants from the town.

The example of Norwich is a reminder of the great antiquity of some of our medical institutions, a conclusion which will be further reinforced by Chapter 2. Even more remote history sometimes impinges on our consciousness.

For instance, the often-mentioned **Hippocratic oath**, although not an original Hippocratic writing, provides a link with medicine as it was practised around 400 BC and with ideas that were current in both the Near and Far East (see Figure 1.3). Although often invoked as if everyone was familiar with its contents, the Hippocratic oath is little known, even among doctors, and it is not well understood. The oath itself is a complex text of some three hundred words. The following is a representative extract:

> I will apply dietetic measures for the benefit of the sick according to my ability and judgment; I will keep them from harm and injustice. I will neither give a deadly drug to anybody if asked for it, nor will I make a suggestion to this effect. Similarly I will not give to a woman an abortive remedy. In purity and holiness I will guard my life and my art. (Edelstein, 1967, p. 6)

The Hippocratic oath has assumed permanent importance because it is taken as a statement of the fundamental obligations of doctors to their patients. The need for this oath at such an early stage in the development of Western civilisation indicates that doctors faced real difficulties in gaining the trust of their patients. The Hippocratic oath

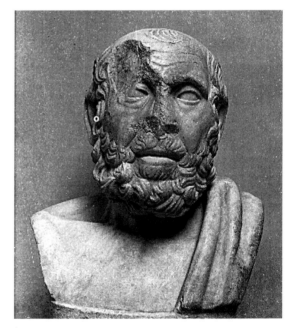

Figure 1.3 *Roman bust of Hippocrates. Hippocrates of Cos (c. 460–c. 380 BC) was a celebrated physician and founder of a school of medicine which flourished in Greece and Rome. The body (or corpus) of writings attributed to Hippocrates are in reality the product of his followers: his contribution is a matter of supposition. Indeed, the Hippocratic corpus breaks down into at least three components, stemming from rival Hippocratic sects, which drew together ideas in medicine from all parts of the Near East. (Source: Deutscher Archaeologischer Institut, Rome)*

attempted to bring the ethical standards of secular practitioners into alignment with those of the most revered sects of religious healers. Doctors in modern times have invested much energy into perpetuating this idea of lofty altruism.

By contrast, also inherited from the ancient world is the notion that an elaborate body of arcane knowledge was cultivated by the higher echelons of the medical profession as a vehicle for the exploitation of a vulnerable public. Thus, according to the respected authority of Pliny the Elder (AD 23–79), the realities of the medical profession were something of a departure from the ideals of the Hippocratic code:

> Pliny deplores the rise of the medical profession, which he regards as having come to Rome through an invasion of crafty, unscrupulous Greek charlatans. Instead of relying on the traditional natural remedies which he admires, the so-called medical art has taken over, which is 'lucrative beyond all the rest'. (Kee, 1986, p. 5)

The two texts from the ancient world quoted above indicate strikingly different views of the integrity of the medical profession. This book takes a more recent starting point—the year 1500—but you should note that the ambivalence about health care in antiquity has persisted and the questions raised by the ancient authorities are as valid today as ever they were.

The scope of *Caring for Health: History and Diversity*

In this book we aim to provide a review of health care in the United Kingdom in particular, but more generally in Western Europe and the European colonial sphere of influence from 1500 to the present. Within the United Kingdom, in order to avoid repetition of detail, most of the specific examples will relate to England. But the general aim is to shed light on the system of health care evolved in modern Western industrialised society and the impact of this system in the wider world. 'Western society' is the term applied to the general sphere of European culture, embodying traditions and institutions influenced by Greek and Roman civilisation. The values of modern Western society extended to regions dominated by settlers from Europe, and they were imposed on indigenous inhabitants where Europeans chose to colonise. Western society provided the environment for the development of modern industrialised economies. As indicated below, advanced Western economies drew the entire world into their orbit of influence.

European colonial expansion began in the sixteenth century, as did the revolution in science, technology and medicine. Thus the foundations for European domination and the beginnings of modern knowledge and institutions can be traced back to an early date. Nevertheless, the period before 1750 was essentially a pre-industrial age. Consequently, consideration of the period between 1500 and 1750 in Chapter 2 provides an insight into health care before the great changes that took place during the Industrial Revolution.

Chapter 3 embraces the catastrophic impact on health care brought about by the first phase of industrialisation in Western Europe (1750–1848). Chapter 4 covers the long period during which control of the environment constituted the first priority in the field of health intervention (1848–1918). Chapter 5 deals with the phase of expanding competence of curative medicine, and includes the shock of two World Wars, and the intervening depression. This period involved some consolidation of the commitment to positive welfare policies (1918–48).

Chapter 6 is concerned with the vast expansion of state-sponsored forms of health care within the context of rising expectations and general support for the substantial development of social services (1948–74). Chapters 7, 8 and 9 consider the changed situation of health care following the oil crisis of 1973, which precipitated reversal of policies concerning state support for social services. Economic constraints were reinforced by a general loss of confidence in existing forms of health care. Chapter 7 concentrates on the efforts made to shore up the British health services. Chapter 8 considers the troubled process of evolving appropriate forms of health care in the vulnerable context of the Third World. Chapter 9 examines trends in health service provision world-wide from the quantitative and economic perspective.

Five themes

Five themes have been selected for special attention. They will occur to some extent in all the chapters, and are the subject of separate sections in Chapters 2–7.

(a) The contribution of informal health care and boundary movements between the informal and formal sectors.

This theme reminds us of the continuing importance of the informal sector, regardless of the expansion in the capacities of modern medicine and the extension of health services. In every period the role of women has been crucial in informal care. Elevation of the status and education of women is recognised as one of the major factors in the improvement of family health and in the reduction of infant mortality (see Figure 1.4).

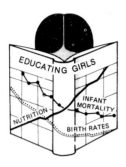

Figure 1.4 *Rising female literacy is closely associated with falling infant mortality and birth rates, and improved nutrition. (Source, Morley, D., Rohde, J. and Williams, G., 1983,* Practising Health for All, *Oxford University Press, Oxford; reprinted 1989; Figure 5.2, p. 77)*

(b)   Environmental health problems and the public health movement.

Public health is the medical specialism that deals with the health problems of the community as a whole, by contrast with other medical specialisms which are chiefly concerned with individual illness. Some of the interventions of public health (e.g. vaccination) are specifically medical in character, whereas others (e.g. environmental controls, water supply, sewerage) are not exclusively medical. The latter form an inevitably vague boundary between the health-care system and the multiplicity of other agencies which impinge on health care. You will notice in Chapters 5–7 that the nebulousness of public health contributed to a crisis of identity in this specialism in the twentieth century.

(c)   The professionalisation of health-care occupations.

The process of professionalisation has developed in parallel with the extension of the formal sector of health care. As noted elsewhere,[3] and re-emphasised at the end of this chapter, professionalisation has entailed benefits but also disadvantages connected with medicalisation and social control.

[3]See *Medical Knowledge: Doubt and Certainty.*

(d)   The health-care system within the emerging structure of state involvement in social welfare, with particular emphasis on the expansion of institutionalised services, the hospital and high technology medicine.

It can be seen that advances in medical knowledge, innovations in medical technology, and the impact of mortality, morbidity and malnutrition, take their place alongside social, economic and political forces, as determinants of the character of formal systems of health care. The complex hierarchical system of health services developed in the twentieth century, by analogy with education, is described in terms of three levels: **primary**, **secondary**, and **tertiary health care**. The primary level of organisation is nearest to the community. In the United Kingdom this comprises primary health-care teams led by general practitioners, while the analogous teams in the Third World have less conspicuous medical practitioner involvement. Secondary health care relates to the activities of district hospitals which provide acute care services, while tertiary care is centred on regional hospitals concerned with more advanced specialist treatment, teaching and research.

(e)   The impact of European models of health care in other continents, with examples of reciprocal influence, where appropriate.

This theme deals with the escalation of Western dominance, beginning with minor trading relations, continuing into colonisation, and culminating with exercises in integration under imperialism. In order to give sufficient prominence to the attempt to evolve appropriate forms of health care since independence from colonial rule, the whole of Chapter 8 is an expanded treatment of Third World health care.

The remainder of Chapter 1 introduces or reminds you about some important social science concepts and terminology that will reappear in later chapters, or that are taken as assumed knowledge.

The modern world system

You will notice that *Caring for Health: History and Diversity* avoids giving the impression that societies and their health-care arrangements in the Third World have existed, like some exotic species, in a state of primitive isolation. Through international trade, colonisation, and exploitation, Western capitalism rapidly extended its influence to all parts of the world. Thus, the entire world system is caught up in a process of reciprocal interaction and interdependence.

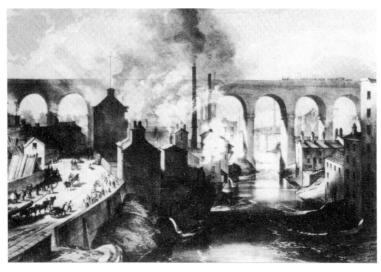

Figure 1.5 *Stockport viaduct, c.1850, lithograph by A. F. Tait (owned by The British Railways Board). (Source:* Charles Dickens: An exhibition to commemorate the centenary of his death, *June–September 1970; exhibition catalogue, Victoria and Albert Museum)*

A reminder of this interdependence is provided by the mills that are such a ubiquitous feature of cotton towns in Lancashire, and that provided the basis for their prosperity. The wealth of estate owners in the West Indies and mill owners in Lancashire was gained at the cost of untold misery and disease among native populations in West Africa, imported labourers in the West Indian plantations, and workers in mills and related industries in Britain. The factory system resulting from this international transaction created a multiplicity of threats to health, stemming from conditions within the factories, the dangers of the various occupations, or the effects on the levels of subsistence within the community. Thus the engine of the Industrial Revolution was responsible for a health crisis in different societies separated by vast distances.

Edwin Chadwick, the Victorian pioneer of public health, drew attention to the similarity of the causes of suffering of the poor in the most deprived colonial territories and in the British conurbations:

> The disruption of the Mexican populace (sunk in the lowest vice and misery amidst the means of the highest abundance) will recall features characteristic of the wretched population in the vast parts of Glasgow, Edinburgh, London, and Bath, and the lodging houses throughout the country. (Chadwick, 1842, p. 247)

Figure 1.5 gives an impression of the wretched industrial landscape of Stockport, near Manchester, the area which inspired Frederick Engels in 1844 to write his book *The Condition of the Working Class in England* (published in 1845).[4]

☐ Itemise some likely threats to health illustrated in Figure 1.5.

■ Smoke; pollutants pouring into the river; obviously unhealthy working and living conditions.

Industrialisation,[5] as one of the major components in the developing world economy, has added enormously to the scale of health problems. The capacity of uncontrolled industrialisation to damage health on a vast scale became apparent in Eastern Europe with the collapse of the Soviet bloc. Even the remotest regions have not been immune from the depredations of industrialisation. For instance, Donald Denoon, an Australian expert on health care in Papua New Guinea, points out that the supposedly enlightened colonial administration introduced only in

[4]An extract from Engels' book, entitled 'Health: 1844' appears in *Health and Disease: A Reader.* It is set reading for an earlier book in this series, *World Health and Disease* (Open University Press, 1993). It would be beneficial to read this extract again now.

[5]Discussed in *World Health and Disease,* especially Chapters 5–8.

resent century had failed to arrest the deterioration in th consequent upon industrialisation and other forms abour exploitation.

> Colonialism did not simply permit the introduction of entirely new diseases (tuberculosis, smallpox, measles and others) but also allowed the more even redistribution of endemic infections into enclaves which had hitherto been isolated. The mechanism for the introduction, dissemination, and redistribution of infection was the mobilisation of labour for mining, for plantation work, and for general employment by the colonists and their government. And that mechanism was much more effective than the frantic attempts of the health authorities to stamp out epidemics once they occurred …Colonialism itself was a health hazard, which colonial medical services were ill-equipped to suppress. (Denoon, 1989, pp. 31–2)

The changes taking place in the Western economy, and in its political and social structure in the period discussed in this book are often called **modernisation**. From the perspective of analysing major trends in welfare, the Dutch social scientist Abram de Swaan has listed some key features of modernisation in the following terms:

> State formation, the development of capitalism and the processes of urbanization and secularization which went with them…established bureaucratic networks linking people together as taxpayers, recruits, students, patients, claimants, voters, thus shaping them into citizens in the modern sense. Equally competitive, capitalist entrepreneurs organized manufacture and constituted markets which connected people in networks of production and exchange as workers and consumers. All this meant increasing interdependency and new, further-reaching external effects of one person's deficiencies and adversities upon others.
>
> …the poor were seen as a threat to public order, to labour harmony and also to public health, while at the same time they constituted a reserve of potential labourers, recruits, consumers and political supporters. (De Swaan, 1988, pp. 2–3)

The above extract introduces some important terminology, which is used repeatedly in discussion of modernisation. De Swaan identifies three important dimensions of modernisation: urbanisation, secularisation and bureaucracy.

Urbanisation is the drift of population from village to town communities, and from a rural to an urban way of life. Urbanisation introduces a multiplicity of threats to health, but it also provides a convenient basis for organisation of such institutions as hospitals.

Secularisation involves the shift from a social system in which religious values and institutions associated with religion perform a dominant role in all aspects of the life of the community. Secularisation also involves a move away from a charismatic and non-rational ethos, to a society where rational and routinised functions are allegedly dominant. Because religious bodies were traditionally closely bound up with the care of the poor and the sick, the escalation of these problems beyond the scope of the church created a major vacuum in welfare provision.

Bureaucracy is a necessary consequence of secularisation. Bureaucrats are the lay officials and professional personnel who take on the tasks of an advanced society requiring the employment of expertise. Recruitment of bureaucrats requires a higher degree of literacy within society, moves towards universal education, training, examinations, certification, etc. The more advanced the economy, the greater the development of hierarchies of bureaucrats. The proliferation of occupations associated with health care is an ideal example of the growth of a bureaucracy.

In this book you will find the term **elite** frequently introduced to describe the group which dominates any particular hierarchy. For instance doctors have constituted an elite with respect to other health workers; but within the medical profession hospital consultants have formed an elite over general practitioners; while, finally, among consultants, specialisms connected with general medicine or surgery have constituted an elite compared with those of geriatrics, psychiatry, or public health.

The problem of equality

It is obvious from the above discussion of industrialisation and modernisation that the great majority of problems of ill-health are rooted in economic inequalities (see Figure 1.6). The correction of these inequalities is clearly beyond the competence of the health services alone. Accordingly, no realistic programme for correcting *health* inequalities can be evolved without attention to reducing *social* inequalities. Therefore any meaningful conception of health care must allow for the application of correctives from any other relevant social service.

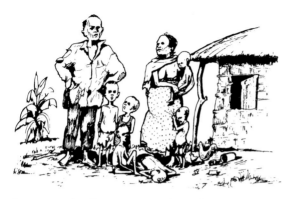

Figure 1.6 *This illustration comes from a low-cost book on practical strategies for achieving the World Health Organisation's target of 'Health for All by the Year 2000'. The original caption reads 'Today's poor are caught in a trap from which, without help, they cannot escape'. (Source, Morley, D., Rohde, J. and Williams, G., 1983,* Practising Health for All, *Oxford University Press, Oxford; reprinted 1989; Figure 4.2, p. 52)*

Formal **equality** (equal share to each individual) has been regarded as a utopian goal, but steps have been made to reduce inequalities and the principle of more equal **access** to resources, employment, social security, education, housing and health care has been the major priority of the modern welfare state. Health services have therefore been provided on a more *universal* basis (that is available to everyone), and the services are more *comprehensive* (covering all eventualities), and they are *free at point of delivery*, sometimes financed through direct taxation, which maximises the redistributive effect, i.e. the poor benefit most because the rich pay the highest tax.

However, events have shown that such measures have not brought proportionate benefits to the most needy. In practice, the more prosperous classes have displayed superior capacity to annex the resources of welfare, thereby merely exacerbating the problem of inequality of access. The perverse tendency of the system to operate in the opposite direction to its professed intentions was noted by the British sociologists Peter Townsend and Nicholas Bosanquet:

> ...the problem has already shifted from establishing services which are designed to be used more or less evenly by most groups in the population to that of preventing the more prosperous sections from benefiting disproportionately from increases in public expenditure. Some of the fastest growing areas of social spending have been in fact for services which are little used by the poor.... There was and is a growing conflict of priorities between providing social services for the poor and providing them for the middle classes. Yet society is largely unconscious of the growth of services for the latter and, by operating means tested schemes for the former is ensuring that many of them do not in fact receive certain services to which they would be entitled. (Townsend and Bosanquet, 1972, p. 8)

Efforts to shift resources to give more meaningful access to services for the most disadvantaged groups began in the 1970s, when it was recognised that positive inducements were needed to provide **equity**—a share of resources according to need. Identified among the vulnerable groups requiring positive discrimination were working-class women, minority ethnic groups, elderly, mentally handicapped, mentally sick, and physically disabled people. These, of course, represented a substantial segment of the population. The final chapters of this book will consider the degree of success of these efforts.

Collectivisation and medicalisation

One of the striking features of modernisation has been the enormous expansion of organised provision for welfare. This process is termed **collectivisation**. The state has become increasingly involved in supervising and even directly organising the collective agencies of welfare. This tendency has brought about the enormous growth of bureaucracies. Medical bureaucracies have come to dominate the **hierarchy of resort** described below.

Most illness is contained within the informal circle of family and friends, and it involves no steps beyond self-medication. In this sphere, women have traditionally played a dominant role. An intermediate level of care involves resort to folk or alternative healers, individuals who specialise in healing, but who lie outside the officially sanctioned medical system. These healers play a leading role in the Third World, and in Western society they are more significant than is customarily assumed. The professional or formal level of health care represents the summit of the hierarchy of resort. At this level responsibility for care is taken over by an elaborate structure of professions, which itself has assumed an hierarchical character. This hierarchy within medicine has resulted in great coherence within the professions and occupations involved in health care, with the result that the medical bureaucracy has come to exercise enormous influence and authority.

You should already be familiar with the idea that professionalisation has entailed the emergence of *social control, medicalisation, surveillance* and *incarceration.*[6] This book will outline in more detail the historical pathways by which these developments have come about. You will see that over the last two hundred years doctors and their ancillaries have built up bureaucratic structures of a kind which scarcely existed before 1800. The nineteenth century witnessed the enormous growth of hospitals and asylums of many types, and the twentieth century has seen both the consolidation of the hospital and the intrusion of medical values into numerous spheres of social existence.

Summing up these trends, the medical sociologist Bryan Turner suggests that:

> ...the emergence of the medical classification of deviance, the growing importance of the doctor as a professional man, the development of medical institutions around the hospital, the clinic and the examination, and the organization of medical surveillance of society represent components of a secularization of western cultures. Put simply, the doctor has replaced the priest as the custodian of social values; the panoply of ecclesiastical institutions of regulation...have been transferred through the evolution of scientific medicine to a panoptic[7] collection of localized agencies of surveillance

and control. Furthermore, the rise of preventive medicine, social medicine and community medicine has extended these agencies of regulation deeper and deeper into social life. (Turner, 1987, pp. 37–8)

The vast increase in the scale of medical intervention has only been rendered possible by the transformation of collective arrangements for health care, and this change reflects tendencies occurring throughout all areas of welfare provision. The modern state has gradually seen the replacement of small-scale, local agencies, often with religious affiliations and depending on the vagaries of charitable subscription, by nation-wide, compulsory structures, involving a high degree of state intervention. Haphazard services, available to narrowly entitled groups, usually conditional on subscription, have been replaced by comprehensive services, available universally, without imposition of subscription criteria.

The latter changes describe the features customarily associated with the welfare state, where the recognition of unrestricted *entitlement* to benefits, as a basic right of citizenship, has conferred on the community a degree of protection from the hazards of the working of the economic system and the chance effects of certain diseases. Assessment of the degree to which collectivisation and medical intervention have in reality fulfilled their intended purpose will be addressed in the following chapters.

[6] These terms and concepts are extensively discussed in *Medical Knowledge: Doubt and Certainty.*

[7] The term 'panoptic' is taken from Jeremy Bentham's idea of a panopticon, an ideal institution in which complete surveillance was possible, and which was most realised in prison building. Bentham was a nineteenth-century social reformer whose contribution to British health care is discussed in Chapter 3.

OBJECTIVES FOR CHAPTER 1

When you have studied this chapter, you should be able to:

1.1 Demonstrate the value of the historical approach towards present-day dilemmas concerning health care.

1.2 Discuss the idea that both patterns of disease and health-care systems are products of the underlying economic and political system.

1.3 Discuss the limitations of medical intervention in attempting to correct the major problems of ill-health stemming from such factors as economic inequality.

1.4 Define and use correctly the following concepts from the social sciences relevant to the interpretation of developments in health care: collectivisation, industrialisation, urbanisation, secularisation, bureaucracy, access, equality, equity, medicalisation, social control, surveillance.

QUESTIONS FOR CHAPTER 1

Question 1 (*Objective 1.1*)

Examine Figure 1.2 again and in particular study the captions relating to each of the institutions pictured. What can you learn about the social and religious values which led to the foundation of these institutions simply by looking at their pattern of distribution in Norwich and their size and appearance?

Question 2 (*Objective 1.2*)

According to modernisation theory:

> Third World countries are under-developed because they are culturally traditional and economically backward. The public health version holds that as 'backward' countries develop, they too will experience the chronic diseases associated with later stages of industrialisation and urbanisation…modernisation theory is patently flawed…[and] the public health version is equally faulty. Not only have diseases such as schistosomiasis, leprosy, venereal disease, and tuberculosis been wrongly labeled…but epidemics of occupational accidents, injuries, and illness would probably be found to occur more commonly in the South than in the North, if anyone kept track of them, as would hypertension and diabetes. (Turshen, 1989, p. 27)

Does this suggestion that the diseases of industrialised society are endemic both in the Western world (the North) and the Third World (the South) necessarily mean that the idea of modernisation is false? Or can it be modified to meet the objections raised by Turshen?

Question 3 (*Objective 1.3*)

In 1938, Richard Titmuss observed that at least 500 000 excess deaths had occurred in the deprived regions of Britain over the previous decade of the Depression, and that this was only the tip of the iceberg of disease attributable to 'the presence of intense poverty on a scale so considerable and so widespread' that it was scarcely conceivable in the 'heart of the British Empire in the twentieth century' (Titmuss, 1938, p. 308). To what extent do such findings suggest that the problems of disease could be largely eliminated without recourse to medical intervention?

Question 4 (*Objective 1.4*)

You are now familiar with many social science terms and concepts relevant to the interpretation of developments in health care. To what extent do these terms and concepts contribute to a view that the expansion of modern medicine and the growth of collectivised health-care systems have resulted in some adverse consequences?

2 Pre-industrial health care, 1500 to 1750

This and the following chapter deal with the more distant periods from 1500 to 1848. They make reference to periodisations of history according to criteria which can be mainly cultural (e.g. Renaissance, Enlightenment), religious (e.g. Reformation), or economic (e.g. Industrial Revolution). We refer to the term most relevant to our context. These terms must be used flexibly because they relate to complex developments, which vary in their character and chronology according to their location.

This chapter assumes that you are already familiar with the changing patterns of health and disease in England from 1500 to 1750, which were described and discussed in **World Health and Disease, Chapter 6.**

Pre-industrial society: chances and changes

Has our own society altered more rapidly than any in the past? Many of those living in the sixteenth and seventeenth centuries had in common with us the sense that their world was changing with terrifying speed. Europe experienced a major shift in the balance between East and West, persistent religious conflicts, emergent nationalisms, and the founding of new colonial empires. The establishment of a Turkish European empire, by blocking the land route to India, prompted the 'discovery' of the New World of the Americas, and led to fateful biological and cultural exchanges between peoples hitherto kept apart. The fall of Constantinople to the Turks in 1453 drove the last custodians of the classical learning of the Byzantine empire to Italy and the West; these refugees, and the manuscripts they brought with them, encouraged new ideals of human potential based on the rediscovery of the world of ancient Greece and Rome.

The new ideals, which stressed the role of the intellectual in organised society, became known as *humanism*. Though very different, all these changes proved relevant for health and disease.

Many saw this period of change optimistically, as one of 'rebirth' of the individual human spirit and rediscovery of the physical world—hence *Renaissance*—a term first applied to a broad shift in cultural outlook at its peak between about 1450 and 1550. A central aim of the Renaissance was to study and then surpass the achievements of ancient Greece and Rome. There was however a dark side of the Renaissance, of which disease represents only one aspect. This sense of a new (and perhaps final) age of corruption was balanced by fresh religious impulses and the search for greater powers over nature. Traditional beliefs in magic and astrology were reinforced at the level of *elite culture* by the rediscovery of ancient learning and 'secrets'. The period saw repeated (and conflicting) attempts to reinterpret human destiny in terms of a reconciliation of Christian and pagan philosophies.

If every age has its disease—as ours may be AIDS, or cancer—then this period is best represented by *syphilis*. Possibly introduced by contact with the New World and trading in slaves, syphilis was given various nicknames like 'the French pox', and 'mal de Naples', because of its association with the movement of armies in Europe. The more learned name of syphilis comes from a character in a Latin narrative poem about the disease, composed by a humanist physician in 1521. Syphilis was treated (drastically but successfully) with mercury (see Figure 2.1).

The search for alternative cures led to the trial of many novel imports from the New World, including tobacco, sarsaparilla, and the wood guaiacum (a monopoly of which by the Fugger banking family helped finance European wars). During this first outburst in Europe, syphilis prevailed in a more infectious form and caused hideous effects on the surface of the body. As a 'new disease' connected with sexual behaviour, it became a major element in satire, slander, social criticism, and fear of marginal groups in society.

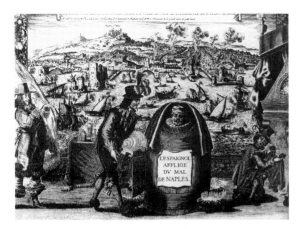

Figure 2.1 *A syphilitic suffering the dangerous treatment of fumigation with mercury. This well-known but deplorable fate is here used as a vehicle for political satire, following the revolt of Naples against Spanish domination in 1647. (Source: Bibliothèque Nationale, Paris)*

Periods of change often lead to periods of reaction. For instance in England, after the melting pot of the Elizabethan period, crisis under the early Stuarts, the turmoils of the Civil War, and the 'Glorious Revolution' of 1688, society in the later seventeenth century sought to damp down 'enthusiasms' and to accentuate social and gender distinctions. At the same time religious and political divisions became institutionalised as different parties and churches. Given this kind of separate development, no single institution was likely to be able to exert an overall control. Each group in society was concerned to defend its own religious and social status, and to implement its social outlook.

The renewed growth of towns as service and leisure centres, and what has been described as a *commercialisation* of society—an accelerated shift to a cash economy, and greater consumption of material goods—reflected the increased need to express fine gradations in social differences. In the earlier half of the period, we can see medicine as a source of consolation for all classes, like alcohol; in the latter, medicine is more obviously being bought in quantity by those who could afford a higher standard of living.

Population and family structure

People's chances in life can often be related to overall population distribution and demographic structure. Compared with the city-states of continental Europe, England presented the paradox of a *one-city nation*: its numerous centres of population were long-established, but small, with the sole exception of London, which by 1750 had grown to be the largest city in Europe, and the fourth largest in the world. London's population increased by immigration, particularly of young people of both sexes, many of whom travelled from remote counties and fell victim to the city's diseases. Although English society remained predominantly rural over the period, there was a gradual shift towards *urbanisation*: the percentage living in towns rose from around 6 per cent in 1500 to around 18 per cent in 1700. The old *corporate* towns—those which had gained some control over their own affairs—were concentrated in East Anglia, the South-east, the North-east, and the West Country. The focus of economic development did not shift to the Midlands and the North until the end of the period.

Population change can take many forms:[1] for example, the age-structure of populations can vary considerably. The Elizabethan period was dominated by young people; over half the population was under 25. Average life expectancy was affected by the great loss of infant lives: a person surviving to the age of thirty could expect to live another 30 years. Changes in age-structure notwithstanding, the English family in the pre-industrial period followed the pattern for northern Europe generally. Although households could be *extended* by the presence of servants, apprentices, journeymen, children being wet-nursed, and relatives temporarily accommodated, it was unusual for a family unit to contain more than two generations. Except among the elite, households were small and *nuclear*.

They could, however, be complicated by the effects of mortality—remarriage was common, especially among men—and by the driving force of poverty. The elderly poor for example often had to live alone, but also followed 'survival strategies' involving living with others who were not their own children. The population as a whole was relatively mobile, travelling to enter service or apprenticeship or to marry, for betterment, or simply in desperation. In northern Europe generally, the supposed 'golden age' of families rooted to the soil with all duties of care carried out by extended kinship networks, turns out to be a myth. On the other hand, though highly stratified into a hierarchical social order, this was still recognisably a 'face-to-face' society, except perhaps in London. Although it may still have had its 'neighbourhoods', London was perceived as a place of bewildering complexity in which appearances were deceiving and it was hard to know people for what they were.

---

[1]Changes in population structure are discussed in *World Health and Disease*, particularly Chapter 2.

Death and disease

What diseases affected people most?[2] We have already mentioned sexually transmitted disease as a major—though unquantifiable—factor affecting society from around 1500. In the early sixteenth century this sense of a crisis in public health was sharpened by the outbreak of another new disease, the 'English sweat', which alarmed because it seemed particularly to affect the elite. Dearths, or 'crises of subsistence', were probably one cause of high mortality, and were feared not least for their effects on political stability. *Plague* broke out repeatedly until the 'Great Plague of London' of 1665–6, and travelled through rural as well as urban areas. The early seventeenth-century epidemics, like those of the 1590s, coincided with economic decline. Although plague retreated from Europe, smallpox and then typhus seemed to increase in importance, contributing to the major peaks in English mortality in the 1680s and 1720s.

Less obvious to us, but of great concern at the time, were: scurvy; rickets (newly identified in the seventeenth century); rheumatism; eye diseases; skin diseases; parasitic infections; occupational diseases, especially rupture and infection following injury; fractures; unhealed wounds and ulcers, especially of the legs; 'the stone' (kidney and bladder stones); complications of pregnancy and childbearing; 'melancholy' (called 'the English disease'); tuberculosis; and conditions which killed infants, like diarrhoea.

Poverty and poor law

In the early sixteenth century, England followed other European countries in introducing ecclesiastical registration of births, marriages and deaths, primarily to detect excess mortality caused by plague. Summary *bills of mortality*, sometimes collating causes of death other than plague, were later instituted in London and other major centres. Surviving an epidemic also involved measuring (and increasing) available resources, so that 'numbering the people' for tax purposes intensified. Moreover, humanist ideals suggested that in a city—or 'commonwealth'—leaders should be responsible and all citizens contributory according to their degree.

The problem of *poverty* became a major aspect of social policy, with suspicion first concentrated on the vagrant, 'sturdy' poor. Parish and town authorities subjected the vagrant poor to deterrent punishments like

badge-wearing, whipping, forced labour and compulsory medical treatment, mitigated on occasion by local discretion, inefficiency, or lack of resources. 'Censuses of the poor' revealed to municipal authorities the extent of poverty and disease among 'respectable', as opposed to vagrant poor. The following quotation shows census-takers' descriptions of a few households out of 2 359 poor people identified in Norwich in 1570—around a quarter of the English-born population of the city. The Norwich Census is the best surviving example of a 'census of the poor', but other English towns carried out similar censuses, probably after precedents set by towns in continental Europe. The references to alms indicate the extent of support from the poor rate (see p.21) then being levied, which the census revealed to be quite inadequate (Norwich, the second city after London, was unusually early in making the poor rate compulsory). Note especially the different compositions of the households, and the recording of sickness and disability, even among children.

Entries from the Norwich Census of the Poor, 1570

Thomas Ellmere of 36 yere, laborer & in no worke, & Alyce, his wyfe, of 30 yer, that spyn & washe etc., & 4 chyldren, theldest 7 yers & is sykly, & have dwelt her 9 yer & cam from Cambrydge. *Mrs. Felixe house. No allms. Veri pore.*

John Drane of 64 yere, gardener in work, and Thannzen, his wyfe, of 40 yeris, that spyn white warpe, & a systers daughter of 15 yere that spyn also, & hath dwelt here 40 yer. (hable) [i.e. able] *The Church house. No alms. Pore.*

Thomas Barthlett of 50 yeris, with one hande, that worke nott, & Jane, his wyfe, of that age, that use to go abrode & peddle; & 3 children of 8, 6, 3 yer, and a deaf wenche that begge, and have dwelt here 7 yer, & cam from the northe. *John Goses house. No allms. Veri pore.*

Gilion Tivet of 60 yeris, wedowe, that knytt, & have dwelt here ever. (hable) *No allms. Veri pore.*

Robert Trace of 80 yere, past work & a deafe man, & Margaret his wyfe, of 60 yere, that spyn white warpe; & a sons child of 10 yere that spyn, & have dwelt here 6 yer, & cam from Walsham. *Hable. Ther house for lyfe. No allms. Pore.* (Pound, 1971, pp. 51, 54, 55, 61, 88)

In the context of economic difficulties, population growth, and crisis mortality it became clear not only that

---

[2]The epidemiology of this period is discussed in *World Health and Disease,* Chapters 5 and 6.

sickness led to poverty but that many of the poor simply lacked employment. Prompted by a range of crises including epidemic disease, dearth and economic decline, English towns could identify as poor over 20 per cent of their populations. Local experience of the problem of the poor accumulated during the sixteenth century and was ultimately codified in the national legislation of 1598 and 1601. This Elizabethan framework endured— eventually becoming known as the **Old Poor Law**—until the New Poor Law of 1834.

The fundamental principle laid down by the Elizabethan law was that a parish should support its own poor on the proceeds of a compulsory **poor rate**, set by, levied upon, and administered by the parish's more prosperous householders. Elizabethan parish officials recognised both demographic and economic realities in instituting a system dependent on *community* rather than family support. In practice, even the closest relatives could be assisted by the parish to care for an infirm family member. As you will see in more detail later in this chapter, the Old Poor Law included medical care, but as one aspect of social welfare.

Lay care: anxiety and expertise

You have seen that this period was marked by the irruption of new and frightening epidemic diseases, which coincided with religious, economic and demographic changes, suggesting to contemporaries the destruction of the existing order. Some historians—Lawrence Stone and Philippe Ariès being among the most eminent—have suggested that people's response to such insecurity was fatalism, reflected in a lack of affection even within the family circle. The barrage of evidence used to counter these views, drawn from such sources as diaries, includes attitudes to health and illness. It can be shown that people worried constantly not only about major, but about minor threats to health. One reflection of this was the widespread resort to health care to monitor and maintain health, even in the absence of illness.

You will already be aware that many modern health surveys depend for their data on how much people use health services, rather than on whether people see themselves, or are seen, as ill. This is a limited way of measuring health, but the information is at least accessible. For similar reasons, more historical attention has been given to doctors than to the sick, and the extent of *lay care* in the past has been greatly underestimated. Where historians have recognised the role of women, for example, it has been mainly in terms of the charitable role of gentlewomen among their dependants. This is seen as

a redeeming feature of a situation in which skilled professional services were unavailable to most of the population. Lay care thus appears in a negative light, as a function of the *absence* of doctors.

This has particular relevance with respect to *children*: few doctors seem to have treated children in this period, and it has been inferred that parents were resigned or even indifferent to their loss. (Here we could remind ourselves that even today up to 90 per cent of children's illnesses are dealt with by *lay* carers.) In fact, parents seem to have assumed that professional care was inappropriate and even dangerous for the majority of children's complaints. The care of children was, then as now, primarily the responsibility of women. Lay nursing care naturally played an even greater role in a medical system in which *symptoms* were treated rather than the underlying disease.

Family and community

Until recently, it had been assumed that formal welfare systems became necessary as a result of the breakdown of the 'extended family'.

□ What demographic realities have we looked at for much of northern Europe in the pre-industrial period which undermine the basis of this assumption?

■ For most of the population, extended families of the kind assumed did not exist. Families were small, especially among the poor; widows and old people often had to live alone; the population was mobile rather than settled.

Thus, although care within the family was important, we need to stress the extent of informal consultation and assistance provided *within communities*—examples being the persistence of folkloric and magical beliefs, the resort to 'cunning' (i.e. knowing) men and women, the role of clergy and parochial assistance, the passing-on of remedies by letter, word of mouth, and recipe book, the survival of local traditions such as holy wells, the origin in popular knowledge of practices as important as inoculation and vaccination (discussed later in this chapter), and the respect given in agricultural communities to those skilled in treating animals. The self-sufficient household was less and less a reality, but most forms of production were still organised on the domestic level. Thus, when we note the importance of 'kitchen-physic', we should remember not only that the workplace was more like a kitchen, but also that the kitchen was more like a workplace, with implications for people's knowledge of processes and materials.

We should, however, avoid idealising lay care, just as we should realise the extent to which health care provided (and provides) a form of psychological support.

Lay and formal care: blurred boundaries

A more revealing historical picture of health care in the pre-industrial period has been achieved in recent years by abandoning definitions of the medical practitioner which derive from the modern idea of **professionalisation**. These modern definitions lay stress upon extensive training, academic qualifications, autonomy, vocational commitment, recognition by the state, and the restraint of groups of inferior status.[3] Even today, some of these criteria are professional *ideals*, rather than realities. In the pre-industrial period, such levels of regulation and institutionalisation did not exist. Nor was full-time salaried employment the way in which people gained their livings. As you will see later in this chapter, many practitioners of all kinds, for a variety of reasons, practised medicine on a *part-time* basis, and learned by experience; community approval could play a decisive role in legitimating a practitioner's activities. Consequently, lay and formal care are often very difficult to distinguish.

It is also right to emphasise how difficult it was for any kind of practitioner to claim a *monopoly* of relevant knowledge. Ill people were, in general, both sceptical and discriminating in their choice of practitioner, and the relationship between practitioner and patient was more evenly balanced than it is now. One reason for this is that practitioners did not then occupy a fixed and relatively advantageous position in the social hierarchy, as they do today, but occurred in all walks of life.

The conventional account of the growth of medical knowledge might suggest another reason: you might expect that traditional practitioners were not cut off from their patients by a massive body of scientific information accessible only to themselves, as is the case today. There is some truth in this, but it is an oversimplification. Three objections to this interpretation can be raised. First, 'special knowledge' is, in all health-care systems, claimed by the practitioner and/or attributed to the practitioner by the patient. Second, we should avoid the idea that there 'wasn't much to know'. There were major bodies of knowledge then seen as relevant to medicine, but at the elite as well as the popular level, relevant knowledge was not confined to practitioners. Third, a plurality of medical philosophies was available: this increased the grounds of choice between practitioners, but also threw patients back on their own judgement. All of these factors enlarged the potential for lay care, and blurred the boundaries between lay and formal care.

A good example illustrating these points is provided by *midwives* (see Figure 2.2). It is rare in most formal records of the period to find women designated by the occupation of midwife, yet women prepared to act as midwives were possibly better distributed in both rural and urban parishes than any other class of practitioner. Women's skills in midwifery were gained on the basis of occasion, example and experience. Community—that is, lay—sanction played the major role in their definition as practitioners. Attempts at ecclesiastical regulation of midwives were uneven and inconsistent.

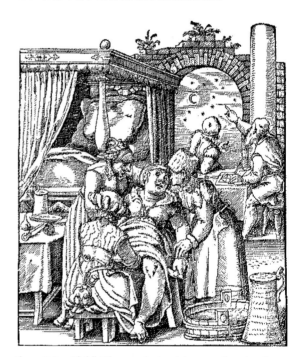

Figure 2.2 *Childbirth scene by Joost Amman, from Jacob Rueff's* De generatione hominis, *1580, a well-known handbook for midwives (and for those who, in northern European towns, were officially responsible for supervising midwives), first published in 1554. (Reproduced from* Medicine and the Artist (Ars Medica) *by permission of the Philadelphia Museum of Art)*

---

[3]The professional status of modern medical practitioners is discussed in Chapter 7 of this book, and in *Medical Knowledge: Doubt and Certainty*, Chapters 2 and 7.

The cleanliness of our ancestors

Until recently, little interest has been taken in the environment of pre-industrial societies in relation to health. It has simply been assumed that our ancestors were dirty. Increasing awareness of the environmental problems caused by post-industrial society, as well as better research, may well remove some of our easy sense of superiority about earlier standards of sanitation and personal cleanliness.

People of this period very frequently expressed disgust, either about their neighbours' habits as compared with their own, or about the habits of other nations. However, living and organic matter of all kinds—urine, for example—was, because it had practical uses, also more intrusive than now. The relationship with the natural world may have been closer and more casual—but this did not preclude cruelty, fear, or distaste:

A 'judgement of God' recorded by the Puritan artisan, Nehemiah Wallington, in the early seventeenth century

The Templers found tow [two] Sargents at a tavarne neare the Temple. And they toke them out. And set them in a kinde of a valt [vault] (where their felth [filth] runeth) up unto the anckels, then they drew their Swords. And said they would rune them through if they did not Shave off halfe one anothers head and halfe the other side of their beard then they did so: then they caused them to take some of the felth and rube one a others face with it then they cut a peace of their eares off and hurled them into the Theams [Thames] and dowssed them…But marke the hande of God upon on [one] of the cheefe actors of this Cruel mischife…Hee boosting of this his cruelty…at the Tavarne hee being drunke went to the house of office [latrine] and fell in to the valte and was there halfe an houre before he was mist, and when they had found him they tooke him out, and laid him upon the grasse, and there he died presently [immediately]. (Quoted in Jenner, 1991, p. 227)

In the medical theory and natural philosophies of the time, odour was an active substance and was consequently taken seriously both as a cause of disease, and a means of its prevention or cure. Similarly, bathing the body had *high* status, not as an everyday procedure, but as one with important consequences for health. Different waters had different (and potent) properties, a belief which is perhaps best known as leading to the development of spa towns—named after Spa, in Belgium, one of the most successful examples.

Threats to health: public and private

The German sociologist Norbert Elias, in his account of the 'civilising process' in Western Europe, has formulated a major shift in attitude from the communal habits of the Middle Ages—for example in eating and bathing—to the emergence in the eighteenth century of sharply defined distinctions between the public and private domains. Obviously such a shift can be detected only among those classes of society with the economic resources to express it, and it could be seen as an inevitable adjunct of periods of increased material consumption. One such period was the 'great rebuilding' which began to change the man-made environment of Tudor England in the later sixteenth century. Permanent materials such as brick were more widely used, and the space within dwellings gradually became more subdivided and less communal. We might also note the increased acquisition of linen and textiles, furniture (including chamber pots and close stools) and items relating to personal appearance such as looking glasses.

At the same time, while their comforts and possessions increased, the Elizabethan elite saw around them a 'crowded society', threatened in an unprecedented way by population increase, social mobility, poverty, and disease. Although the 'sweating sickness', bubonic plague, and syphilis are not 'filth diseases' in the nineteenth-century sense, sixteenth-century authorities did develop a fear of situations in which disease might be engendered by putrefaction. Both people and places could be dangerous—as, for example, when beggars congregated together, strangers used the same utensils in alehouses, or butchers threw offal into a town ditch. Although plague had a more obvious effect in redefining social administration—as, for example, in quarantines or the collection of mortality statistics—the contagion of syphilis was also a factor in Tudor and Stuart social policy, and may have been even more important than plague in prompting the sense of estrangement from 'other people' suggested by Elias.

After the 1660s, plague became an exotic disease, and hence an aspect of relations with other countries. Domestic policy was influenced more by endemic diseases such as typhus, smallpox and syphilis. These diseases affected relations within households and between social groups. Smallpox, for example, which particularly affected young migrants to towns, became a factor in the agreements between masters and apprentices.

Inoculation,[4] a traditional practice observed in the Eastern Mediterranean, was introduced into Britain by the elite in the early eighteenth century to protect their children, and was soon extended to servants and the poor.

A rural society and its environment

When considering environmental effects on health we tend to think of towns rather than the countryside. However, local conditions were first determined by local geography. Classical tradition and folk experience affirmed the influence of airs, waters and places on health. A disease which very much underlined these traditional beliefs was *malaria* (then called ague or marsh fever), which was endemic in the Fen country and low-lying parts of south-east England, as well as in similar regions throughout continental Europe.

The countryside was, of course, increasingly shaped by human activity, such as deforestation. Major projects in fen drainage and water supply were begun for economic reasons in the sixteenth and seventeenth centuries. It is important to note not only the influence of agricultural labour on health in this period, but also the effect of agricultural practices on the environment. In arable areas, according to the nature of local industries, animal hair, bone, dung, decaying fish, offal, blood, sawdust, malt dust, soot, soap ashes, leather scraps, and rags were used to condition the soil. Agriculture thus provided some incentive for the removal of wastes from towns and villages. Research is beginning to reveal the extent of 'recycling' in the economies of this period. Sometimes (as in the trade in second-hand clothes and left-over food) this would have had adverse consequences for health.

The responsibilities of towns

We should not assume that the development of relevant services such as street cleaning and paving had to await the emergence of strong centralised government, although we should acknowledge the piecemeal nature of improvements—like paving in main streets—carried out in the interests of 'polite' society. The changing prosperity of a town could produce considerable variation in its physical condition, and a town's representatives would complain of defects in drainage, paving and cleaning as proof of decline.

In older towns, the detailed regulation of markets included constant attention to the quality, honesty and price of provisions exposed for sale—especially staple commodities such as meat, grain, bread, and ale or beer. Fairly consistent concern was felt by parishes, occupational gilds, and town corporations for the effects on the public health of the activities of butchers, fishmongers, curriers, dyers, tanners, and other trades producing 'annoying' wastes, or contaminating large volumes of water. Such tradesmen were normally restricted in certain ways, for instance in being allowed to burn or transport their waste only at night, or to operate only outside city walls.

During this period, hitherto small-scale or domestic industries, such as brewing, soap boiling, distilling, and even baking, were moving on to an industrial scale of operation, to use coal or charcoal rather than wood as a fuel, and thus to change the character of urban pollution. The medieval legal concept of 'nuisance', which was still a major feature of public health legislation in the nineteenth century, enshrined the conviction that offences against the environment were injurious to neighbours or to the community at large.

Two examples follow, from different levels of the legal system, of action taken to control noxious trades in seventeenth-century London. Note that James Farr provides an instance of a barber diversifying into a new branch of the food and drink trades.

> ### A justice giving his view in the case of Jones vs. Powell, heard in the court of King's Bench in 1629, and concerning complaints over pollution from a brewhouse
>
> I have known someone indicted for making candles, namely for using the trade of tallow-chandler, whereby he annoyed his neighbours; and yet that is a trade necessary for the common wealth, but because it was so obnoxious to men and so noisome, being in an inapt place for such a trade, he was indicted...one may use a trade that is lawful in itself in such a way that it shall be noxious and unlawful. Thus if a butcher (which is a trade lawful and necessary for the public good) uses his trade in Cheapside, certainly an action lies against him by those that live there. There is a lawful place for such noisome trades, as the Shambles at Newgate, and therefore no action lies against a butcher who occupies his trade there, since it is a proper

[4] See also the discussion of the slave trade later in this chapter. Inoculation at this period involved the deliberate introduction of smallpox matter through the skin or mucous membrane. A variety of methods were used. This would frequently, but not invariably, result in a milder case of the disease which conferred immunity from subsequent infection. (As indicated in Chapter 3, inoculation was superseded by vaccination. The terms 'vaccination' and 'immunisation' are explained there.)

place for it. The makers of hats and beavers have a lawful trade; yet one was indicted for setting up and using such a trade at Ludgate Hill. But we all know that on the back side of Bridewell there is a great number of this trade; and surely they may lawfully use it there. (Quoted in Jenner, 1991, p. 34)

A prosecution for nuisance by the wardmote inquest of the parish of St Dunstan's in the West, London, in 1657

[James Farr, barber, is presented] for makeing & selling of a Drinke called Coffee whereby in making the same he annoyeth his neighbors by evill smells & for keeping of ffier for the most part night & day whereby his Chimney & Chamber hath ben set on fier to the great danger & affrightment of his Neighbours. (Quoted in Jenner, 1991, p. 37, note)

Utopia: a healthy city

Some of those facing the realities of human society also tried to imagine ideal states, or to find good models elsewhere. A number of writers in this period produced **utopias**, beginning with Utopia, the ideal Christian city imagined by Sir Thomas More in 1516. A noticeable characteristic of utopias is that they addressed themselves to the problems of urbanisation, postulating planned environments which ensured a high standard of hygiene and fostered the prolongation of life. More was influenced by humanist ideals of civic responsibility but also by the model architectural designs of the Italian Renaissance. There was consequently little resemblance between More's highly planned Utopia and the organic growth of the countrified towns of provincial England. More's authoritarian prescriptions for the public health are likely to have been based on the quarantine regulations and public health boards of the cities of northern Italy, which developed from temporary measures prompted by the Black Death in the fourteenth century.

One such board (Venice) wrote to another (Bologna) in 1630:

With letter from Your Lordships, we received the box containing the drugs against the current disease. We shall dispatch them to the pest-house in order to have them tested. We shall keep you informed of the results… (Quoted in Cipolla, 1976, pp. 51–2, note)

The quotation shows these boards taking an active role in medical care and investigation, yet they were an arm of civic rather than medical administration, and in time of plague had very major powers over medical personnel. Compared with this level of development, in terms of institutions, personnel, and the built environment, English public health remained in a state of nature.

Medical practitioners: many and varied

People of this period suffered a high level of anxiety about health and disease. This in turn created demand for health care, which was met, once the decision was made to look outside the resources of the family and the community, by an extremely wide range of healers. Medical practitioners existed in large numbers as well as great variety, and there is ample evidence of their activities in a broad range of sources. As you have seen earlier in this chapter, modern criteria of professionalisation are inappropriate for analysing medical practice in the pre-industrial period. To do justice to the historical picture, we adopt here the term **medical practitioner**, to cover all forms of practice, by women as well as men, and we define a practitioner as one whose contemporaries saw him or her as pursuing the occupation of caring for health and of healing the sick.

> ☐ Can you think of any objections which could be made to this definition?

> ■ You may feel that, since we are referring to an early period, the definition is too inclusive—that we should include only those practitioners who were effective, and should also exclude those who were dishonest.

These are, of course, essential issues in relation to any service provider. However, both criteria are very difficult to apply historically, and the first is not applied directly even to modern health-care workers. It is best to adopt a critical approach to the claims made in *any* historical context, and to assume also that 'gullibility' is a danger at all periods, because of patients' need to believe in their practitioners. Similarly, 'effectiveness' must be judged relative to the standards of the time.

The tripartite division: physicians, surgeons, and apothecaries

Medical polemics can be highly misleading. For example, in different historical contexts critics and apologists alike tended to claim the existence of a rigid (and male-dominated) **tripartite division of medicine** into *physicians*, *surgeons*, and *apothecaries*, in descending order of status (each occupation is described below). For England, however, the occupational structure of medicine, looser and more competitive than in continental Europe, meant that the divisions between types of practitioner were by no means clear cut. In the pre-industrial period, the tripartite division was an *ideal* transferred from the highly organised city states of continental Europe. Not surprisingly, this was an ideal which appealed particularly to the physicians, who claimed pre-eminence on the ground of their lengthy formal education in humanistic learning as well as medicine. We will return to this ideal in the next section, but here we need to ask what relation it bore to the reality of the occupational structure of medicine in this period.

A rough version of the tripartite structure did exist in pre-industrial towns, but had far less meaning for patients in rural areas. Many high-status university-trained **physicians** based themselves in towns, and patients often travelled long distances to consult them. But in other ways physicians did *not* dominate urban medical practice. Their numbers were small; only two English towns possessed universities, and only London, which had no university, developed an organisation for physicians. The English elite lived as much in the country as in the town, and physicians usually had to do the same. These factors help to explain the frequent presence of academically qualified physicians in the countryside, although it is harder to determine whether such men practised extensively. Probably more numerous, and certainly more accessible, were the *practitioners of physic*, who were rarely university-trained but saw themselves as qualified by reading or experience in this 'internal' part of medicine.

Paradoxically, the anxiety of English physicians to maintain their status could make their practice more rigid than in countries where medicine was actually better regulated, as the report of one late-sixteenth-century traveller, Fynes Moryson, indicates:

> The Universities...espetially of Padoa...have yielded famous phisitians who in Italy are also shirgians [surgeons] and many of them growe rich for all that have any small meanes will in sicknes have their helpe, because they are not prowde but will looke upon any ordure and handle any sore, but espetially because they are carefull for their patients, visite them diligently and take little fees which make heavy purses. (Quoted in Cipolla, 1976, p. 107)

☐ What does the quotation suggest were the virtues of the surgeon-physicians of Italy—and, by implication, of surgeons in general as compared with physicians?

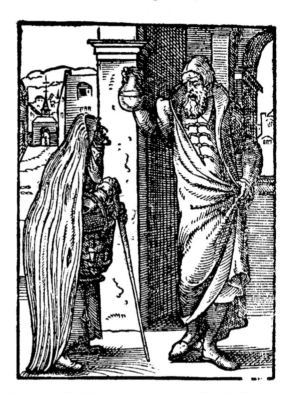

Der Doctor.

Figure 2.3 *Physician, by Jost Amman, in Hans Sachs, Beschreibung aller Stande, 1574. This belongs to a genre of 'galleries of characters' from the trades and professions (see also Figure 2.8). There is often an element of caricature. Sachs added a poem (of earlier date, c. 1520) which translates, 'I am a doctor of medicine. From the urine I can determine exactly what illness befalls a person, whom I can help, with God's grace, through a syrup or recipe which counteracts their malady. In order that the person shall again be in good health—with medicine taught by the Arabs'. Note the poem's emphasis on prognosis and internal remedies—two major areas of physic. The old woman is likely to be the patient's servant; she has brought the urine to the doctor, rather than the doctor going to the patient. (Reproduced from* Medicine and the Artist (Ars Medica) *by permission of the Philadelphia Museum of Art)*

■ The Italian practitioners were well-trained, with a wide range of skills—but just as important, from the patient's point of view, they did not charge prohibitive fees, they provided careful attention for all but the poorest, and, rather than diagnosing or prescribing from a distance (see Figure 2.3), they were prepared to come to the patient and with their own hands treat even the more revolting conditions.

Moreover, Moryson suggests that the Italian practitioners also reaped material rewards by their absence of pride—they became rich, even though they often charged small fees.

Medical organisation in Scotland more closely resembled that in continental Europe, especially France, and surgery was consequently of higher status than in England.

The **barbers** and **barber-surgeons**, who offered the greatest range of personal services, from beard-dyeing and toothscraping to blood-letting (see Figure 2.4), surgery, and the treatment of sores, were more popular than the physicians, as well as better integrated into urban life. Although of only middling status, they were among the most numerous of urban trades, and could be found even in villages. The barber-surgeon is the nearest equivalent in this period to the modern general medical practitioner (GP), and can be seen as providing the bulk of formal health care in towns (see Figures 2.5 and 2.6, *overleaf*).

Living over (or in) 'the shop' was then the norm in medicine as in most other trades, and some barber-surgeons (as did other kinds of practitioner) took in patients as lodgers. Different notions of privacy meant that the barber-shop could offer treatment and yet be a place of semi-public resort, involving attractions such as drink, musical instruments and the exchange of news.

Under such influences as the campaign for the 'reformation of manners' from the later seventeenth century—an aspect of the changing attitudes identified by Elias—and the association of barber-surgeons with the treatment of sexually transmitted disease, the barber-shop connection became, by the early eighteenth century, one which higher-status surgeons wished to shed as thoroughly as possible. At the same time, surgeons wished to retain the advantage of being seen by patients as both useful and effective.

By the early seventeenth century, some **apothecaries** as well as some barber-surgeons in towns were beginning to call themselves 'doctor', and we also see the emergence of the **surgeon-apothecary** who is usually regarded as the true ancestor of the modern GP. It is, however, mistaken to see apothecaries as humble tradesmen who climbed in status as a result of intruding into medicine. From the medieval period, apothecaries were more often traders in expensive commodities (drugs and spices) who ranked in the higher-status retail sector of urban occupations, with other merchants and holders of capital such as goldsmiths. It is at least arguable that apothecaries *lost* status as their numbers expanded and they increasingly

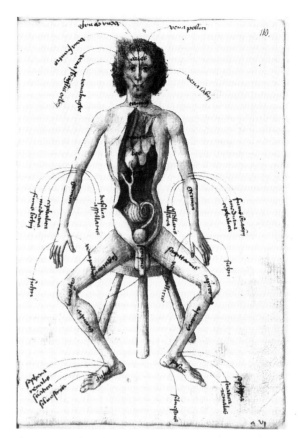

Figure 2.4 *Blood-letting man, from a sixteenth-century manuscript, showing the points at which to let blood from veins. This figure belongs to a tradition which often also conveyed correspondences between the body and the cosmos by means of astrological signs. The upper part of the body and the extremities are fairly naturalistic; the internal anatomy is somewhat behind the knowledge of the time. (Source: Herzog August Bibliothek, Wolfenbüttel, Cod. Guelf. 18.2 Aug 4, fol. 10r)*

adopted roles within medicine. As London grew as a centre of distribution, apothecaries were able to set up shops in smaller towns (see Figure 2.7, *overleaf*).

Specialists and itinerants

Because pre-industrial populations were comparatively mobile, and tireless in their pursuit of health care, the services of physicians, surgeons and apothecaries were not limited to those living in towns. People also travelled to resort to such specialists as bonesetters, cutters for

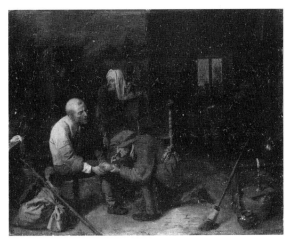

Figure 2.5 *Village barber-surgeon, by Adriaen Brouwer (d. 1638), in the Alte Pinakothek, Munich. (Source: Bayerische Staatsgemäldesammlungen)*

cataract, lithotomists[5] and specialists in such deformities as fistula[6] and harelip. These specialties involved high risk and expense for the patient, but existed because the need was correspondingly great. The useful bonesetter existed in both rural and urban versions. Not surprisingly, some specialists travelled from centre to centre, but acquired as much accreditation as possible from patients to distinguish themselves from unscrupulous itinerants (see Figure 2.8).

The spread of remedies associated with a particular healer began early in this period and these, whether *specifics* ('sovereign remedies' for particular diseases) or *panaceas* (cure-alls), had all the ambiguous attractions of metropolitan or continental sophistication.

Numbers and distribution of practitioners

It does not follow, of course, that all classes of practitioner are equally visible in the historical record—or that those for whom we have the most evidence were necessarily the most numerous or even the most important in terms of contemporary health care.

---

[5]Before anaesthesia, lithotomy or 'cutting for the stone' was, after amputation, the most frequently performed major operation and a traditional specialty. It usually involved the removal of calculi or stones from the bladder via a cut in the perineum (the area between the genitals and the anus).

[6]Fistulae could occur anywhere in the body and were in effect drainage holes caused when wounds and ulcers would not heal. Before antibiotics they could be extremely difficult to treat and were a major cause of long-term distress.

□ What kinds of practitioner would you expect to be least visible, and which most visible?

■ Women practitioners (including midwives), and practitioners serving small rural communities are less likely to be visible. Most visible are elite university graduates such as royal physicians—and notorious 'quacks' who succeeded in advertising their activities in urban centres.

Intensive local surveys aimed at including all kinds of practitioner except midwives have suggested that the ratio of practitioners to population in England around 1600 may have been as high as 1 : 200 in major towns, and 1 : 400 in well-populated rural areas. By contrast, a GP's 'list' in England and Wales in 1948 was 2 400, and in 1990, 1 700. This striking comparison might suggest that modern populations are *less* well provided for than those of the past.

□ Why might such a direct comparison be misleading?

■ There are several reasons:

1   The ratio for the pre-industrial period was probably much lower for sparsely populated rural areas.

2   The ratio for the pre-industrial period refers to all kinds of practitioner: the modern GP is expected to provide *comprehensive* primary care, but with the help of the primary care team, which includes several kinds of health-care worker.

3   The modern model of effectiveness in treatment requires less time to be spent by the GP with each patient.

4   A modern GP works full time in medicine, whereas the majority of practitioners around 1600 (and probably much later) almost certainly did not.

Occupational diversity: a means of living, not a way of life

Today we stress the vocational aspect of medicine, even though it is frequently chosen as a dependably lucrative career. It is important to realise that in the pre-industrial period, even for the educated elite, medicine was a useful means of subsistence and people drifted in and out of it as their needs required. For example, religious upheavals meant that many of the educated elite could find themselves unable to hold an ecclesiastical benefice and had to earn a living by other means. Medicine could also be a useful resort for those wanting to do something else that society would not pay well for, such as satirists and

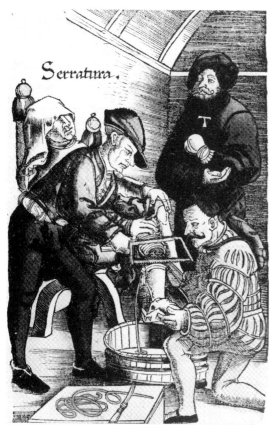

Figure 2.6 *Surgeons at work. An illustration of amputation by Johannes Wechtlin in Hans von Gersdorff's textbook,* Feldtbuch der Wundartzney, *1540. Note that the patient undergoing surgery appears to be unconscious. (Reproduced from* Medicine and the Artist (Ars Medica) *by permission of the Philadelphia Museum of Art)*

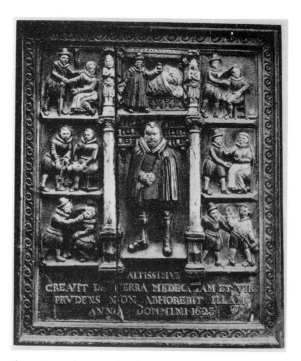

Figure 2.7 *This carved and painted signboard, dated 1623, shows the various services available from the Dorset (surgeon-)apothecary who displayed it. (Source: Wellcome Institute Library, London)*

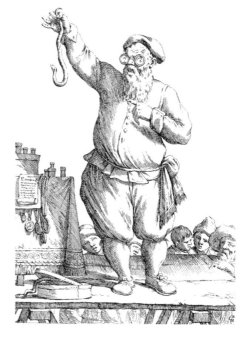

Figure 2.8 *'The Quack', after Annibale Carracci (1560–1609), in a set of street characters of Bologna, published in 1660. Italy, which provided models of medical organisation, also supplied striking images of quackery— including the terms 'mountebank' and 'charlatan'. (Source: Wellcome Institute Library, London)*

writers. Among the less literate, medicine could combine well with a range of other trades, especially those connected with food and drink, and the production of such substances as dyes and cosmetics.

This tendency was denounced (and exaggerated) by propagandists like the London surgeon William Clowes who, in 1585, deplored the intrusion into medicine of good trades and bad, such as painters, glaziers, tailors, weavers, cooks, bakers, tinkers, toothdrawers, pedlars, sow-gelders, horse-leeches, witches, rat-catchers, and 'such other like rotten and stinking weeds' (quoted in Webster, 1979, p. 186). Medicine, as a portable skill much in demand, was also a useful occupation for those wishing or needing to travel. These social and economic factors increased the difficulties of regulating the practice of medicine.

A health-care system outside institutions

In previous sections, we have outlined a system including a high consumption of medical care and a high per-capita incidence of medical practitioners.

> ☐ From what has been said, can you suggest how pre-industrial society was able to sustain such a system?
>
> ■ Much medical care was provided by family or community members on an exchange basis; most medical practitioners did not practise full-time but followed other occupations as well.

The costs of medical care: community provision

Practitioners in pre-industrial England offered a scale of treatments, and a scale of charges, according to what the patient was likely to be able to pay. With respect to adolescents and young adults, the potential burden was spread in that masters were expected to take responsibility for servants or apprentices if they fell ill. Nonetheless, families could be rendered destitute by the high cost and protracted nature of medical care, and this was also a factor in the gradual breakdown of apprenticeship. Recognition of the catastrophic effects of ill-health or disability, together with the community's fear of disease, produced a range of systems in which the community contributed to the costs of medical care.

Medical poor relief

In England the basis of most of these systems was the parish, although major towns evolved a more elaborate and centralised system of medical poor relief involving payments (sometimes on a 'retainer' or contract basis) to a wide range of both male and female practitioners. By the eighteenth century, parishes were also employing practitioners on a contract basis. This was in addition to occasional payments by towns or parishes for individual parishioners to seek expensive cures, 'go to the Bath' (i.e. Bath Spa), or be sent to 'Bedlam' (Bethlehem), London's hospital for the insane.

As we noted earlier, the financial basis for poor law provision (also known as poor relief) was the poor rate, although charitable doles and endowments made an important contribution in many parishes. Parish officials decided on pensions to single-parent families, the infirm elderly, and those disabled for work, and made temporary grants in time of sickness and to large families. These officials also provided for improved levels of clothing, heating, and nutrition, paid the expenses of childbirth or burial, and supported children into service or apprenticeship. Single payments for medical treatment could be extremely high, and officials certainly saw medicine as a worthwhile investment, transforming the impotent into the able-bodied, that is, able to work. Overall, however, the bulk of parish expenditure on poor relief was in the form of income support.

Most forms of support for the sick poor involved an expedient which was to prove very enduring: the able poor were employed to look after, nurse, or even treat the sick poor. Typically, a woman needing support herself would be paid as a nurse, 'watcher' (i.e. night-nurse or sick-minder), or child-minder. Although sometimes coercive, this practice can be seen, in this period at least, as increasing the resources of informal care within the community.

The importance of lay care notwithstanding, it may seem from this that the poor were offered only a very 'second-class' service. The evidence suggests the contrary: town and parish authorities did, according to need, select practitioners from among the whole range of those available, including high-status physicians. Notable aspects are first, the lack of reference by such authorities to any system of licensing or regulation of practitioners, and second—since parish officials were laymen—the primacy of lay control.

Hospitals and other institutions

It may have surprised you that we have made no mention so far of hospitals, almshouses, or other institutions. Except for London, the hospitals familiar today date only from the 1730s, and will be dealt with in the next chapter; but, in general terms, hospitals were not central to health care in Britain until the twentieth century (unlike the rest of Europe; see Figure 2.9).

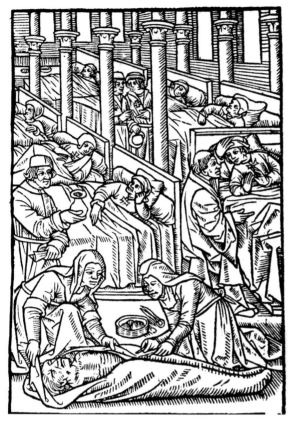

Figure 2.9 *Woodcut from Saint-Gelais,* Le vergier d'honneur, *c. 1500. This rare depiction is not so much a literal representation of a hospital interior, as an image of the cycle of life and death which took place there. (Reproduced from* Medicine and the Artist (Ars Medica) *by permission of the Philadelphia Museum of Art)*

The poor relief system just described was gradually built up following the Reformation,[7] although its roots go back much earlier. As a one-city nation, England was unusual even before the dissolution of the monasteries in its lack of major institutions for the sick poor, just as it was unusual in the elaboration of its system of parish administration. This was primarily a system of *out-door* relief,

---

[7]The Reformation refers to the fragmentation of the church which occurred in Europe in the first half of the sixteenth century. The breakaway movement is known as Protestantism. Acceptance or rejection of Protestantism in any state usually involved a lengthy power struggle. Only gradually were the dominant traditions of Protestantism, linked with such figures as Calvin or Luther, consolidated into national and international church organisations.

involving forms of community care which did not entail entering an institution.

The City of London refounded five monastic hospitals for the custody and regulation of the poor in the post-Reformation period, but only three of them (St Thomas's, St Bartholomew's, and Bethlehem) had any major responsibility for the *sick* poor. Christ's Hospital was refounded for orphans; Bridewell for the summary punishment and work-training of rogues, prostitutes, and vagabonds. London also used, in a more *ad hoc* way, an outlying circle of smaller institutions, once leperhouses, to treat or segregate chronic or threatening cases.

Other towns seem at times to have made equivalent use of the same range of institutions but, as in London, the numbers institutionalised were very small compared with the scale of need, and the initiatives involved were often short-lived. Sick people (including lunatics) crop up in almshouses, prisons, 'houses of correction' or 'bridewells' (named after the London institution), and (especially from the early eighteenth century) workhouses, and relief could be provided for these individuals on an occasional basis. As the names suggest, the primary aim of houses of correction and **workhouses** was to instil work-discipline or, more positively, to provide work and train the poor to be self-supporting (see Figure 2.10, *overleaf*).

□ Overall, what would you see as the disadvantages and advantages of these provisions for the sick poor?

■ Relief was not systematic or comprehensive; it could be punitive; and it depended upon the presence and goodwill of prosperous householders. But, especially at the parish level, it could also have the flexibility to meet individual needs possible only in a 'face-to-face' society; and it did not require massive investment in institutions such as hospitals.

Medicine and the 'common weal'

What responsibility did society take for the *quality* of medical care? In this period, relations between patient and practitioner seem often to have been governed by conditional contracts, including an element of payment by results. What was bargained for was not cure, but 'a cure', a balance between what the ill person wanted and what the practitioner was prepared to predict as the outcome of his or her treatment. Pre-industrial society was highly litigious and dissatisfied patients readily took legal action. Both the highest- and the lowest-status practitioners tried to bypass this system, physicians by stressing their role in prognosis and by charging standard fees for advice, and quacks by minimising follow-up contact with their patients.

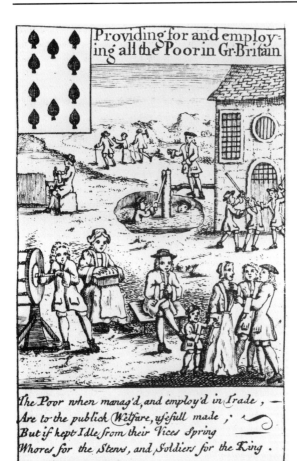

Providing for and employ-
ing all the Poor in Gr·Britain

The Poor when manag'd, and employ'd in Trade , —
Are to the publick Welfare, usefull made ; —
But if kept Idle, from their Vices spring
Whores for the Stews, and Soldiers for the King .

Figure 2.10 *A workhouse depicted on a playing card of 1720. Note the emphasis on productive forms of labour. The late seventeenth century brought renewed interest in work training and workhouses for the poor. (Source: Hulton/Deutsch Picture Collection)*

Even in a highly competitive situation, in an emergent capitalist economy, 'buyer beware' was not the only law. By around 1600, the medieval town gilds had evolved into **companies**, controlled and manipulated according to changing economic and social conditions by civic authorities—a form of devolved economic planning. Companies supervised training, inspected merchandise, and exerted a 'right of search' over premises, apprentices and journeymen. These standard functions could take different forms according to the trade in question: for example, a responsibility of the officebearers of barber-surgeons' companies was to supervise contracts for 'cures' made with dangerously ill patients by less-experienced members. Separate barber-surgeons' companies, which could include physicians, existed in the

largest towns. Apothecaries were commonly in companies that included grocers and other merchants.

The nearest approach to a *national* system regulating medicine was represented by the licences to practise issued by bishops, after 1511, to physicians, surgeons and midwives, but this system was only patchily administered. The humanist *College of Physicians of London*, founded in 1518, differed from the *London Barber-Surgeons' Company* (reorganised in 1540) and the *Worshipful Society of Apothecaries of London* (separated from the Grocers' Company in 1617) in aspiring to national control. However, although it sought to prosecute unlicensed practitioners, the College was limited in its effectiveness even within London. Municipal authorities, and under them the companies, seem to have been the most effective regulators of crafts and trades in this period, including the different branches of medicine.

Later in this book you will compare this situation with that in advanced modern societies, in which the ideals of professionalisation are firmly established. Expectations tend now to be high, but we also find that successful outcomes are not guaranteed, and redress for the individual is often a lengthy and much-obstructed process.

Empires and exchanges: the first phase of expansion

Systems of health care in Western Europe did not develop in isolation. The beginnings of European expansionism mentioned at the outset of this chapter, and the increasing frequency of maritime trade with distant parts of the globe, resulted in a series of pathogenic and cultural exchanges which proved deadly to both colonisers and colonised, and which had lasting consequences for the development of both Western and indigenous medical systems. The establishment of territorial and commercial interests overseas was central to the consolidation of European nation states also referred to earlier.

The impulse for English overseas expansion began during the reign of Henry VIII and gathered momentum under Elizabeth I, with the voyages of Drake, Frobisher, and Ralegh. By the mid-seventeenth century, England had established colonies and trading posts in Ireland, the Americas, and in India, but England was still in its infancy as a colonial power. Foremost among the expansionist powers were Spain, which held sway over much of South and Central America, and Portugal, with footholds in South America and the East Indies.

The medical and demographic impact of European expansion is one of the darkest but now, also, one of the best-known chapters in imperial history. The unparalleled savagery of the Spanish *conquistadores*, in particular, has attracted a good deal of attention from historians.[8] So too has the decimation of the native American population by epidemic diseases, like smallpox, brought from the Old World—a process which the American historian Alfred Crosby has referred to as the 'Columbian exchange'. The horrific effects of smallpox were chronicled in accounts written by the Spanish and depicted in illustrations such as Figure 2.11. The importation of these diseases, which might more generally be referred to as an **epidemiological exchange**, precipitated a demographic decline which greatly facilitated the European conquest of the Americas, although the role of technology and military force in establishing European domination should not be underestimated.

The slave trade

The birth of the Atlantic slave trade in the seventeenth century also had terrible medical consequences for those black Africans who were enslaved, and for those who were left behind. The slave trade, which involved the capture of indigenous peoples in West Africa for work on European plantations in the Americas, and which in turn provided the raw materials for industrial expansion in Europe, provides one of the most vivid examples of the pervasive and deadly influence of Western capitalism. By forcibly bringing together slaves from all over Western

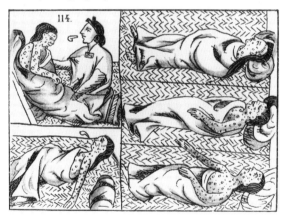

Figure 2.11 *Various stages of smallpox among Aztec victims of the disease in the sixteenth century, illustrated in a manuscript,* Historia de las Cosas de Nueva Espana. *(Peabody Museum, Harvard University)*

[8]The effects of European colonisation of the Third World are discussed in *World Health and Disease*, Chapter 7.

Africa, the slave trade blended the varied and hitherto distinct disease environments of different parts of Africa with 'new' European diseases. Impounded in overcrowded 'barracoons' on the African coast, and in the cramped and ill-ventilated conditions on slave ships, smallpox, dysentery, and eye diseases spread like wildfire. Just how crowded slaving vessels were can be appreciated from the diagram in Figure 2.12 (*overleaf*).

On arrival, conditions at the plantations were little better, with people, plants and animals concentrated in lowland areas ridden with vector-borne diseases such as malaria and yellow fever, imported from Africa by the slave trade. This trade, then, not only facilitated the geographical spread of infectious disease, but greatly favoured its multiplication.

Initially, little thought was given to the health of slaves, but the appallingly high mortality among them led to some attempts to contain disease in order to increase the profitability of the trade and the plantations. One of the most successful measures introduced was the practice of inoculation against smallpox. Inoculation was practised in India, North Africa, and the Middle East, from where it was introduced into Britain in 1717 by the wife of the ambassador to Turkey, Lady Mary Wortley Montagu.

The same desire to increase economic efficiency lay behind other medical provisions for slaves on plantations, including the establishment of 'slave hospitals' staffed mainly with black attendants, and the occasional employment of European doctors in cases of last resort. Western medical care and the slave hospitals were usually distrusted by slaves, who had good reason to be suspicious of the intentions behind such arrangements, and who generally preferred to consult practitioners of African medicine, which was closely intertwined with their religious and cultural practices. Given this cultural distance, 'the white doctor could only practise medicine as if he were a veterinarian' (Sheridan, 1985, p. 355). Limited medical provisions on plantations had little effect on the health of slaves while they continued to be subject to over-work, poor diet, and poor housing.

'The white man's grave'

Yet the 'epidemiological exchange' was not as one-sided as Alfred Crosby and others have suggested.

☐ Can you recall an example given earlier in this chapter?

■ It was widely believed that syphilis was introduced into Europe from South America or Africa.

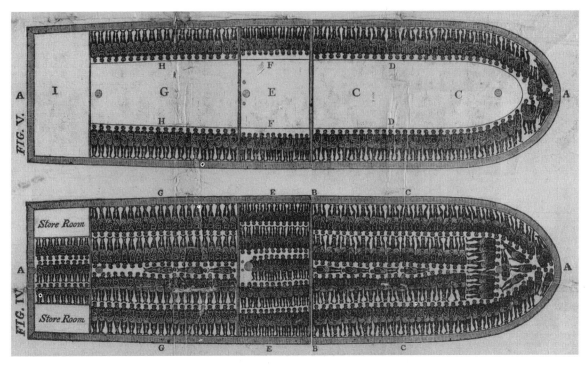

Figure 2.12 *Plan of two lower decks of the slave ship* Brooks, *supplied to the House of Commons in 1788 by Captain Parrey. AA lower deck. BB beam on lower deck. CC men's room on lower deck. DD platforms in men's room. EE boys' room. FF platform in boys' room. GG women's room. HH platforms in women's room. I gun room on lower deck. The space allowed to each category of slave in this plan is 'To the Men 6 feet by 1 foot 4 inches. Women 5 feet 10 in. by 1 foot 4 in. Boys 5 feet by 1 foot 2 in. Girls 4 feet 6 in. by 1 foot', providing room for 482 slaves in total. The actual figures for slaves carried by this ship as supplied by the slave-merchants to Captain Parrey were 351 men, 127 women, 90 boys and 41 girls, a total of 609; the report notes how much less space they had to lie in, how the men were chained together, and the 'horrible mortality'. The report also notes: 'Besides the time spent on the coast to complete their cargoes, which sometimes lasts several months, the slaves are from six to eight weeks on their passage from thence to the West Indies…when to a long passage are added, inhuman treatment, scanty and bad provisions, and rough weather, their condition is miserable beyond description'. (Wilberforce House Museum, Hull City Museums and Art Gallery)*

The first English writer on so-called *tropical medicine*, Thomas Trapham, believed that the disease was a form of divine punishment for the 'sexual transgressions' of black and native American peoples, and that its increasing incidence among the Spanish was a sign that they were becoming morally and physically unfit to rule their vast conquests. Equally, in the colonies, and especially in West Africa (the 'white man's grave'), Europeans experienced levels of mortality far higher than indigenous peoples. In the early eighteenth century, troops stationed in the colonies suffered much higher death rates than those who remained in Britain, as Table 2.1 shows.

Table 2.1 Death rate of British troops stationed in Britain in the early eighteenth century, compared with those stationed in the colonies

Troops stationed in	Death rate per 1 000
Britain	just over 15
India	30–75
West Indies	85–138
West Africa	483–668

Data from Sheridan, R. B. (1985) *Doctors and Slaves: A Medical and Demographic History of Slavery in the British West Indies 1680–1834*, Cambridge University Press, Cambridge, p. 12.

Indigenous medical systems

European medical practitioners, having made only limited progress in alleviating the burden of sickness in their own countries, found themselves virtually powerless in the face of 'new diseases' and more familiar afflictions which seemed to increase in virulence in the tropics. It was not long before they began to solicit information from indigenous practitioners of medicine, who had a superior knowledge of local medicinal plants. This was particularly true of Europeans in India, who were confronted by two highly sophisticated traditional medical systems: the Hindu or *ayurvedic* system, and the Islamic *unani-i-tibb*. Surgeons of the English East India Company incorporated many Indian drugs into their pharmacopoeia, and practitioners of Hindu and Islamic medicine (*vaidyas* and *hakims* respectively) found employment with the Company as apothecaries and, from the 1660s, as assistants in its hospitals.

The Spanish, too, employed Aztec medical practitioners to tend their sick and wounded, while some European practitioners in the West Indies and North America were intrigued by the folk medicine of slaves and native Americans. Indeed, indigenous medical practitioners, or 'medicine men', frequently captured the imagination of Europeans, and were often depicted in illustrations accompanying travellers' accounts (see Figure 2.13).

The use of indigenous medical knowledge by Europeans was by no means confined to the colonies. As trade with the Americas and the Indies became more frequent, indigenous remedies were transported to Europe and were employed increasingly against the maladies of the Old World. The 'voyages of discovery' were bound up with a new spirit of investigation in science and medicine, associated with the rediscovery of ancient learning and 'secrets' mentioned earlier in this chapter.

Trade with the colonies fuelled this new approach to medicine by supplying exotic new remedies attractive to innovative practitioners. The 'new disease' of syphilis, as already mentioned, was treated with the wood guaiacum from South America; while the bark of the Peruvian cinchona tree (from which quinine was later derived) was widely employed in the treatment of various fevers. Opium, together with cinnamon, ginger, cumin, nutmeg and other spices became popular remedies for a wide range of diseases—cinnamon water, for instance, in the treatment of intestinal disorders. Thus, increasing contact with America and the Orient opened up exciting new therapeutic possibilities as well as testing the resourcefulness and resilience of European practitioners.

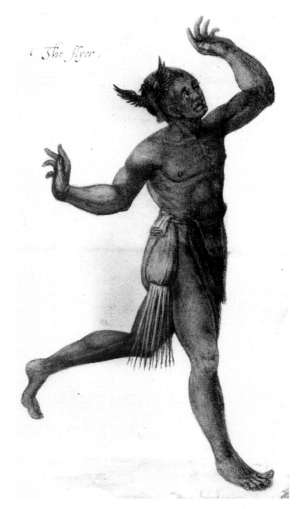

Figure 2.13 *A medicine man of Roanoke, North Carolina, 1585. Watercolour by John White. (Source: British Museum)*

In the long run, however, the most profound consequences for health stemmed from the importation of the potato and of tobacco. The potato (originally cultivated in South America) became one of the principal sources of nutrition for the poor of European countries such as Ireland; tobacco (originally from the West Indies and North America)—a subject of medical controversy from the start—was identified as a major cause of certain cancers and of heart disease in the later twentieth century.

By the end of the seventeenth century, European medical practitioners in India and the colonies were becoming more confident of their ability to treat and to combat diseases in the tropics. Having imbibed considerable local knowledge, their dependence on indigenous practitioners decreased, though cross-cultural consultation did not cease altogether. This tendency was perhaps most marked in Portuguese India, where the municipality of Goa attempted to ban the practice of indigenous medicine.

□ What does the decision of the Goa municipality tell us about the attitude of Europeans to indigenous medical practice?

■ European practitioners exploited indigenous medical knowledge but saw their own system as fundamentally superior to indigenous systems. They may also have been concerned about competition from indigenous practitioners.

European expansion, then, brought only a gradual extension of European systems of health care, but the medical problems and opportunities presented by the encounter with India, Africa, and the New World fuelled important developments in medical knowledge and practice. The fatal consequences of the epidemiological exchange between Europeans and indigenous peoples was matched by an exchange of medical knowledge and expertise.

However, this exchange was, in both pathogenic and cultural terms, an unequal one. The incidence of disease among European colonisers may have been as high, if not higher, than among indigenous peoples, but the devastation of the latter was far more extensive, and played a major part in the process of European domination. Equally, while European practitioners freely plundered indigenous medical knowledge, the benefits of Western health care were distributed only selectively, and with little effect, upon their colonial subjects. This state of affairs was to alter little in the next century of colonial expansion, considered in Chapter 3.

OBJECTIVES FOR CHAPTER 2

When you have studied this chapter, you should be able to:

2.1 Illustrate the difficulties of distinguishing between lay and formal care in the pre-industrial period.

2.2 Briefly describe the principal epidemic diseases and environmental threats to health in this period and estimate the extent of concern about them.

2.3 Explain what is meant by the tripartite division of health-care occupations in this period, indicate the limits of its applicability, and give reasons for the limited role of physicians compared with practitioners of other types.

2.4 Discuss the ways in which the problem of poverty was related to the development of poor-relief systems of health care, supported by public expenditure.

2.5 Demonstrate, by use of appropriate examples, an understanding of the relevance for health of the increasing European domination of the 'New World' of the colonial empires.

QUESTIONS FOR CHAPTER 2

Question 1 (*Objective 2.1*)

In 1601, Lady Margaret Hoby of Hackness, Yorkshire, recorded in her diary:

> This day, in the afternone, I had a child brought to me that was born at Silpho, one Talliour sonne, who had no fundament [anus] and had no passage for excrementes but at the Mouth; I was ernestly intreated to Cutt the place to see if any passage could be made, but, although I Cutt deepe and searched, there was none to be found. (Quoted in Wyman, 1984, pp. 31–2)

Look again too at Figure 2.2. In what ways do women illustrate the roles of both formal and lay practitioners in the pre-industrial period?

Question 2 (*Objective 2.2*)

The following is a lease of property agreed in late sixteenth-century London:

> This daie order is taken by this courte that Humfrey Morrey Inholder shall have the house in Goldinge Lane…being bound to

all reparacions with condition he suffer no butchers to dwell in any parte thereof or usuallye take any sicke people into the house which shalbe diseased of the plague or pox [venereal disease]. (St Bartholomew's Hospital Journal, H/a 1/2, fd. 165 [1581])

What does this tell us about efforts at this time on behalf of the public health?

Question 3 (*Objective 2.3*)

The different behaviour of practitioners in the plagues of the late sixteenth and early seventeenth centuries had a considerable effect on popular opinion at the time. Recalling the crises of the 1590s, the self-taught astrological practitioner of physic, Simon Forman, wrote:

> And in the time of pestilent plague
> When Doctors all did fly,
> And got them into places far
> From out the City,
> The Lord appointed me to stay
> To cure the sick and sore,
> But not the rich and mighty ones
> But the distressed poor.
> (Quoted in Rowse, 1974, pp. 56–7)

Forman's 'poem' says something about the individual sense of religious pre-ordination characteristic of the period. What does it also suggest about the activities and reputations of the different types of practitioner?

Question 4 (*Objective 2.4*)

The historian Paul Slack has estimated for pre-industrial England that 'five per cent was the normal background level of poverty in urban societies'. This however was a minimum. Among other higher contemporary estimates he mentions that:

> The crisis level could go higher still. A listing taken in Sheffield in 1616 counted at least 20 per cent and perhaps as many as 33 per cent of the population as 'begging poor', and there were other householders who '(though they beg not)…are not able to abide the storm of one fortnight's sickness but would be thereby driven to beggary'. When sickness in the form of plague hit Cambridge in 1630, 2,858 people—36 per cent of the population—were thought to require relief. (Slack, 1988, p. 72)

What does this suggest to you about the connections between poverty, disease, and poor relief?

Question 5 (*Objective 2.5*)

Writing of his experiences in the East Indies in 1658, the Dutch physician Jacobus Bontius extolled the medicinal virtues of local plants and medical practitioners; if he himself was ill, he preferred to 'trust himself to one of them' rather than to a European practitioner (quoted in Patterson, 1983, p. 460).

What does this tell us about the nature of the medical exchange which took place in this period between European and indigenous practitioners?

3

The Industrial Revolution, 1750 to 1848

This chapter builds on knowledge of the rate and underlying causes of population growth in the Industrial Revolution in Britain, and the shifts in patterns of disease associated with profound changes in the structure of an industrialising society (discussed in World Health and Disease, Chapters 5 and 6). The articles by Thomas McKeown and Simon Szreter, which were set reading for Chapter 6 of that book (see Health and Disease: A Reader[1]) are particularly relevant here.

The first industrial nation

During the Industrial Revolution, Britain seems to have escaped the Malthusian trap of the pressure of population on resources.[2] The heading of this section, 'the first industrial nation', reflects the essentially optimistic idea that Britain was the first to experience dramatic economic and demographic changes which will, sooner or later, be repeated in the 'undeveloped' world, just as they were in nineteenth-century mainland Europe. In simple terms this view assumes that progress, in the form of unrestricted economic growth, can always be expected to 'trickle down' to raise the standard of living even of the poorest, and thus, eventually, to limit population growth. Commentators are, however, increasingly noting that this process of *modernisation* (defined in Chapter 1) is *not* being duplicated in Third World countries.

This is one reason for the continued interest in the 'standard of living' debate about conditions in Britain in the period after 1750, when modernisation first occurred.

Some historians (the so-called 'optimists') point to certain measurable factors such as economic growth, rising incomes, and falling mortality rates, and conclude that other historians (the so-called 'pessimists') have greatly exaggerated the ill-effects of industrialisation on the condition of the British people at this time. The pessimists, say the optimists, have paid too much attention to impressionistic evidence, such as the 'horror stories' publicised by reformers, or the claims put forward by working-class protesters.

Industrialisation and health

Particularly important in the context of health care is a counter-argument put by one of the pessimists, the social historian E. P. Thompson:

> The controversy as to living standards during the Industrial Revolution has perhaps been of most value when it has passed from the somewhat unreal pursuit of the wage-rates of hypothetical average workers and directed attention to articles of consumption: food, clothing, homes: and, beyond these, health and mortality. (Thompson, 1975, p. 347)

Thompson's main point is that rapid urbanisation and the uncontrolled exploitation of the labouring poor during industrialisation caused a drastic deterioration in living and working conditions; that for many the most basic necessities of life—air, water, food, rest, and shelter—degenerated to an appalling degree; and that these evils could not be remedied by the poor themselves—at least not under the existing system.

Neither the optimists nor the pessimists would see medical advance as making much difference at this time.[3] The only innovation of note was the replacement of inoculation (see Chapter 2) with *vaccination* (a similar procedure using cowpox, a related but lesser disease which experience had shown to confer immunity against

[1]*Health and Disease: A Reader* (second edition, 1995).

[2]Discussed in *World Health and Disease*, Chapter 5.

[3]Discussed in *World Health and Disease*, Chapter 6.

smallpox).[4] The comparative unimportance of medical progress gives added prominence to the role of nutrition and environmental regulation.

Class divisions

Some people, as you will see, gave early warning of the effects of industrialisation. However, the humanitarian principles that inspired some reformers in the later eighteenth century were severely set back by the depressed economic conditions and political repression of the period around the Napoleonic Wars. The term *working class* was first used in the revolutionary 1790s, and was applied by middle-class reformers from around the end of the wars with France in 1814. Many saw a solution in political action, as remembered by one middle-class observer: 'From 1815 to 1830 the question of revolution or no revolution lurked in all our English discussions' (quoted by Weindling, 1980, p. 139). The fear of popular unrest was one motive behind upper-class support of the 'meliorative' social policies adopted in the wake of industrialisation.

What no historian involved in the 'standard of living' debate would deny is the *magnitude* of the changes over this period. The Census of 1851 showed that, for the first time, more people (in Wales as well as England) lived in towns than in the country. In Scotland, the shift of population to the major industrial centre of Glasgow was particularly rapid.

Eighteenth-century *urbanisation* produced different kinds of town, many of which would not be described as industrial. This point is made especially clearly by considering 'pairs' of different towns—as for example, Wakefield and Huddersfield, contrasted by the historian Hilary Marland. Of these adjacent centres in the industrialising north, Wakefield was the 'county' town, the favoured residence of gentry and the prosperous middle classes (particularly doctors and lawyers), while Huddersfield was industrial, highly productive but at the cost of poor conditions among its burgeoning working-class population. There was, however, no simple contrast between such towns in terms of economic growth or mortality: Wakefield had its poor, but they were hidden away in alleys and subdivided tenements.

Much the same point can be made about the debate over the effects of *enclosure of common land* and *agricultural improvement*: these effects varied enormously according to region. Forced emigration from rural

Ireland, for example, not only devastated that country but had consequential effects for major industrial ports in England such as Liverpool. It was not only regionally that experience varied. The 'cellar-dwellers' of Liverpool became a by-word for squalor and depravity—yet Liverpool was also 'the city of millionaires across the Mersey'.

In the previous chapter, we noted a trend towards *social differentiation:* this trend greatly accelerated during the Industrial Revolution, and increasingly came to be expressed in physical terms, so that the poor were even seen as racially distinct. In rural society, the breakdown of the system of 'live-in' service in husbandry increased estrangement between the classes. Even those seeking to understand rural decline could describe the rural labourer as 'a physical scandal, a moral enigma, an intellectual cataleptic' (the *Morning Chronicle*, 1850, quoted by Snell, 1987, p. 7).

Towns enlarged at first by 'in-filling', leading (as in Wakefield) to hidden pockets of poverty; and then by sprawling new terraces, where contact between the different social classes was minimised, and amenities non-existent. In both town and country, the face-to-face society gave way, in the terms of the time, to a society in which one half did not know how the other half lived. Pompous urban architecture expressed social distance as well as civic pride, although there were attempts, as with the voluntary hospitals (discussed later in this chapter), to bring the classes together in a hierarchical way within new institutions.

In 1832, while investigating the cotton operatives, Dr Charles Turner Thackrah of Leeds, the pioneer of industrial medicine, glimpsed the working poor *en masse*:

> I saw, or thought I saw, a degenerate race— human beings stunted, enfeebled, and depraved—men and women that were not to be aged—children that were never to be healthy adults. (Quoted by Thompson, 1975, p. 364)

By the 1830s and 1840s, it could come as a profound shock to the comfortably off that they shared an environment with the 'labouring population', and that the environment in which the poor lived was so physically degraded as to pose a greater threat to society than the 'moral' (or political) condition of the poor. Thackrah was looking at factory workers, but he was well aware that the conditions for those working long hours in slum housing or in cramped workshops could be equally disabling.[5] For different ways of seeing the poor and their conditions, see Figure 3.1(a) and (b) *overleaf*.

---

[4]Edward Jenner published the account of his first experiment with vaccination in 1798. The same term was later used for the similar preventive treatment for tuberculosis; for other infectious diseases the term 'immunisation' was generally applied.

[5]The article by Engels, 'Health: 1844' in *Health and Disease: A Reader* could usefully be consulted again, even if you read it during your study of Chapter 1.

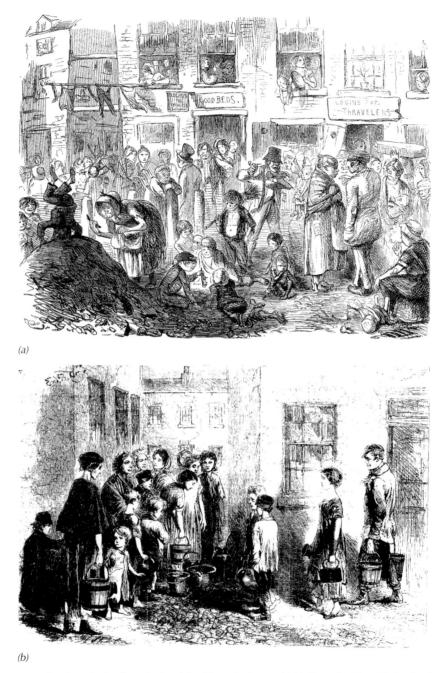

(a)

(b)

Figure 3.1 *Two ways of seeing: the 'undeserving' and the 'deserving' poor. (a) 'A Court for King Cholera', a Punch cartoon by John Leech. (b) Queuing for water in Bethnal Green. In (a), Leech shows the poor as almost sexless, full of low cunning, and as matched to their conditions of life. At the same time he depicts particular targets of sanitary concern: lodging houses, muck heaps, and the 'court' itself—a crowded courtyard squeezed between buildings and almost hidden from the street—a classic 'fever nest' as well as a focus for cholera. In (b), the poor are made to look pitiable rather than depraved, the women are more feminine, and the emphasis is placed on the inappropriateness of the physical burden being imposed on women and children in particular. (Sources: (a) Punch, 25 September 1852; (b) Mary Evans Picture Library)*

Reformers first expressed this revelation in terms of different class-related and district-related mortalities, using local surveys and then the information provided by the *Registrar-General's Office* instituted in 1836 (for an example, see Table 3.1).

However, it is as well to stress that *mortality* is only a rough index to health experience. The argument over the effects of industrialisation can be explained not only in terms of the radically different experiences of different groups in society, but also in terms of *our* inability to

Table 3.1 Life expectancies for different classes in different localities, 1839–40, as set out by Edwin Chadwick

Number of deaths		Average age of deceased/years
Bethnal Green		
101	Gentlemen and persons engaged in professions and their families	45
273	Tradesmen and their families	26
1 258	Mechanics, servants, labourers and their families	16
Leeds Borough		
79	Gentlemen, etc.	44
824	Tradesmen, farmers, etc.	27
3 395	Operatives, labourers, etc.	19
Liverpool		
137	Gentlemen, etc.	35
1 738	Tradesmen, etc.	22
5 597	Labourers, mechanics, servants, etc.	15
Unions in the County of Wilts.		
119	Gentlemen, etc.	50
218	Farmers, etc.	48
2 061	Agricultural labourers, etc.	33
Kendal Union		
52	Gentlemen, etc.	45
138	Tradesmen, etc.	39
413	Operatives, labourers, servants, etc.	34

Data from Flinn, M. W. (ed.) (1965) *Report on the Sanitary Condition of the Labouring Population of Great Britain, by Edwin Chadwick, 1842*, Edinburgh University Press, Edinburgh, pp. 224–5, based on the earliest returns of the Registrar-General's Office. Note, however, that in all areas each class is present in very different proportions, and that the table has not been corrected for the age-structure of the population in question.

measure *morbidity* as accurately as we can mortality. Extreme disadvantage, even protracted suffering—suggested by the quotation from Thackrah—may occur without being reflected in mortality statistics.

It is necessary too to take note of what people themselves regarded as making the difference between subsistence and despair. In the rural context, this could be the loss of such entitlements as bed-and-board, gleaning and the right to keep livestock. A similar point can be made about the abandonment in towns of controls on the price and quality of staple foodstuffs such as bread (which we mentioned in Chapter 2)—what has been referred to as the displacement of the *moral economy* by the rise of *economic liberalism* during the eighteenth century.

The New Poor Law

Above all, it is issues of *entitlement* which are at stake with respect to the Poor Law. The **New Poor Law** of 1834 targeted the *able-bodied*; it stressed *deterrence* rather than entitlement, *institutionalisation* rather than 'outdoor' mechanisms of relief such as pensions, and sought to replace haphazard localism with the ugly **principle of 'less-eligibility'** (explained below).

The main aim behind the New Poor Law was to reduce public expenditure, and in particular to reduce the supplementation of depressed wages in the agricultural south of England. In order to eliminate this form of out-door relief, the **workhouse test** was instituted: to obtain assistance, the poor person had to be desperate enough to enter the workhouse (*in-door relief*). In-door relief had to be 'less eligible' (more distasteful) than any work available *outside* the workhouse—and there were no minimum standards governing conditions of employment at this date.

The 15 000 autonomous parishes of the Old Poor Law could not be expected all to have workhouses, so economies of scale were achieved by creating fewer and larger organisational units (the *Poor Law Unions*), which were accountable to a central administration, and which were better able to provide large institutions (see Figure 3.2, *overleaf*).

Rather than appearing to the poor as a source of assistance at times of their lives when they needed it most, the New Poor Law created a new underclass, the *paupers*, which the poor had to join before any assistance was offered. While designed to reduce the dependency of the poor by deterrence, the harshness of the New Poor Law was intended to be balanced by the preventive principles of *sanitary reform*, and by a system of *medical poor relief*. We will look at these later in this chapter.

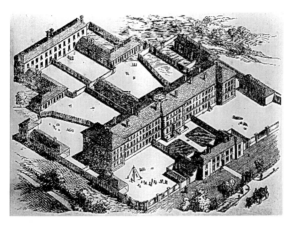

Figure 3.2 *'Economies of scale': an aim of the New Poor Law, in amalgamating 15 000 very different parish units into fewer than 600 Poor Law Unions, was to make it possible to construct large workhouses with purpose-built infirmaries. Some Unions did so (though many did not, especially in rural areas): this vast new workhouse, opened on 4 August 1849, was for the United Parishes of Fulham and Hammersmith. The largest workhouses not only segregated the poor according to age, sex, and health, but provided separate accommodation for each of the sexes according to 'good' and 'bad' character. (Source: Hulton/Deutsch Picture Collection)*

Lay care: urbanisation and self-help

Many aspects of lay care show remarkably little change into the industrial period and beyond, in spite of major social and economic dislocations. The wealth of sources (letters, diaries, pamphlets) produced by a literate (male) population, and the flourishing of a less-restricted press, increased the 'noise level' of lay interest in health, but it should not be assumed that such interest was new. Charles Waterton, eccentric naturalist and Squire of Walton Hall, near Leeds in Yorkshire, for example, came from a long line of busy gentry, advocating long-established remedies as well as adapting to new emergencies:

> [Waterton] recommended that travellers should carry with them bark [cinchona, the source of quinine], laudanum [tincture of opium], calomel [chloride of mercury]...and, most important, a lancet...He had his own prescriptions and Mr Waterton's Pills were famous in Walton and the neighbourhood. During the 1849 cholera epidemic Waterton gratuitously distributed amongst the poor of Leeds and adjoining townships a powder which he claimed was highly beneficial in cases of cholera. (Marland, 1987, pp. 214–15)

The example of Squire Waterton suggests that it is not necessarily the case that lay knowledge was falling behind professional knowledge. This is partly because medical practice itself continued to be traditional in content. The interconnected phenomena of *population growth*, *social dislocation*, and *class differentiation* did, however, create a mass of conflicting claims affecting the possession and diffusion of knowledge. This is one aspect of what is called **the Enlightenment**—a set of ideas and political beliefs stressing the power of reason (and therefore of information) and the perfectibility of 'man'. The Enlightenment particularly expressed the interests of the middle classes, speaking on behalf of the working class.

Useful knowledge

Although the ideas behind it seemed mainly to have spread from other countries—especially France, America, and Scotland—the Enlightenment in England was also a revival of grievances left over from the Civil War period (approximately 1640–60). These grievances had included criticism of the monopoly of knowledge by doctors and lawyers, as well as assertions of the unity of spiritual and physical life. Thus we find that much lay interest in health and healing was allied to movements in popular religion—just as, for more established denominations, subscribing to a hospital had religious as well as medical justifications.

These different trends are illustrated in this period by the two most successful medical manuals written for the laity—*Primitive Physick* (1747) by John Wesley, the founder of Methodism, and William Buchan's *Domestic Medicine* (1769), which was based on a French handbook. These provided new resources for local figures traditionally inclined to take an interest in medicine, such as the clergy and schoolmasters. Here is a nineteenth-century writer recalling a late-eighteenth-century Scottish schoolmaster:

> He was very useful in the parish, for he could let blood, and was a daily reader of 'Buchan's Domestic Medicine', all whose instructions he rigidly, and often successfully, practised. (Quoted by Lawrence, 1975, p. 32)

By the time editions of Buchan's book ceased appearing, in the early nineteenth century, the four major movements in popular medicine were well-established: *medical botany* or *herbalism, homoeopathy, hydropathy* (a system of cure based on water), and *mesmerism* (a form of hypnotism combined with magnetism). In this period these 'alternatives' are best seen as self-help systems, appealing to a wide range of classes in society (including medical men), and offering a rich mixture of traditional concepts, modern science, and spirituality. These eclectic systems were essentially urban growths, imported from mainland Europe or America. They were not simply updated versions of traditional indigenous folklore about herbs, magic, and holy waters, although there was a stress on a 'return to nature' which we also hear today. The proliferation of spas in this period further shows how readily the traditional could combine with the scientific, the fashionable and the entrepreneurial.

In addition, we can see provincial towns experiencing, on a variety of scales, the diversity—and insecurities—of urban life as it was previously known only in London and the provincial capitals. The irrepressible lay interest in health and disease had many new outlets for its expression, as well as new sources of concern. The outlets included book clubs, circulating libraries, publication by subscription, mechanics' institutes, and lectures on such subjects as chemistry and phrenology.

It is characteristic of this period's methods of communication—and of the difficulty of separating lay care from qualified practice—that both medicines, and information about practitioners, were sold and distributed by booksellers, circulating libraries, printers, and publishers (who could also be the proprietors of newspapers carrying medical advertisements). These links were *in addition to*, rather than instead of, medicine's older occupational diversifications, such as those involving traders in food and drink, or farriers, blacksmiths, and others dealing with animals.

Druggists: further steps in the commercialisation of self-help

Two other developments can be mentioned to illustrate the theme of self-help. The first is the rise of the **druggist**, who in this period displaced the apothecary and the grocer as the shopkeeping source of medication and advice. (The apothecaries were tending to run practices rather than shops.) By the 1840s, according to census information, there were in England and Wales about two druggists to every three qualified medical practitioners. Like the barbers' shops in pre-industrial towns, the druggists were well-distributed, and could be up-market or down, able to cater for high levels of self-medication among the better-off as well as the poor. Here is a druggist targeting the middle-class market in Wakefield:

> Those Families who may honor him with their Commands, may depend upon having every Article in the Medical Department, as Genuine as at the Apothecary's Hall, London. (Quoted in Marland, 1987, p. 217)

□ The druggists were very like today's pharmacists—but does the quotation suggest any differences?

■ Their main business in medicine was not filling the prescriptions of doctors, but filling the orders and making up the recipes brought to them by their (lay) customers.

Druggists also sold *proprietary remedies*, which began to be patented in the seventeenth century, and had swelled to become a useful source of tax revenue by the late eighteenth. The better-known of these medicines differed little in composition from the official versions listed in pharmacopoeias. Many of them (patented and otherwise) also dated from the seventeenth century rather than the eighteenth, although they multiplied during the period of industrialisation according to increased demand, improved distribution, and the beginnings of the pharmaceutical industry—an area in which Nonconformists such as Quakers were highly successful, as they were in the food industry.

Friendly societies

The second development is the emergence of the **friendly societies**—self-help organisations which developed in the industrial North to meet the three main threats to working people and their families: sickness, unemployment, and death. A society might maintain a subscription to an institution such as a hospital, but its main function was to pay out benefits to members according to their contributions. Unlike the gilds and their successors the companies, which had been broader organisations, taking some responsibility for sick and aged members, the friendly societies were organised by wage-earners for wage-earners. They were often the only safety-net for working men and women affected by long-term, seasonal, and chronic illnesses.

□ Can you think of factors likely to limit the success of societies dependent upon the contributions of wage-earners?

■ The societies could be affected by: the age-structure of their membership; prolonged slumps in employment; a decline in mortality not associated with a decline in morbidity. Dependants could benefit only indirectly.

In this section we have concentrated upon lay care as an aspect of self-help (and self-expression) in an urbanising society. We should also stress here how elites among the laity not only continued to control previously established systems of health care, such as the Poor Law, but also dominated the new urban systems, such as the hospitals, the dispensaries, and other forms of medical charity. This will be further examined later in the chapter.

Public health: a shared environment?

Most public health issues involve a practical idea of the common good. Listen to Samuel Johnson, condemning schemes to pipe water from Plymouth to the adjacent industrial sprawl of Dock (now Devonport):

> No, no! I am against the *dockers*; I am a Plymouth man. Rogues! let them die of thirst! (Quoted by Corfield, 1989, p. 46).

Old corruption

Johnson's hyperbole encapsulates the successes and failures of the impulse to environmental improvement in this period. Local initiatives and Improvement Acts— enabling legislation specially applied for by a locality— achieved benefits for certain parts of certain towns, but the public good tended to be very narrowly defined. This reflected the extremely inconsistent and undemocratic structure of eighteenth-century English local government, which was only partially rectified by Bills passed in the 1830s aimed at eliminating corruption and extending the franchise.

The idiosyncrasies of local custom were an impossible basis for managing social and economic crises of mounting scale. Population growth and industrialisation could mean gross mismatches between changing local needs and traditional political structure and representation. Local bodies such as Boards of Commissioners multiplied on an *ad hoc* basis to take separate responsibility for services like street paving, nuisance removal, lighting, highways, sewerage, and burial grounds, but only for limited areas and with minimal accountability.

All such services were dependent upon a narrow rate base, restricted borrowing powers, or on local philanthropy. Above all, they were dependent upon the honesty and goodwill of a few individuals, in a situation where conflict of interest was inevitable. Gas lighting and the extension of water supplies were left to market forces: private water companies were active in this period, but tended to compete for the same few profitable customers. Industrial change provided potential for improvement but new standards had to be enforced: for example, iron rather than wooden piping for water systems was made compulsory in 1827.

Fever: the diagnosis of social evils

The disease that lay at the heart of the dominant approaches to public health in this period was *fever*—in particular, *typhus* (an infection carried by the body louse), with an increasing admixture of *typhoid* (a water-borne disease), and *relapsing fever* (a disease exacerbated by famine). These diseases were only gradually distinguished from each other during the first half of the nineteenth century. They were known collectively as 'continued fever' (as distinct from ague or intermittent fever—that is, malaria).

During the eighteenth century, typhus became recognised as a disease of the poor and of crowding— notable outbreaks occurred in ships, prisons, and military camps. Hospitals and factories were also observed to become foci of infection. Hospitals generally excluded fever cases for fear of concentrating infection. Investigators, for example the prison reformer John Howard, concluded that these epidemics could be prevented by such measures as improving ventilation, reducing overcrowding, and strengthening the constitutions of those at risk.

An even broader diagnosis of the causes of continued fever was made by Thomas Percival (1740–1804), a Unitarian physician and intellectual, who was central to pioneering initiatives undertaken in England's 'first industrial city', Manchester. Percival and his associates saw children as especially sensitive to industrial conditions; they condemned child labour and advocated universal education. Percival's comprehensive reforms included local boards of health given wide regulatory powers by national legislation. The hostility of industrialists blocked most of his ideas; one of the model institutions to survive was the *fever hospital*. The major outbreaks of fever in Ireland in the early nineteenth century also led to some experimentation with institutions like fever hospitals.

New arms of government

As you have seen, health-related administration was at its most fragmented just when the environmental crises of industrialisation and population growth became most acute. Apart from quarantine and other emergency provisions, no responsibility was taken for public health at the national or even regional level. Late in the period, the Unions of the New Poor Law in England and Wales provided for the first time a national system of larger units of civil administration; Poor Law authorities, notably the *Board of Guardians* elected by each Union's ratepayers, were subsequently expected to take on other responsibilities—civil registration, sanitary improvement, and vaccination, for example.

☐ Can you see a disadvantage in this use of the Poor Law authorities for public health administration and health education?

■ Health-related functions became associated in people's minds with the New Poor Law—and suffered from its unpopularity.

As already suggested, the connection between sanitary reform and the New Poor Law goes even deeper than this.

Benthamism and sanitary reform

The **sanitary movement**, launched in the 1820s, became a broadly-based campaign aimed at cleansing, watering, sewering, and rehousing—and thus preventing disease among—neglected human populations, especially in large towns. Britain was the first country in Western Europe to approach the urban environment in this way because it was the first to impose unrestricted industrial development on an entirely inadequate system of local administration.

The immediate inspiration of the sanitary movement was provided by the **Benthamites**—followers (notably the lawyer Edwin Chadwick) of the lawyer and philosopher Jeremy Bentham (1748–1832) (see Figure 3.3). Bentham's ideas became the main means by which the Enlightenment belief in reason and the perfectibility of man was preserved for nineteenth-century reformers. Bentham's 'constitutional code' placed considerable stress on health and *disease prevention* as responsibilities of the state, along with complementary functions such as education and the gathering of statistics.

The Benthamites emphasised the need for the role of the qualified expert in the service of government—for example, in factory inspection. In economic matters, they saw the function of government as one of regulation,

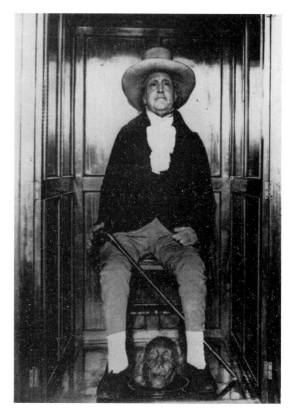

Figure 3.3 (b) *Jeremy Bentham died in 1832, aged 84 years. In his Will he left his body for public dissection by his friend and fellow-campaigner for sanitary reform, Thomas Southwood Smith, 'with the desire that mankind may reap some small benefit in and by my decease'. Bentham's private papers included a pamphlet on 'Auto-Icons'—dehydrated human corpses, preserved for posterity and recognisable as individuals. Southwood Smith had an Auto-Icon made from Bentham's skeleton (pictured here), stuffed to fit his clothes, but his attempt to dehydrate the head did not preserve the features and it was replaced by a wax model. (Source: University College Library)*

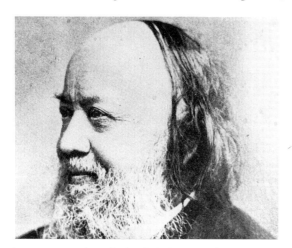

Figure 3.3 (a) *Edwin Chadwick, the lawyer and lifelong campaigner for sanitary reform, died in 1890 at the age of 90 years. (Source: The Londoners; The Pilot Press)*

rather than direction. In practice, Bentham's view of the collective functioning of individual self-interest tended to be taken out of context and combined with the prevailing climate of liberalism or *laissez-faire*, which minimised the role of government with respect to the economy.

In 1842 Chadwick wrote with typical trenchancy:

The expenses of local public works are in general unequally and unfairly assessed, oppressively and uneconomically collected, by separate collections, wastefully expended in separate and inefficient operations by unskilled and practically irresponsible officers. (Quoted by Simon, 1897, p. 193)

☐ What features of the Benthamite approach does this suggest to you?

■ Particularly characteristic are the stresses on: efficiency; equity of taxation and representation; co-ordination of administrative functions; accountability; and professional qualifications.

Both the New Poor Law and sanitary reform were designed to reduce wasteful expenditure, to induce labour to move to where there was employment, and to prevent the diseases which so reduced the earning capacity of the labouring classes. A major point of the Benthamite inquiries was to establish that epidemic disease struck *unnecessarily* at the *able-bodied breadwinner*, rather than 'conveniently' removing the weak and unproductive (see Table 3.2).

The *preventable* diseases were traced to the influence of local causes of pollution—impure or inadequate water supply, accumulated sewage, contaminated air, overcrowded housing, overcrowded graveyards, industrial waste and decaying organic matter generally. Other commentators pointed to the broad range of factors behind poverty; still others blamed the conditions in which the poor lived on their own habits or lack of moral education.

For the Benthamite sanitarians, moral effects were defined as having physical causes. Intervention in 'social wrongs' was seen as imperative; the most efficient way of intervening in this case was to remove the physical causes of preventable disease, and the most efficient means of intervention was by government action. In this, as in other areas of social policy, the Benthamites formed a model pressure group committed to national legislation.

As you might be thinking, not even the Benthamites could move the mountains of filth by themselves. **Sanitarianism** became a broadly-based creed, having as its unifying principle the reduction of environmental pollution in the interests of human health. The 'health of towns' was a major political and social issue in the 1830s and 1840s, leading to local initiatives such as the appointment of the first *Medical Officer of Health* or MOH (Liverpool, 1847), national pressure groups such as the Health of Towns Association, and national legislation, culminating in the Public Health Act of 1848. This Act set up England's first central health department—the short-lived *General Board of Health*, of which Chadwick was the dominant member.

In continental Europe as well as in Britain, public health reformers increasingly saw *infectiousness*—and therefore 'excess' or preventable disease—as dependent upon environmental factors, rather than being a fixed property of a given disease. The 'sanitary idea' pushed by the Benthamites from the late 1820s onwards was based on experience of *fever nests*—pockets of urban degradation, inhabited by the poorest, from which disease could spread, not by the movement of infected individuals, but through the widespread prevalence of insanitary conditions. (Look again at Figure 3.1.)

These ideas were adapted to include *cholera*, which first extended to Europe in the 1820s, reaching Britain in 1831. Cholera gave impetus to sanitary reform, but being an occasional invader it was not the most important cause of death. One effect of cholera was to limit initiatives to temporary or emergency provisions.

Sanitarians continued to stress the cost to society of endemic, indigenous disease, with continued fever as the best example, and called for a central, permanent Board of Health. But Chadwick's General Board foundered in 1854, owing to pressure from vested interests and political opposition to centralised health administration.

Partly professionalised: the general practitioner

Medicine lagged well behind the Church and the law in its achievement of middle-class respectability. Whether this status was gained during the process of 'gentrification' in towns in the eighteenth century, or as a result of the 'multiplication of intellectual callings' in the nineteenth, has been a matter of debate. Historians have also suggested that medical practitioners in this period were 'marginal men' who took on a range of high-profile social roles in provincial institutions and societies in order to establish their professional position.

What does seem clear is, *first*, that the rank-and-file 'regular' practitioners managed to redefine themselves somewhat, a change signified by the deployment of the term **general practitioner** around 1820; *second*, that the new ideals of respectability increased the pressures of competition for 'respectable' patients among regular practitioners, even though middle-class demand for medical services also increased (Figure 3.4 (p. 48) suggests the working conditions that many were trying to get away from, and Figure 3.5 (p. 48) that even middle-class practice could be less than rewarding, at least intellectually); *third*, that medical practitioners remained extremely various, and critical of each other; and *last*, that it is unhistorical to regard medical practitioners even of this period as behaving first and foremost as medical personnel, defined in their outlook only by purely professional considerations—as if, for example, they were not also motivated, like their contemporaries, by different religious or political beliefs, which determined their alliances and position in society.

Table 3.2 'Pecuniary burdens created by neglect': extracts from a table of Poor Law returns for a lead-mining area in Cumberland as presented by Chadwick in the 1842 Report, highlighting the deaths of breadwinners.

Alston with Garrigill Parish

Number of widows, and children dependent upon them, in receipt of relief in the above parish; age of husband at death; and the alleged cause of death

Initials of widows	Number of children dependent at the time of husband's death	Occupation of deceased husband	Age at death	Years' loss by premature death	Alleged cause of death
R.W.	–	miner	83	–	decay of nature
M.B.	–	miner	73	–	not stated
M.L.	–	miner	64	–	influenza
J.P.	–	labourer	62	–	consumption
H.T.	2	mason	62	–	asthma
S.H.	2	miner	60	–	rupture of blood-vessel
M.P.	1	turner	57	3	consumption
H.S.	3	miner	57	3	influenza, terminating in dropsy
M.J.	3	blacksmith	55	5	asthma
S.M.	–	miner	55	5	inflammation of lungs from cold
J.W.	2	miner	54	6	pleurisy
H.P.	5	miner	48	12	typhus fever
E.H.	6	miner	48	12	killed in lead-mines
M.A.	7	miner	48	12	consumption by bad air in the pit
H.P.	3	miner	45	15	scarlet fever
M.S.	2	miner	45	15	inflammation of bowels
H.M.	7	miner	43	17	asthma, which terminated in consumption
A.J.	2	miller	42	18	found drowned
M.R.	–	shoemaker	40	20	injury from fall of a cart
E.R.	7	joiner	38	22	affection of the liver
J.B.	5	miner	38	22	consumption
A.P.	7	miner	37	21	asthma
E.H.	3	miner	35	25	killed in coal-pit
M.L.	2	miner	35	25	water of the head
S.H.	7	miner	34	26	accident in coal-mine
E.A.	2	miner	30	30	consumption
A.W.	2	miner	28	32	cholera
J.M.	2	miner	21	39	small-pox
89	**242**	–	**4418**	–	**Totals listed in unedited table**
		Average age at death of each below 60 years of age: } 45			Total no. of orphans by deaths caused below 60 years of age: } 236

Chadwick added: 'This premature widowhood and orphanage is the source of the most painful descriptions of pauperism…it is the source of a constant influx of the independent into the pauperised and permanently dependent classes'. (Data from Flinn, M. W. (ed.) 1965, *Report on the Sanitary Condition of the Labouring Population of Great Britain*, by *Edwin Chadwick, 1842*, Edinburgh University Press, Edinburgh, pp. 258–60, 255)

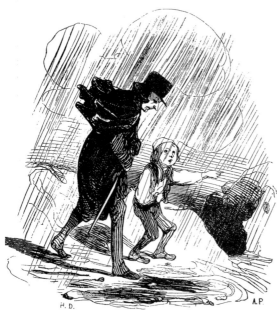

Figure 3.4 *The country doctor: wood engraving after Honoré Daumier. (Source: A. F. H. Fabre,* Némésis médicale illustrée, *revised edition, Paris, 1840)*

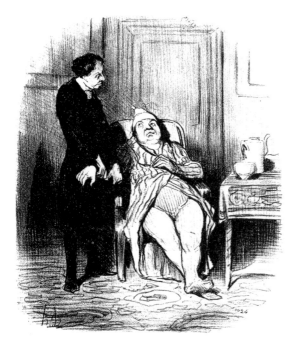

Figure 3.5 *'Oh, doctor, I'm sure I'm consumptive': lithograph by Honoré Daumier. (Reproduced from a series by Daumier,* Tout ce qu'on voudra *('everything one would want'), Paris, 1847)*

Doctors, in effect, did not 'hang together' just because they were doctors. It might be more important to an individual practitioner that (for instance) he was Unitarian in his religious beliefs, or that he had read an influential philosophical work at an impressionable age. Religion was important for a variety of reasons—for example, many able Nonconformists went into medicine, because their religion debarred them from other means of advancement.

The sporadic attempt at national regulation of physicians, surgeons and midwives, made through the ecclesiastical licensing system of the sixteenth century, faded out during the eighteenth century, as did the provincial barber-surgeons' companies, except where they became small, privileged enclaves dominated by certain families. Apprenticeship for barber-surgeons and apothecaries continued, but on an individual basis, as the system of apprenticeship in general was broken down. Personal knowledge was more than ever the patient's best security in choosing a practitioner. In an urbanising society such knowledge was harder to come by, and so was valued accordingly; this helped to shape, for the middle classes at least, new ideals of the private relationship between practitioner and patient.

At the same time, in the urban setting, if a practitioner did not have good connections he might gain acceptance by other means (for example, a striking physical presence, or public appearances, such as lectures), which could equally well be exploited by his rivals. As you will recall from earlier discussion, the necessary techniques of self-assertion, such as advertisement in newspapers, were also increasing.

Consequently it is difficult to define a 'regular' practitioner in this period, although this adjective (and its opposite, 'irregular') were beginning to be used (perhaps derived from military service). It should not surprise you that itinerant practitioners were probably more numerous (in proportion) before 1800 than at any other time; and that the laity were still ready to assume the medical role—even though, for example, the aspiring middle-class family might decide to patronise a *man-midwife*, rather than a more traditional female attendant (compare Figure 2.2 in Chapter 2 with Figure 3.6).

The first of the nineteenth-century national Censuses to include detailed occupational information (1841) showed that, even when only main occupations were asked for, the *regular* practitioners—defined by then in terms of formal qualifications—were still considerably outnumbered by the *irregulars*, by a ratio of 1 : 3. The irregulars included particularly the druggists, whom we discussed earlier.

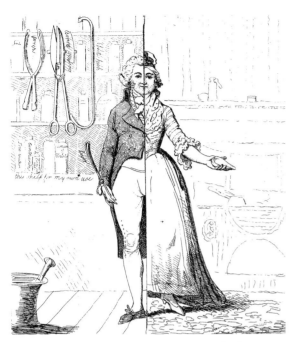

Figure 3.6 *Cartoon from S. W. Fores,* Man-Midwifery Dissected, *1793. The term 'man-midwife' was in use in England by 1625, and such work seemed for a time likely to become a largely male preserve (as it did in the USA). Behind the male half-figure are bottles of 'love water' and other potions allegedly used as sexual stimulants. (Source: Wellcome Institute Library, London)*

As in the pre-industrial period, the numbers of regular practitioners actually practising only physic, or only surgery, were extremely small, even in the London hospitals, where you might expect demarcation lines to be most precise. The hospitals offered an opportunity for professional self-definition, but were also an arena for religious, political and professional conflicts. A hospital connection, for reasons we shall look at later, was honorary or unpaid, but it offered rewards to be competed for in the form of social contacts, which increased private practice, and large fees or premiums from pupils.

Medical reform: divided in diversity

Regular medicine at this time was hierarchical but far from orderly. Entry to the pinnacles of practice was guarded in London by the *Royal College of Physicians* and the *Royal College of Surgeons* (which had abandoned the Barbers in 1745, and obtained new charters in 1800 and 1843). These two London medical colleges, by withholding recognition of the courses offered by private or provincial medical schools—as opposed to pupilage in the London hospitals, or degrees from Oxford or Cambridge—also restricted access to the higher levels of qualification (the medical colleges' licentiateships, memberships, or fellowships).

Pressure on the London medical colleges, especially the Surgeons, came from the increasing minority of regular practitioners who were university-trained—not by Oxford and Cambridge, which produced only tiny numbers of medical graduates throughout the period and imposed religious tests—but in the Netherlands (especially Leiden), in Scotland (especially in Edinburgh and Glasgow), in Dublin, and, after 1828, by the non-denominational University College London (which became the University of London in 1836). A minimum qualification by examination was first introduced with the LSA—*Licence of the (London) Society of Apothecaries*—in 1815.

The favoured credentials for the ambitious new 'general practitioner' were *'College and Hall'*, meaning respectively the MRCS (Membership—not Fellowship—of the Royal College of Surgeons), and the LSA ('Hall' because the Apothecaries' Society, being one of the old London companies, still had its 'gild hall'). Box 3.1 (*overleaf*) shows how, by 1847, the emergent GP could make his credentials contrast with those of some of his competitors.

However, because educational options had multiplied, and there was no effective overall regulation, even formal credentials remained very confusing. 'The legal titles of medical practitioners', as one experienced critic put it, 'were as various as the names of snuffs or sauces' (Simon, 1897, p. 269). In the period from around 1800 to the Medical Act of 1858, between 15 and 20 bodies could offer different qualifications to someone wishing to practise in England.

This, the period of the *'Medical Reform'* movement, was one of campaigning and conflict. The main ingredients were attacks by rank-and-file practitioners on the London royal colleges and the London medical elites (study the distinguished example given in Box 3.2, *overleaf*, now), and the founding in 1832 of a rival pressure group representing general practitioners, the Provincial Medical and Surgical Association (later the *British Medical Association* or BMA). In many respects, the failure of the London medical colleges to adapt was no bad thing, as it preserved both pluralism and independence in the broader reaches of the profession.

BARRETT, John, Orange-grove, Bath—Surg.; F.R.C.S. (by exam.) 1846; Surg. to Western Dispensary; to St Michael's Lying-in Charity; to Great Western Railway (Bath District); Vaccinator, and Registrar of Births and Deaths for Abbey District.

BATTEN, Thos., Coleford, Monmouthsh.—General Pract.; M.R.C.S. 1827; L.S.A. 1826; Surgeon to eight collieries in the district.

BEASLEY, John, Oadby Blaby, Leicester—Gen. Pract.; In practice prior to the Act of 1815.

BEDINGFIELD, James, Stowmarket, Suffolk—Gen. Pract.; M.D.; In practice prior to the Act of 1815; formerly Apoth. to the Bristol Infirmary; Surg. to the Hundred of Stow, and the Dorcas Society; Mem. of the Council of the Prov. Med. and Surg. Association, and of the Nat. Instit.; Author of "The Enemy of Empiricism", and of a "Compendium of Medical Practice"; Contributor of numerous Papers to the *Lancet, Provin. Med. and Surg. Journal,* and *Dublin Med. Press,* on Medicine, Surgery, and Midwifery, on Medical Reform, and on the New Poor Law.

FERNELEY, Charles, Denton, near Grantham, Lincolnshire—Gen. Pract.; M.R.C.S. 1833; Med. Officer to Grantham Union. Author of "Lectures on Nutrition of Plants". Contributed to *Med. Gaz.* a paper "On certain Medical Laws which obtain in the Animal Economy", Jan. 1840.

MOTT, William Hadley, Kemp Town, Brighton—Surgeon; in practice prior to the Act of 1815; formerly Surgeon in the Army.

Box 3.1 *Selected entries from the* Provincial Medical Directory, 1847, *London, John Churchill (pp. 20, 23, 98, 200). Although inspired by the 'Medical Reform' movement, the 1840s directories were essentially commercial enterprises which preceded the* Medical Register *resulting from the Act of 1858. The publisher put together the* Directory *of 1847 from Census-related information collected by the District Registrars, supplemented with other sources. Note that not all those who might have done so, wished to call themselves 'General Practitioner'; and that those giving themselves this description were still very diverse. Note also that publications on almost any scientific subject could be regarded as improving a practitioner's status, and that practitioners already lived on connections with a wide range of institutions (the army, mines, the Poor Law, etc.).*

Philanthropy: the role of bricks and mortar

Major changes in 'bricks and mortar' provision took place in the period covered by this chapter—in Britain, the spread of 'voluntary' hospitals and other medical charities, and in continental Europe, the reshaping of the large institutions dating from earlier periods. However we should stress that the bulk of medical care—even *formal* medical care—continued to be provided *outside* institutions. Only small select categories of poor people were treated in British hospitals. The intake of the new lunatic asylums seems to have been broader in social terms, as a reflection of demand for that kind of custodial institution from families of all classes.

Voluntary hospitals and reforming dispensaries

The **voluntary hospitals** were 'voluntary' rather than 'chartered' because they were initially supported not by endowments but by annual donations from subscribers, who administered the institution and also had the right to sponsor patients for admission. This amounted to a system of lay control, although the medical and surgical staff normally had the same rights as subscribers, and, as another indication of a shared social outlook, gave their services free. As we mentioned in the previous section, these honorary posts rewarded their holders indirectly.

The voluntary hospitals probably owe their origins in the early eighteenth century to a new form of piety, which stressed philanthropy as a common ground on which Anglicans and Nonconformists could work in the interests of social harmony. There was also continued interest in what was called 'political arithmetic'—the relevance to government of the structure, wealth, health, and earning capacity of the nation's population, particularly with reference to colonial expansion.

As in the Civil War period, hospitals were advocated as only one element in schemes outlining systems of medical provision for the whole population. These ideal hospitals were intended to have a major role in the improvement of medical knowledge, and were inspired partly by continental European examples (especially in the Netherlands). In the event, no comprehensive systems were created, and the hospitals which began with the Westminster Infirmary in 1720 were designed to be charitable rather than useful to the state.

GUY'S HOSPITAL

THE OPERATION OF LITHOTOMY BY MR BRANSBY COOPER, WHICH LASTED NEARLY ONE HOUR!!

…It will, doubtless, be useful to the country 'draff', to learn how things are managed by one of the privileged order—a Hospital surgeon—nephew and surgeon, and surgeon because he is 'nephew'.

The performance of this tragedy was nearly as follows [there followed a dramatic eye-witness account of the bungled operation by Cooper, after which the patient died; another patient ran away from the hospital]:

> …When Cooper's *nevey* cut for stone,
> His toils were long and heavy;
> This patient quicker parts has shown,
> He *soon cut* Cooper's *nevey.*

…Such are the men who style themselves the heads of the profession! such is the race of hospital apprentices, *neveys* [nephews] and noodles, who insolently domineer over the great body of the profession! What, it has been asked, must the priests have been in a country, where the god was a monkey? If such men were at the head of the profession, who could be at its tail? The truth is, we repeat, that the highest degree of professional knowledge and skill, as well as the greatest amount of intelligence and activity, is to be found among that enlightened, though hitherto degraded class, which has been stigmatised by the corrupt few, as a *subordinate* department of the profession. In conclusion, we earnestly impress it as a rule of conduct, subject to a few, and very few exceptions, on all who value the health and lives of those who are near and dear to them: '*So long as the present corrupt system of patronage continues*', avoid the men who style themselves the heads of the profession; above all, avoid the metropolitan hospital physicians and surgeons'!

Box 3.2 *Extracts from a campaign in the* Lancet, *conducted by its founder and first editor, the radical surgeon and Member of Parliament, Thomas Wakley. (Lancet, 1827–8, i, p. 959; ii, p. 88; 1828–9, i, pp. 535–6. Quoted in Brook, 1945, pp. 52–63.) During its first years, Wakley's journal waged a fearless and uninhibited war against incompetence and nepotism among the London medical elites. Wakley championed a range of radical causes (including the Tolpuddle martyrs, transported for the equivalent of trades unionism), but his view of the profession was meritocratic, rather than democratic. He pushed the claims of the increasing numbers of well-educated medical men, particularly in the provinces, who reflected most credit upon the new category of 'general practitioner'.*

Entry to the voluntary hospitals was restricted to 'deserving Objects' (i.e. objects of charity—the term often used for patients) who had managed to bring themselves to the favourable notice of a subscriber. The procedure for admission by subscriber's letter involved close personal contact between rich and poor, with the poor entirely dependent upon the goodwill of the rich. (You may like to reflect on how little—or how much—this resembles the modern system of referral to hospital by GP's letter.) This procedure was more appropriate for paternalistic relationships within a traditional 'face-to-face' society, than for large urban populations where the different social classes were increasingly divided. Take the 'domestic' note sounded in the following advice, given as late as 1816:

> A lady visitor in an hospital or Asylum, should
> be to that institution what the kind judicious

Mistress of a family is to her household,—the careful inspector of the oeconomy, the integrity and the good moral conduct of the housekeeper and other inferior servants.
(Quoted in Prochaska, 1980, p. 141)

This quotation illustrates the way in which the voluntary hospitals attempted to display, in a very different context, a set of social relations modelled on the traditional, pre-industrial extended household—that is, the kind of household likely to have included servants and apprentices. The geographical distribution of hospitals was also related to concentrations of middle-class medical practitioners and clergy.

The maps shown in Figure 3.7 (*overleaf*) show you in two stages the dates and places of voluntary hospital foundations in the eighteenth century, alongside population growth and urbanisation.

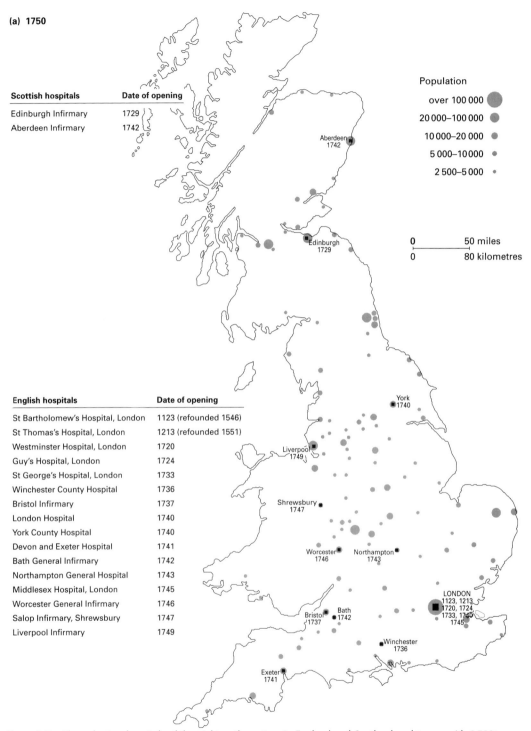

(a) 1750

Scottish hospitals	Date of opening
Edinburgh Infirmary	1729
Aberdeen Infirmary	1742

Population

over 100 000

20 000–100 000

10 000–20 000

5 000–10 000

2 500–5 000

English hospitals	Date of opening
St Bartholomew's Hospital, London	1123 (refounded 1546)
St Thomas's Hospital, London	1213 (refounded 1551)
Westminster Hospital, London	1720
Guy's Hospital, London	1724
St George's Hospital, London	1733
Winchester County Hospital	1736
Bristol Infirmary	1737
London Hospital	1740
York County Hospital	1740
Devon and Exeter Hospital	1741
Bath General Infirmary	1742
Northampton General Hospital	1743
Middlesex Hospital, London	1745
Worcester General Infirmary	1746
Salop Infirmary, Shrewsbury	1747
Liverpool Infirmary	1749

Figure 3.7 *The voluntary hospitals of the eighteenth century in England and Scotland and towns with 2 500+ inhabitants in (a) 1750 and (b) 1801. Note that we are equating population growth with industrialisation. (Population figures from Corfield, P. J., 1982,* The Impact of English Towns, *Oxford University Press, Oxford, esp. pp. 13–14; Mitchell, B. R., 1988,* British Historical Statistics, *Cambridge University Press, Cambridge, pp. 25–7;*

(b) 1801

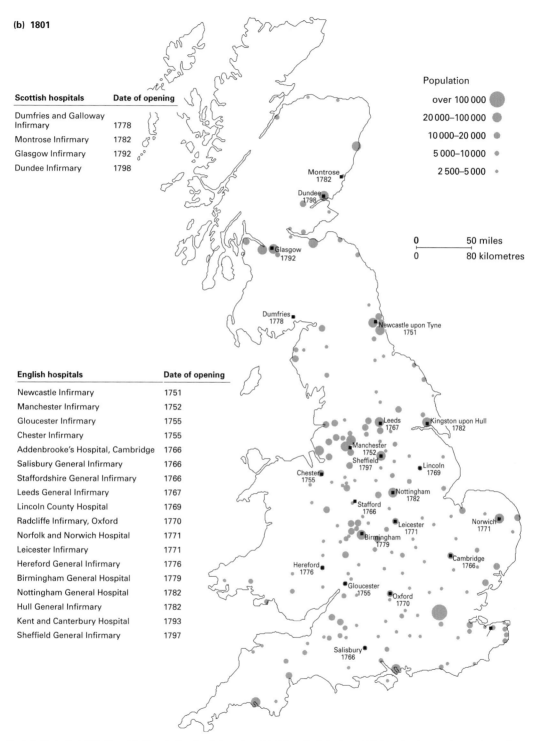

Scottish hospitals	Date of opening
Dumfries and Galloway Infirmary	1778
Montrose Infirmary	1782
Glasgow Infirmary	1792
Dundee Infirmary	1798

Population

- over 100 000
- 20 000–100 000
- 10 000–20 000
- 5 000–10 000
- 2 500–5 000

English hospitals	Date of opening
Newcastle Infirmary	1751
Manchester Infirmary	1752
Gloucester Infirmary	1755
Chester Infirmary	1755
Addenbrooke's Hospital, Cambridge	1766
Salisbury General Infirmary	1766
Staffordshire General Infirmary	1766
Leeds General Infirmary	1767
Lincoln County Hospital	1769
Radcliffe Infirmary, Oxford	1770
Norfolk and Norwich Hospital	1771
Leicester Infirmary	1771
Hereford General Infirmary	1776
Birmingham General Hospital	1779
Nottingham General Hospital	1782
Hull General Infirmary	1782
Kent and Canterbury Hospital	1793
Sheffield General Infirmary	1797

Kyd, J. G. (ed), 1952, Scottish Population Statistics, Scottish Historical Society, Edinburgh; data on hospitals, with amendments, from Woodward, J., 1974, To Do the Sick No Harm: A Study of the British Voluntary Hospital System to 1875, Routledge, London, Appendix 1)

□ Look carefully at Figure 3.7 and note when and where the hospitals were founded, remembering that the effects of industrialisation belong to the second rather than the first half of the century. What strikes you about the pattern of foundation?

■ It is not closely related either to the pace or to the location of industrial change. The foundations began in the old 'corporate' or county towns (mentioned in Chapter 2), especially in the South and West of England, and the rate of opening slackened just when the demands of industrialisation began to increase in the later eighteenth century.

Admission policies varied, but most hospitals tried to *exclude* major categories of those in need, such as young children, pregnant women, *domestic* servants (as opposed to apprentices or journeymen), the incurable or terminally ill, consumptives, epileptics, the mentally ill, and those suffering from infectious diseases, especially sexually transmitted disease. These policies differed little from those of the poor-relief hospitals of the Reformation period. Accident cases might obtain admission without a letter, the main problem for the patient very often being one of reaching the hospital in time.

The few hospitals that were founded in industrial centres, such as Manchester (1752) and Birmingham (1779), had huge catchment areas. As in the earlier period, many hospitals were small, even those in industrial towns. The Leeds Infirmary had only 27 beds in 1771; it had reached 128 beds by 1802, for an estimated population of 53 000.

When hospitals extended their functions, it tended to be with the aim of attracting middle-class interest and support. They therefore diversified into lunatic asylums, baths and balneotherapy (therapeutic bathing), 'medical galvanism' (a form of electrotherapy fashionable at the time), and 'pneumatic medicine' (a by-product of interest in gases). Some unmet need was catered for by hospitals which had an active policy towards outpatients. Home visiting, however, was extremely rare, which restricted knowledge among practitioners of the living conditions of poor patients.

The limitations of the hospital system, as to both function and geographical distribution, led to the founding of **dispensaries**. These were more modest institutions than the hospitals, less well known, but in many ways more significant in health-care terms. They gave out free medicine and advice to all comers. A few tried to provide food, by prescription. The charitable dispensary as an adjunct of a hospital or medical college had existed since the Renaissance, but the British movement, in which the dispensary was usually an independent institution, effectively began in the 1760s. The following appeal to dispensary subscribers was made in 1816:

> If it be our Duty to guard the Poor from the frequent ill Effects of defective Food and Clothing, of ill ventilated Abodes, or dangerous Callings; as well as our Interest as much as possible to arrest the spread of Infection, which commonly has its rise in the Abodes of Poverty, this Charity imperiously calls for your Support. (Quoted in Marland, 1987, p. 128)

□ What does this suggest to you about the aims and concerns of the dispensaries?

■ The quotation concentrates on the *living conditions* of the poor, and in particular the problem of infection. The voluntary hospitals generally excluded infectious diseases.

Dispensary staff carried out home visits, and attempted to restrict the spread of infection in poor housing. Like the fever hospitals, some dispensaries tried to deal with changing epidemiological patterns. They had an important role in the measurement of disease, and in medical education. Dispensaries were diverse in character. They were often sectarian (especially Quaker) in inspiration, they found it hard to attract subscriptions, they could be disliked by the subscribing classes because they gave benefits to the poor with no strings attached, and they required a high degree of idealism in their medical staffs.

By the early nineteenth century, a high take-up by the lower classes of the services of the medical charities was coming to be seen, not as success, but as a sign of growing dependency or exploitation. In this altered political climate, 'provident' dispensaries became more popular. These required regular contributions from their beneficiaries, on the insurance principle. Some dispensaries from this period (like that of Newcastle-upon-Tyne) continued to function up to the foundation of the National Health Service, in 1948.

Besides the fever hospitals and the dispensaries, other forms of medical charity evolved to cater for some of the groups excluded by the hospitals. These included *lying-in* charities (for pregnant women), vaccination charities, children's hospitals and dispensaries, and hospitals for the control of prostitution and sexually transmitted disease. The early nineteenth century was a major growth period for small 'specialist' hospitals.

Medical poor relief and the Old Poor Law

The hospitals, although intended for the poor, in no way removed the need for other forms of provision. Under the Old Poor Law, many parishes paid subscriptions to hospitals, dispensaries, and friendly societies, as one means of providing for their sick poor. Otherwise, parish overseers continued the range of expedients adopted in the earlier period.

□ Can you summarise the principal features of medical poor relief under the Old Poor Law?

■ You could have selected five features:

1   one-off payments to a wide range of practitioners, from lay healers, local midwives, and bonesetters, to physicians and surgeons;

2   paying the poor to care for the poor;

3   paying for the poor to be kept in private houses;

4   'buying in bulk' by contracting with practitioners on an annual basis;

5   paying pensions.

The following extracted account-book entries show payments made to one family during a particular period of need:

1784

May 9	John Marshall Wife midwife for Nat. Hudson Do. [ditto, i.e. 'wife']	2s 0d
May 16	Rachel Hudson Going to Church after Lying in	9d
	Rachel Hudson shoes	3s 6d
May 30	Itch Salve & Brimstone for Nat. Hudson	7d
July 25	A Godfrey Bottle for Rachel Hudson Child	6d
Aug 15	Natt Hudson to Whitworth Doctor	5s

(Quoted in Marland, 1987, p. 69)

The quotation illustrates the wide range of specific necessities which could be provided in some cases. Directly provided medical poor relief—as here, to Nathaniel Hudson and his wife Rachel—remained a *minor proportion* of total parish expenditure on the poor, but could be a *major investment* at any given time. Even before 1834, many sick, aged, or lunatic poor were accommodated in *workhouses*, which began to be purpose-built from about 1760, financed by the poor rate. By the early nineteenth century however, the Old Poor Law, 'the largest branch of public administration', had come to be seen as *creating* paupers, rather than relieving them.

Health care and the New Poor Law

As you saw earlier in the chapter, the economic assumptions of the New Poor Law (1834) were deeply flawed. It assumed, for example, that there would always be enough employment to go round, and that it would be well-enough paid. The Law was also not as originally envisaged by the Benthamite reformers who helped to shape it. The compensating *collateral aids* envisaged by Chadwick—for example, the improvement of health by investment in housing—were dropped, and almost no attention was paid to the implications of the new Law for medical poor relief. This had to be defined in further directives in the 1840s.

True to the Benthamite belief in professionalism in the service of the state, the New Poor Law prohibited the employment of unqualified practitioners. Each Union was to have a contracted, qualified surgeon, who had to supply all drugs as well as attendance, and to whom midwifery cases had also to be referred. This looks like a more powerful role for the professional practitioner—except that the Poor Law surgeon, in addition to being low-paid, was also *subordinate* to the Relieving Officer, a *lay* employee of the Guardians of the Union, who decided on all applications for relief.

In principle, paupers were to be admitted to a large workhouse organised on 'scientific' principles of classification: instead of the hugger-mugger approach of the Old Poor Law, women, children, the mentally ill, the sick, were to be catered for separately. *In practice*, many Unions avoided building large-scale institutions, and coercive segregation, because of the expense. (Look again at Figure 3.2.)

Forms of out-door relief (such as pensions) continued, especially in the North, where mass *seasonal* lack of employment made the new law inoperable. In sickness, the poor of the Northern industrial areas continued to depend on friendly societies or sick clubs, and on the wide range of resources of 'irregular' medicine.

Lunacy

There was one major exception to the continued piecemeal approach of most Unions. Institutional provision for the mentally ill and mentally disabled grew relatively rapidly. Under the Old Poor Law, provision for lunatics tended to be the largest single item of expenditure on medical poor relief. As you have seen, the distancing of all classes from these groups had led to the building of lunatic **asylums** in conjunction with the hospitals, as well as to the proliferation of private madhouses.

By the early nineteenth century, lunatic asylums were seen as being as much in need of reform as prisons. Legislation permitting counties to build large asylums at public expense was followed by efforts to make such provision (and a system of inspection) compulsory—efforts which finally succeeded in 1847. As with other forms of institutional provision, the county asylums did not necessarily appear where need was greatest. Both workhouses and asylums housed a miscellaneous population of poor people perceived as deviant, and tended to be concerned with custody rather than rehabilitation.

The intention of the new system was that the sick poor would benefit from organised access to qualified practitioners, and from purpose-built workhouse infirmaries. In practice, the more formalised—and more professionalised—medical services of the New Poor Law were slow to develop, even to the extent intended. The old outdoor practices were discouraged, but were not compensated for by enforcement of the new standards. At the same time these services fell under the shadow of the workhouse, which became a thoroughly detested institution (see Figure 3.8).

Continental Europe: medical police or social medicine?

You have seen how Enlightenment ideas, current in a number of countries, combined with the social and economic factors behind Britain's status as 'first industrial nation' to produce a particular kind of health-care system. What was happening in continental Europe, which (especially in the eighteenth century) had slower rates of industrial and population growth than in Britain?

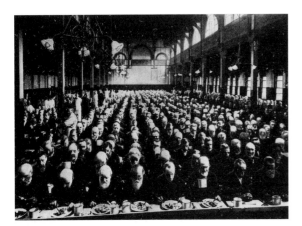

Figure 3.8 *Christmas dinner, Marylebone Workhouse, c. 1900. (Source: Mary Evans Picture Library)*

The period saw a series of confrontations (often in the same country) between two divergent models of health care. State-administered systems—in theory covering all aspects of health care—emerged under rulers who, although politically *absolutist*, harnessed the Enlightenment faith in human reason to promote educational and economic reforms. These hierarchical health-care systems conflicted with more modern notions of health care as a *democratic right*, arising from the post-1789 revolutionary movements. We will look at each system in turn.

Medical police

The aim of the absolutist rulers of the eighteenth century was to boost population numbers and so ensure a fit labour force and plentiful military conscripts. The notion of **medical police** was promoted from 1779 by the physician Johann Peter Frank, to assert state omnicompetence in the medical sphere. That Frank was partly educated in France, but had administrative roles in various German-dominated states, is indicative of the widespread European influence of Frank's system of state-administered preventive and curative medicine. For example, a treatise on medical police was published in Edinburgh in 1808. The policing model of public health was to remain influential in Britain: for example with the factory inspectorate from the 1830s, and John Simon's vision in the 1850s of a universal system of Medical Officers of Health (MOHs) with compulsory powers under the criminal law. (We will be looking further at MOHs in Chapter 4.)

A distinctive feature of absolutist states was massive metropolitan hospitals. These were crowded institutions with vast numbers of patients (the General Hospital in Vienna, for example, had an annual turnover of 14 000) and consequent high mortality.

Enlightenment rulers like Joseph II, the Habsburg emperor, pressurised monastic religious orders to adopt a useful *secular* role, to establish hospitals and to provide nursing: indeed, the formally recognised *priest-physician* was an innovative feature of rural health care in Austria and Sweden. The elaborate state-supervised hierarchies of physicians, surgeons, and midwives were intended to eliminate unlicensed practitioners, who were branded as 'quacks'. We find here a strong contrast with Britain, where there was a greater emphasis on medicine as a free trade.

Medicine and revolution

Turning to the second model of health care, the French revolutionary ideals of liberty, equality, and fraternity stimulated movements for the emergence of a unified medical profession, for state control and reform of hospitals, and for the application of science to clinical medicine. An example of an innovation disseminated to the general population in the wake of the French armies was vaccination against smallpox from 1800.

The full working-out of revolutionary ideals for health care—with their inevitable clash of social interests—occurred in the period before 1850. The French Revolution of the 1780s and 1790s enhanced the prestige of the bourgeois medical profession, freed from absolutist regulation. Concepts of *social medicine* were introduced in France in the 1830s and disseminated more widely in Europe, but the notion of health care as a democratic right only emerged in the German medical reform movement during the revolutions of 1848–9. Reacting against state policing systems, revolutionary doctors argued that diseases were caused by political repression, and economic and educational deprivation. In 1847, Salomon Neumann, a poor-law doctor in Berlin, defined health as 'the highest individual right of every person'.

However, the medical revolutionaries clashed over the principle of the public accountability of the medical profession. The radical German pathologist, Rudolf Virchow, resisted demands for a democratically accountable health-care system. Reflecting science's perceived role as a secular faith and source of ethical standards, he argued that the doctor's scientific credentials were a basis for professional autonomy, without need of state regulation. He was criticised by other radicals, including Neumann, who responded that doctors should be accountable to workers subscribing funds in democratically organised workers' health-care associations.

□ In your view, was the doctor the 'best friend of the poor', as Virchow claimed in 1848?

■ Doctors helped the poor by showing how social and economic factors (like malnutrition and poor housing) caused the spread of disease, and by arguing the need for education. But doctors were reluctant to allow medical systems to be subjected to democratic controls.

Reviewing Virchow's influential position in the revolutionary medical reform movement, the historian Erwin H. Ackerknecht commented, 'the patient remains silent'. Ackerknecht's verdict leads us to ponder the question: did demands for professional autonomy from state regulation help legitimate a fully medicalised and coercive new form of authority over the patient? If so, what are the implications for patients' rights today?

British India: the costs of colonialism

Just as rapid and unregulated industrial development posed serious threats to health and labour efficiency in Britain, so British overseas expansion, too, presented a series of medical problems which threatened the profitability of colonial rule and the lives of both colonisers and colonised.

In India, which was the main focus of European expansion in this period, the London-based *East India Company* (EIC) was rapidly expanding its territorial and commercial interests in the Subcontinent, bringing it into conflict with Indian princely states and its imperial rivals the French (see Figure 3.9 *overleaf*).

By the end of the eighteenth century, French influence had been confined to several enclaves in the south, and vast areas of India, such as Bengal, had been subordinated to Company rule. The Company's increasing administrative functions swelled the ranks of its bureaucracy, while its army grew to become one of the largest in the world. At the same time, the disruption caused by war, and increasing population movement within India, facilitated the spread of epidemic diseases like cholera and smallpox, resulting in several devastating epidemics in the early- and mid-nineteenth century.

Medicine and military considerations

From the mid-eighteenth century, war in India placed a severe strain on the EIC's medical services. More surgeons had to be recruited from Britain and from other European countries, and all Company surgeons were required to serve at least two years with the *military* before becoming eligible for the *civil* medical service. In 1763, a permanent Medical Board was established to coordinate the civil and military branches of the medical service in Bengal, and similar organisations were set up in Bombay and Madras a few years later.

The conflicts of the mid-eighteenth century also highlighted the need for more hospital assistants and orderlies—posts which were often filled by Indians trained in the rudiments of Western medicine. The Company increased its recruitment of Indians and organised them into a separate *Military Subordinate Medical Department*. By comparison with those in the 'superior' service, which offered a serviceable if unremarkable income, these men were poorly paid and often complained bitterly of their position.

Military considerations were also dominant in the growth of institutionalised health care in eighteenth-century India. War against France provided the stimulus

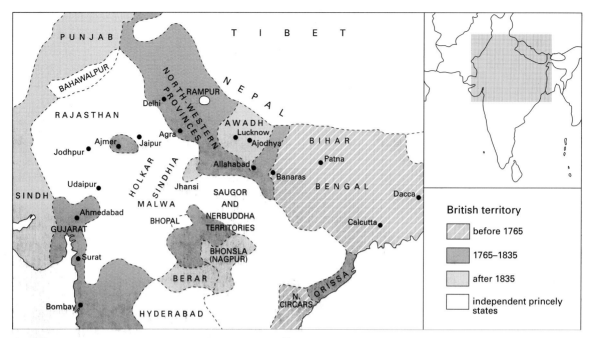

Figure 3.9 *British expansion in Northern India, 1750–1860. (Data from Bayly, C. A., 1988,* Indian Society and the Making of the British Empire, *Cambridge University Press, Cambridge)*

for the construction of the Royal Naval Hospital at Madras, and the British conquest of Bengal resulted in a hospital in Calcutta. In Bombay, by 1784, there were three large hospitals—two for British and one for Indian troops—whereas there had been only one before 1750.

The need for such institutions was acutely felt, since mortality among British troops in India continued to be high throughout the eighteenth and nineteenth centuries.

☐ Look at Figure 3.10. In what ways might the conditions depicted in this barrack room be thought conducive to the spread of disease and the poor health of soldiers in India?

■ The barrack room is ill-ventilated, having to rely on the *punkah* (fan) shown on the right, rather than on open windows. The same room is being used both for washing and for recreation. The beds are crowded close together.

Dragoon guards stationed in Britain, for example, suffered an average annual mortality of 14 per thousand in 1830–6, while British troops in the Bombay area suffered an annual mortality of over 47 per thousand between 1830 and 1849. The high mortality among British soldiers in India at this time was partly a consequence of the spread of cholera throughout India following the

British military conquests of the eighteenth and early nineteenth centuries. Anxieties about health, and the lower social prestige of the Indian services, deterred many Britons from seeking a career in India.

Medical practice in India

The EIC's increasing administrative commitments at the end of the eighteenth century presented both medical opportunities and medical problems. Company surgeons were quick to exploit the growing market for health care and many lucrative private practices were established in the three largest cities: Bombay, Madras, and Calcutta. As early as 1752, there were complaints in Madras that hospital surgeons paid more attention to their private practices than to their hospital patients.

However, as in Britain, *self*-treatment remained an important component of health care until well into the nineteenth century. 'Self-help' manuals for Europeans remained popular in India until the 1880s, some years after their appeal had waned in Britain. In the eighteenth century, and early years of the nineteenth century, it was not uncommon for these to be modelled on indigenous customs such as the avoidance of meat, alcohol and undue exercise. Translations of indigenous medical texts, by William Jones and other 'orientalist' scholars, had also enhanced European knowledge of Indian pharmacology.

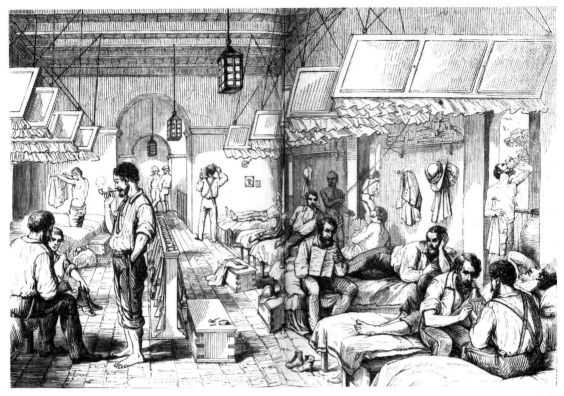

Figure 3.10 *From Florence Nightingale (1863)* Observations on the Sanitary Conditions of the British Army in India. *(Source: British Library, London)*

The health of Indians

By comparison with the health care lavished on European civilians and troops, provisions for the indigenous population outside the armed forces remained meagre throughout this period. This apparent lack of concern with the health of Indians provides a point of contrast with the increasing interest taken in the 'political arithmetic' of health in Britain. There were, however, some notable exceptions. At the beginning of the nineteenth century, an 'Infirmary and Native Poor Asylum' was opened in Madras, under the auspices of a charitable fund raised by subscription among Europeans and wealthy Indians.

The EIC also played a role in institutional health care. In Bombay, for example, a 'native hospital' partly funded by the Company opened in 1809, and a dispensary some years later. By the middle of the nineteenth century, Indian gentlemen, like the Parsi philanthropist Sir Jamsetji Jejeebhai, were taking an active interest in Western medical care and funding the building of hospitals for the use of Indians. Charitable donations also funded the growth of the dispensary movement in India from the late 1830s; a movement which was to grow considerably in the second half of the nineteenth century, aided by the injection of funds from provincial governments and municipalities.

However, it is not easy to assess the level of demand for such institutions among Indians. The historian David Arnold has shown that considerable suspicion of hospitals remained into the late nineteenth century. They were unable to escape their association with an alien and often oppressive regime, and the very concept of hospital treatment was foreign to the majority of Indians who were traditionally treated at home. But the dispensaries, or at least their out-patient clinics, proved far more popular, and became one of the principal outlets through which indigenous Indians encountered Western health care in the later nineteenth and twentieth centuries. Yet Indian women, bound by the Indian custom of *purdah* (the seclusion of women), continued to be ill-served by these dispensaries, which were only rarely supplied with female medical personnel.

Public health in India

The early nineteenth century also brought the first moves in the direction of public health in India. For the most part, sanitary reforms such as those begun in British cities from the 1830s, were confined to military cantonments and to the European quarters of Indian cities. The vast majority of Indians remained untouched by these reforms until the twentieth century.

Vaccination against smallpox was the only exception to this rule. This began in India in 1802 and was performed on Indians at a relatively early stage. Like hospital provision, the vaccination of Indians was supposed to be read as a sign of the Company's good intentions and of Western cultural superiority. Perhaps more important, however, was the concern with economic efficiency, which, as you should recall from earlier in this chapter, was a guiding principle of sanitary reform as espoused by Chadwick and other Benthamite reformers in Britain.

The extension of vaccination to rural areas of India in the 1820s and 1830s, similarly, occurred amidst reforms of India's administration, and was promoted by Benthamite administrators like Lord Elphinstone, Governor-General of Bombay. However, most of these vaccination programmes failed to meet their objectives. This was due to lack of financial support, and to resistance from the indigenous population, which had developed its own system of inoculation and which, in many cases, regarded arm-to-arm vaccination as ritually polluting because people from whom the vaccine was transferred were usually Untouchables or low-caste Indians. It was not until the late nineteenth century that vaccination programmes began to reach substantial numbers of Indians.

Tropical hygiene

The other principal development in public health in nineteenth-century India was the changing nature and content of *tropical hygiene*. As a consequence of European political domination, reflected in the growing social distance of Europeans, Indian people, their dwellings, and their lifestyle, came to be viewed increasingly as 'reservoirs of dirt and disease'. Whereas Indians had once been consulted and, to some extent, emulated in order to facilitate European acclimatisation to the tropics, Indian culture and the Indian people came to be seen as part of the sanitary *problem* confronting Europeans. Increasingly, European medical texts began to recommend the separation of British from Indian settlements, and to view Indians as physically as well as culturally different. Only the 'martial races' of Northern India, whose military traditions and physical stature endeared them to the British, continued to be viewed in a favourable light.

□ What similarities do you find between colonial attitudes towards the health of indigenous peoples, and the attitude of Benthamite reformers towards the health of the working class in Britain?

■ The 'fever nests' in working-class districts of Britain were viewed as threats to health in the same way as Indian dwellings, and the health of both groups was considered in terms of economic efficiency rather than moral responsibility.

This trend was accompanied by an increasing pessimism about the possibility of European acclimatisation to the tropical environment. In the eighteenth century, many doctors in India and the West Indies believed that, over time, and through the adoption of certain indigenous customs, they would become fully adapted to tropical climates. Some even believed they would acquire the physical characteristics of native peoples. But, in the nineteenth century, with the growing social separation of colonisers and colonised, such views became extremely rare.

The Company surgeon, James Johnson, writing in 1812, maintained that Europeans in India tended to 'droop', and, before long, to seek refuge in their native climate. The offspring of those who remained in India, he believed, would 'gradually degenerate', morally and physically (Johnson, 1812, p. 3). Johnson urged that much could still be done to make the existence of Europeans in India more comfortable but, in later texts, a more fatalistic attitude prevails, and is reflected in the growing interest in *medical topography*—the attempt to locate microclimates most suitable to Europeans.

This concern with medical topography led to two parallel developments: the gathering of medical and meteorological statistics from British military cantonments and towns from the 1830s, and the increasing resort to sanatoria and hill stations with more salubrious climates. At the same time, it became fashionable to send children back to Britain for their schooling. Ironically, with British influence approaching its zenith in India, Europeans had come to regard themselves as exotics, prone to wilt on foreign soil.

It was not until after 1858, with the assumption of government by the British Crown, and in the wake of the Indian Mutiny, that the British administration began to intervene more directly in public health, and then, largely out of concern for the health of British troops. With the exception of smallpox vaccination and the establishment of a few charitable institutions in the larger cities, the EIC showed little concern for the health of the indigenous civilian population. Health-care provisions clearly reflected colonial, and especially military, priorities and, in the early nineteenth century, the increasing pessimism about European acclimatisation to the tropics.

But, although belief in the possibility of bodily adaptation to tropical climates declined considerably in the years after 1830, the potential for transforming the tropical environment remained, and infused the rhetoric of the so-called pioneers of tropical medicine considered in Chapter 4.

OBJECTIVES FOR CHAPTER 3

When you have studied this chapter, you should be able to:

3.1 Identify the principal social and economic factors affecting health during the Industrial Revolution, where necessary relating the content of this chapter to relevant material in *World Health and Disease*.

3.2 Indicate ways in which lay care and self-help changed—and did not change—as a result of industrialisation, urbanisation and Enlightenment ideas.

3.3 Comment on the degree to which different kinds of medical practitioner might have gained (or lost) by the growing professionalisation of medicine, associated with the trend towards formal qualifications.

3.4 Explain why pre-industrial mechanisms of public health were inadequate to deal with threats to the environment associated with industrialisation; and describe the ways in which the sanitarian movement addressed these threats.

3.5 Give examples that show how health-care systems in Britain and continental Europe in this period were influenced by attitudes towards the poor, including attitudes derived from religious belief.

3.6 Describe the origins of British medical intervention in India and explain its limitations.

QUESTIONS FOR CHAPTER 3

Question 1 (*Objective 3.1*)

Here is Samuel Johnson again, in 1776, defending his birthplace, the cathedral city of Lichfield, against charges of idleness:

> We are a City of Philosophers: we work with our Heads, and make the Boobies of Birmingham work for us with their Hands... (Quoted in Corfield, 1989, p. 94)

This is a piece of evidence given to the Commission of 1842 enquiring into children's employment in mines:

> Mr Holroyd, solicitor, and Mr Brook, surgeon, practising in Stainland, were present, who confessed that, although living within a few miles, they could not have believed that such a system of unchristian cruelty could have existed. (Quoted in Thompson, 1975, p. 377)

What do these very different statements have in common? And what can they tell us about social conditions during industrialisation?

Question 2 (*Objective 3.2*)

A local historian wrote in 1898 of the spa baths at Lockwood, near Huddersfield, created in the 1820s:

> The existence of mineral springs had suggested to the speculative mind dreams of an English Baden [Baden-Baden, in Germany, one of the most fashionable spas in Europe in the nineteenth century], or at least of another Harrogate [the spa resort in Yorkshire]. The river was spanned with a rustic bridge, grounds were laid, and a Bath Hotel opened its doors. (Quoted in Marland, 1987, p. 232)

The new baths were on the site of an old sulphur well. What points does the quotation illustrate about the connections between urbanisation and self-help health care at this period?

Question 3 (*Objective 3.3*)

A 'letter to the editor' written in 1827 and signed 'General Practitioner' read in part:

> I am not factious or querulous, but I fearlessly maintain, that the promised rights, which I naturally expected, as a member of the College and Hall, have no existence, and that those who have never been educated have had as many advantages, and much more, than those who qualified and received diplomas in surgery and pharmacy. As the profession is now constituted a man cannot select a worse mode of life than that of a general practitioner. (Quoted in Loudon, 1986, p. 181)

What kind of practitioner was 'General Practitioner', and what grounds were there for his complaint?

Question 4 (*Objectives 3.4 and 3.5*)

In 1839, Dr Southwood Smith reported as follows to the Poor Law Commissioners, who were looking for ways of reducing the 'rate-burden' arising from disease and destitution:

> While systematic efforts on a large scale have been made to widen the streets, to remove obstructions to the circulation...of air, to extend and perfect the drainage and sewerage, and to prevent the accumulation of putrefying vegetable and animal substances in the places in which the wealthier classes reside, nothing whatever has been done to improve the condition of the districts inhabited by the poor. These neglected places are out of view, and are not thought of...Yet in these pestilential places the industrious poor are obliged to take up their abode; they have no choice; they must live in what houses they can get nearest the places where they find employment. By no prudence or forethought on their part can they avoid the dreadful evils of this class to which they are thus exposed. (Quoted in Simon, 1897, p. 183)

What does this suggest about the obstacles to improving the living conditions of the poor?

Question 5 (*Objective 3.5*)

What follows is part of a reply to objections made in the 1730s to the plan to found Winchester County Hospital—which, you may recall (see Figure 3.7) was the first English voluntary hospital outside London:

> It was objected that the poor dislike anything with the appearance of constraint or removal from their families. But any who desire it shall be considered and received as outpatients. Experience tells that whenever a hospital has been erected the poor have esteemed it a blessing and have flocked to it with eagerness; for there they get free air, wholesome and proper diet, clean and constant attendance, the best advice, and no more medicines than are necessary. (Quoted in Woodward, 1974, p. 13)

What does this suggest to you about the functions of the voluntary hospitals—and the attitudes and circumstances of their patients?

Question 6 (*Objective 3.6*)

The following are extracts from the *Medical Topography of Calcutta*, written by the East India Company Surgeon James Ranald Martin, and published in 1837.

> The Bengallee, unlike the Hindu of the North, is utterly devoid of pride, national and individual. His moral character is a matter of history...when we are looking forward with such well-founded hope to the improved results of European knowledge and example diffused among the natives....The natives have yet to learn that the sweet sensations connected with cleanly habits, and pure air, are some of the most precious gifts of civilization. (Martin, 1837, pp. 45, 24)

In what ways do these extracts illustrate the changes that were taking place in colonial medicine in India in the early nineteenth century?

4 The era of public health, 1848 to 1918

This chapter assumes a familiarity with modern evolutionary theory (see **World Health and Disease,** *Chapter 5, and* **Human Biology and Health: An Evolutionary Approach[1])** *and the 'bacteriological revolution' in the later part of the nineteenth century when it was conclusively demonstrated that infectious diseases were caused by micro-organisms (discussed in* **Medical Knowledge: Doubt and Certainty***). In this chapter, these developments in theoretical and practical biology are related to the social and political developments which they helped to fuel.*

Reference is also made to the two Reader[2] articles by Thomas McKeown and Simon Szreter, which you read during your study of **World Health and Disease***, and revised in Chapter 3.*

During study of this chapter, you will be expected to read an article in the Reader, by the historian Rosemary Stevens, entitled 'The evolution of the health-care systems in the USA and the United Kingdom: similarities and differences', first published in 1976.

From sanitarianism to personal responsibility

The failed liberal revolutions of the 1840s in Western Europe were followed by decades of pragmatic politics, economic expansion and competition, the consolidation of nation states and, at the turn of the century, imperialism and World War I. Historians are increasingly finding links between major economic and social changes in this period, and rapidly developing areas of the human sciences, in particular evolutionary biology, sociology, anthropology and genetics. Here is the prominent sanitarian, William Farr, addressing the Statistical Society of London in 1872:

> Politics is no longer the art of Letting things alone, nor the game of audacious Revolution for the sake of change; so politics, like war, has to submit to the spirit of the age, and to call in the aid of science: for the art of government can only be practised with success when it is grounded on a knowledge of the people governed, derived from exact observation. (Quoted by Eyler, 1979, p. 28)

Major shifts in social policy, like sanitarianism, made overt reference to biological principles as applied to human populations—the effects on health and behaviour of crowding, for example. The interdependence of science and industrialisation was rationalised by the French philosopher Auguste Comte, in whose positivist account of human progress the most advanced stage was marked by the rise of the secular science of *sociology* and by successful *social engineering* based on scientific laws.

Darwinism and human society

This inherently optimistic outlook was countered by more pessimistic trends as capitalism failed to ensure benefits for all. The principle, as put forward by Charles Darwin and Alfred Russel Wallace, of *evolution by natural selection*[3] —the so-called 'survival of the fittest'— was in part a further development of Malthusianism,[4] and fostered continued adherence to economic individualism later in the century. Unfettered competition, it seemed, was a 'law of nature', and not to be interfered with.

---

[1] Another book in this series, *Human Biology and Health: An Evolutionary Approach* (Open University Press, 1994).

[2] *Health and Disease: A Reader* (second edition, 1995).

[3] *World Health and Disease*, Chapter 5, and *Human Biology and Health: An Evolutionary Approach*, Chapter 3.

[4] *World Health and Disease*, Chapter 5.

TABLE XVIII.—**Deaths in 30 Large Town Districts** in the 10 Years 1851–60 ; and also the DEATHS which would have occurred in the 10 Years if the MORTALITY had been at the same Rate as prevailed in the 63 HEALTHY DISTRICTS (1849–53).

AGES.	DEATHS in 10 Years 1851–60.	DEATHS which would have occurred in the 10 Years at HEALTHY DISTRICT RATES.	EXCESS of ACTUAL DEATHS in 10 Years over DEATHS at HEALTHY DISTRICT RATES.
ALL AGES -	711,944	384,590	327,354
0— - -	338,990	135,470	203,520
5— - -	31,319	19,290	12,029
10— - -	14,240	11,020	3,220
15— - -	43,807	37,550	6,257
25— - -	48,625	36,150	12,475
35— - -	50,071	30,320	19,751
45— - -	49,638	26,680	22,958
55— - -	49,763	27,020	22,743
65— - -	47,445	31,510	15,935
75— - -	30,583	22,920	7,663
85 & upwards -	7,463	6,660	803

Figure 4.1 *This table, reproduced from William Farr's official report of 1865, illustrates the development of a standard of comparison for healthiness in terms of the rates of the so-called 'healthy districts'. Note also that Farr has corrected for differences in the age-structure of different localities (compare this with Table 3.1). (Source: Supplement to the 25th Annual Report of the Registrar-General, 1865, p. xxvi)*

Natural selection, which depended upon another of Darwin's assumptions, the surplus production of off-spring, encouraged speculation about 'fitness to survive' among human populations. Darwinism was readily deployed to discredit state intervention in the field of social welfare, to oppose feminism, and to defend imperialism and the subordination of 'inferior' races. So-called **social Darwinism**, reinforced by the new 'science' of **eugenics** (the devising of policies to improve the genetic quality of the human race, especially by selective breeding), provided a framework for exaggerated fears, contrasting the declining fertility of the middle classes with high fertility among 'degraded groups' in large industrial towns. This represented the dominant social philosophy among the Darwinists, but it was not the only legitimate construction. For instance, Wallace, co-founder of the theory of natural selection, supported socialism and women's rights. 'Neo-Malthusian' advocates of contraception, and social reformers, also looked to biology to reinforce their arguments.

Sanitarianism—success and failure

Sanitarianism instilled the conviction that epidemic disease acted indiscriminately, and did not in fact remove only the supposedly 'unfit'. Sanitary reform delivered considerable benefits in the course of this period, particularly with respect to water supply, sewage removal, and food production. Nonetheless, implementation was slow; the problem of inadequate housing was particularly intractable; and many reformers were disappointed to find, around the turn of the century, that some mortality rates remained obstinately high. This applied especially to *infant mortality*, and crude mortality rates in areas of *high population density*.

□ Can you think of one reason why both rates remained high?

■ The two were in fact related, in that an increasing proportion of most populations was urbanised—a higher proportion of babies was being born in poor conditions in densely populated areas.

Even now, there are difficulties in accounting for mortality trends in this period, since it appears that first adult and then infant mortality declined in most Western European countries at about the same time. A similar secular decline in fertility can also be detected.[5] Nonetheless, whatever the influences on overall rates, observers of the time were correct in discerning wide differentials of mortality between town and country, and between different social groups (see Figure 4.1).

Imperialism and national deterioration

Towards the end of the century, the balance of economic power was shifting away from Britain and towards Germany and the USA. Fears of economic decline at home, and loss of empire abroad, were sharpened by

[5] *World Health and Disease*, Chapter 6.

revelations of the physical state of the nation's manpower. Industrial supremacy required a fit labour force, and controlling the empire, an effective standing army: yet the examination of Boer War recruits, reinforced by many other surveys, produced a devastating picture of physical inadequacy (see Figure 4.2).

The evidence of these reports was discussed against the background of a changing climate of opinion about the causes of ill-health. Environmental solutions had been downgraded by the *bacteriological revolution,* and

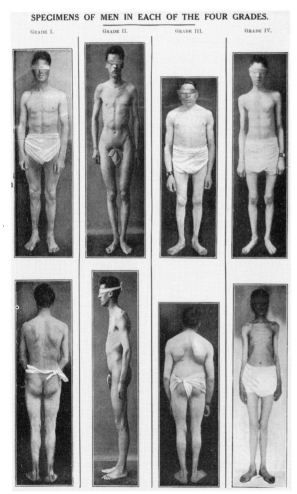

SPECIMENS OF MEN IN EACH OF THE FOUR GRADES.

GRADE I.   GRADE II.   GRADE III.   GRADE IV.

Figure 4.2 *Army recruits in World War I. These photographs underline the physical defects and class disparities in health which were revealed by the World War and previously by the Boer War. (Source: Ministry of National Service, 1919,* Report upon the Physical Examination of Men of Military Age by National Service Medical Boards from 1st November 1917 to 31st October 1918, *HMSO, London,Cmd 504)*

the establishment of the *germ theory of disease*[6] led to what the American historian Paul Starr has called a 'new concept of dirt'. Increasingly the focus was not the broad vision of nineteenth-century public health, but responsibility for health at the *individual* level, and especially at the level of individual mothers. A conviction that **maternal inefficiency** was a serious factor affecting working-class health prompted an armoury of devices aimed at delivering advice to mothers, although there was some realisation, as you will see, that 'efficiency' was severely constrained by housing conditions.

In later life, even John Simon, whose crucial role in mid-nineteenth-century public health will be highlighted later in the chapter, could share in the trend towards personal responsibility:

> Especially it would seem reasonable to connect the principle of Compulsory Insurance with the principle of Free Education; for surely, if the State is to provide gratuitous education for the masses of the people, it may reasonably require, as first-fruits from the receivers of such education, that they shall, as far as practicable, secure themselves against future pauperism, and thus guarantee the community against further costs on their behalf. (Simon, 1897, p. 462)

But services also expanded under the control of local authorities. In the first decade of the century a modest start was made, with child welfare and ante-natal clinics, the provision of school meals, and school medical inspection.

The national system of measures directed at mothers and children was part of a more general system of welfare benefits established under the threat of *national deterioration.* Legislation was passed for old age pensions in 1907, and National Health Insurance in 1911. This embryo *welfare state* was established not just out of humanitarianism, but through a desire to develop *national efficiency.* The modern sociologist Lesley Doyal has called the reforms an 'important element in the attempt to restructure British capitalism' (Doyal and Pennell, 1979, p. 160).

At another level, too, the focus was on individual responsibility. The downturn in infectious epidemic disease at the end of the century brought a shift in patterns of mortality and morbidity towards chronic diseases such as cancer, heart disease, and tuberculosis (TB).[7] Alcoholism, venereal (sexually transmitted) diseases (VD), and mental 'deficiency' were perceived as major problems

[6] *Medical Knowledge: Doubt and Certainty,* Chapter 4.

[7] *World Health and Disease,* Chapter 6.

because of the threat of national deterioration through transmission and inheritance of these disorders of 'degeneration'. These 'diseases' were viewed within an individualistic, moralising framework. Concern about VD peaked during World War I and led to the establishment of venereal disease clinics, but not to other preventive measures. The wider impact of that war on health and health-care practice remains uncertain. Expectations were aroused that World War I would be followed by the creation of a national system of health services. The actual response fell far short of this goal.

The erosion of lay care and lay control

The legal boundaries between qualified and unqualified practice became clearer in this period, and some women carers began to be included in the professional hierarchy. On the ground, however, the informal sector remained strong, stretching from the paupers who continued to serve as nurses in workhouses, to the practitioners of homoeopathy and other 'alternative' systems who were increasingly presenting themselves as part of the formal sector. Examples such as the following show the persistence of the lay carer who was sanctioned by the community and paid in kind, rather than cash.

Praise of Sally Dunkirk, a lay practitioner from Slaithwaite, Yorkshire, around 1860

Any bad case of fever, or lunacy, of exceptional emergency, was a call for Sally's services. In such cases she became general, and house maid, doctor and nurse, friend and physician all in one.... A most useful woman was she for the times in which she lived.... If her treatment failed to restore the patient to normal health it was a case forthwith to be sent to a lunatic asylum. Her fees were never much more than a liberal supply of home-brewed beer, unrestricted stock of good 'bacca', and the indispensable long clay pipe, with a good 'table', and implicit obedience to her orders. (Quoted in Marland, 1987, p. 219)

Commercial growth

Lay care was also construed to be a matter of self-care and self-medication. Although earlier traditions of self-medication remained strong, a *commercial* tendency became increasingly apparent. A fall in the price of drugs was part of a general decline in the cost of raw materials in the 1870s and was accompanied by a rise in the real value of wages. The increased sale of patent medicines was a demonstration of greater prosperity among certain sectors of the working class (see Figure 4.3).

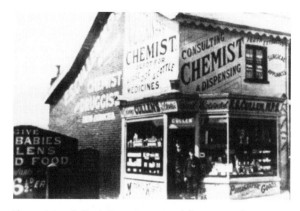

Figure 4.3 *Cullen's Drug Store, Norfolk, 1890s. The services and products offered include: 'Trusses [for rupture] a speciality'; photographic goods; teeth extraction; 'veterinary chemist'. (Photo reproduced by courtesy of the Royal Pharmaceutical Society of Great Britain)*

Newspaper advertising expanded; the advertising expenditure of pharmaceutical entrepreneurs like Holloway (see Figure 4.4) or Beecham reached unprecedented heights (Holloway's jumped from £5 000 a year in 1842 to £50 000 in 1883). Several of the leading proprietors and sellers of patent medicines, like Beecham himself, a herbalist, and Jesse Boot, who was expanding his chain of cash chemists in Nottingham in the 1870s, had strong connections with the earlier traditions of folk medicine and medical botany.

There were many abuses of patent medicine sale and advertisement (see Figure 4.5). Wild claims for efficacy were made, and leading public figures quoted as endorsing products they had probably never heard of. Pharmaceutical composition of remedies was variable.

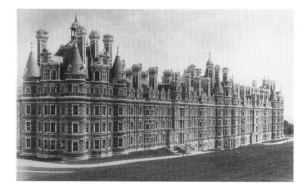

Figure 4.4 *Royal Holloway College, opened in 1886 as a women's college of the University of London: modelled on a French château, and endowed by Thomas Holloway out of the proceeds of his patent medicine empire. (Source: Royal Holloway and Bedford New College, University of London)*

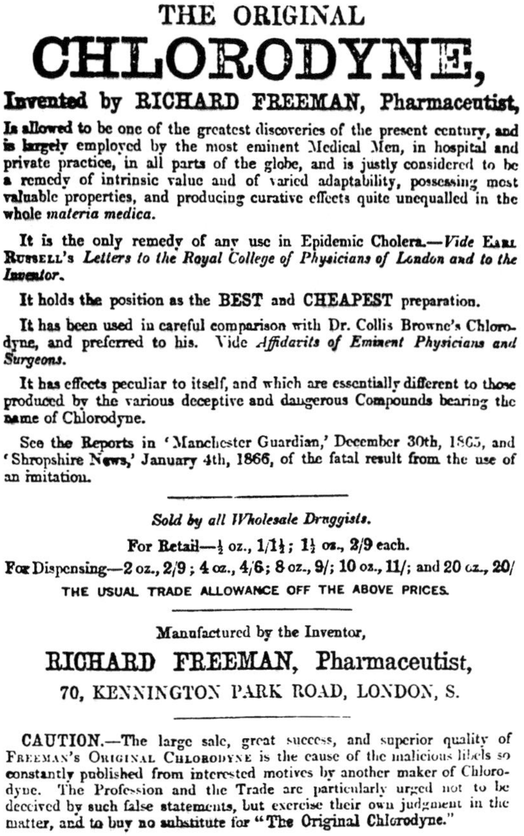

THE ORIGINAL
CHLORODYNE,
Invented by RICHARD FREEMAN, Pharmaceutist,

Is allowed to be one of the greatest discoveries of the present century, and is largely employed by the most eminent Medical Men, in hospital and private practice, in all parts of the globe, and is justly considered to be a remedy of intrinsic value and of varied adaptability, possessing most valuable properties, and producing curative effects quite unequalled in the whole *materia medica*.

It is the only remedy of any use in Epidemic Cholera.—*Vide* EARL RUSSELL's *Letters to the Royal College of Physicians of London and to the Inventor.*

It holds the position as the BEST and CHEAPEST preparation.

It has been used in careful comparison with Dr. Collis Browne's Chlorodyne, and preferred to his. Vide *Affidavits of Eminent Physicians and Surgeons.*

It has effects peculiar to itself, and which are essentially different to those produced by the various deceptive and dangerous Compounds bearing the name of Chlorodyne.

See the Reports in 'Manchester Guardian,' December 30th, 1865, and 'Shropshire News,' January 4th, 1866, of the fatal result from the use of an imitation.

Sold by all Wholesale Druggists.

For Retail—½ oz., 1/1½ ; 1½ oz., 2/9 each.

For Dispensing—2 oz., 2/9 ; 4 oz., 4/6; 8 oz., 9/; 10 oz., 11/; and 20 oz., 20/

THE USUAL TRADE ALLOWANCE OFF THE ABOVE PRICES.

Manufactured by the Inventor,

RICHARD FREEMAN, Pharmaceutist,

70, KENNINGTON PARK ROAD, LONDON, S.

CAUTION.—The large sale, great success, and superior quality of FREEMAN's ORIGINAL CHLORODYNE is the cause of the malicious libels so constantly published from interested motives by another maker of Chlorodyne. The Profession and the Trade are particularly urged not to be deceived by such false statements, but exercise their own judgment in the matter, and to buy no substitute for "The Original Chlorodyne."

Figure 4.5 *Chlorodyne advertising, c. 1870. Rival inventors and distributors of chlorodyne (an opium-based patent medicine used in the treatment of diarrhoea and other ailments) attacked each other's products. This advertisement for Freeman's chlorodyne attacks Dr Collis Browne's remedy. (Photo reproduced by courtesy of the Royal Pharmaceutical Society of Great Britain)*

These abuses were attacked in a campaign promoted by the medical and pharmaceutical professions at the turn of the century.

Lay care stretched beyond its limits

In other respects, self-help systems were giving way under the strain. The friendly societies began to wilt under pressure from the effects of 'unhealthy trades' and the changing demographic regime in which adults lived longer, but were not necessarily in better health. Lay care for the chronically sick was also affected by the absorption of married women into paid work. The position of the elderly had always been difficult, and was worsened by their longer survival. For all but a few groups (for

example, army officers) there was no 'retirement age', and no age-related entitlement, for example to charity or poor relief, until state pensions were introduced in 1907.

Middle-class expectations of the poor were based partly on a hardening attitude to the division of responsibility between the family and the state, and partly on Victorian family ideals relevant only to the more prosperous. Poor households were unable to 'extend' to provide carers for older relatives, and even co-residence with relatives did not mean that the needs of the infirm elderly could be met. This became evident when, during the depression of the 1870s, strenuous attempts were made to force the care of parents on to their children, to avoid paying pensions from the poor rate. The end result of greater stringency was to increase the proportion of elderly in the workhouses (see Figure 4.6).

Institutionalisation and lay control

The rate of institutionalisation also increased for the steeply rising numbers classified as mentally handicapped or insane. That medical men rather than laymen

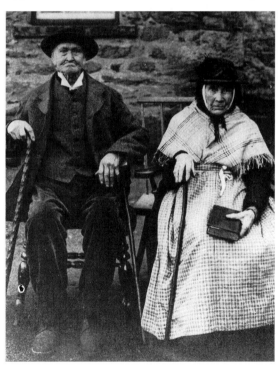

Figure 4.6 *Roland and Betsy Jones of Hen Hafod, Merioneth, in 1870. This self-respecting couple are known only by a Welsh inscription on the back of the original photograph: 'They entered the workhouse at Bala, but instead of separating them the Guardians permitted them to have a room to themselves'. (Source: Gwynedd Archives Service)*

should control and inspect asylums was a well-established principle by the mid-nineteenth century, but as asylums grew to grotesque size and ineffectiveness, this was at best an ambiguous development both for medicine and for the mentally ill. As the following pronouncement suggests, the boundaries between lay and formal care were considerably complicated by status and gender divisions:

> The circumstance of a superintendent's wife acting as matron involves a sacrifice of social position injurious, if not fatal, to success. It is above all things indispensable that medical superintendents of asylums should be educated gentlemen; and if that is to be the case, their wives cannot be matrons. Indeed, it is inconceivable that a man of position and culture would allow his family to have any connection with an asylum. (J. M. Granville, 1877, quoted in Scull, 1979, p. 182)

With respect to lay control of other institutions of medical care, there was some shifting of boundaries. The Poor Law remained under lay control, as did much of the public-health administration evolving under the new structures of local government. Medical authority was increasing, but within, rather than in opposition to, existing lay hierarchies: examples are the army, asylums, and the voluntary hospitals, which we will look at later in this chapter.

Inefficient mothers?

The high, and even increasing, rate of *infant mortality* drew attention to the crucial importance of mothers as carers. Mary Scharlieb, a leading doctor, singled out the relationship between mothers' drinking and poor infant care. Her opinion was that:

> The high death rate amongst English babies is not dependent upon poverty alone.... There is no doubt whatever that the drinking habits of the nation and especially of the women of the nation, are doing more harm to our financial and social position than is any depression in trade or other economic causes. (Scharlieb, 1907–8, p. 59)

□ In what ways is Scharlieb's view of maternal responsibility characteristic of middle-class attitudes to the poor?

■ She was advancing an *individually* focused view of causes, which could instead be ascribed to poverty. Mothers were being blamed for the results of poor social and economic conditions.

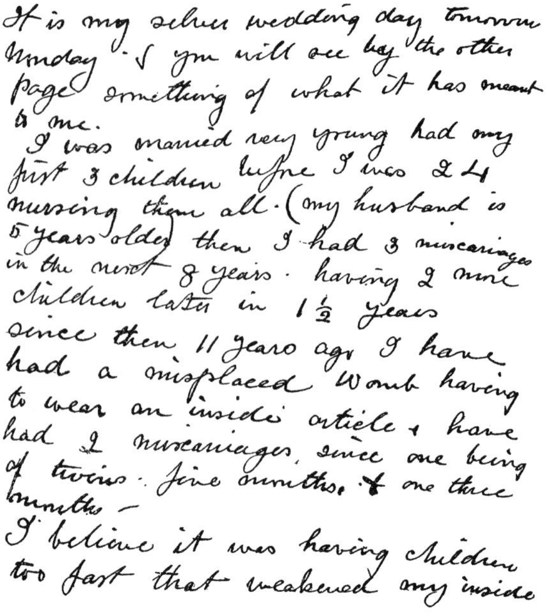
It is my silver wedding day tomorrow Monday. If you will see by the other page something of what it has meant to me.
I was married very young had my first 3 children before I was 24 nursing them all. (my husband is 5 years older then I had 3 miscarriages in the next 8 years. having 2 more children later in 1½ years since then 11 years ago I have had a misplaced Womb having to wear an inside article & have had 2 miscarriages, since one being of twins. five months, & one three months –
I believe it was having children too fast that weakened my inside

Figure 4.7 *A letter written to the Women's Co-operative Guild describes the burden of unwanted births and untreated health problems for women who did not have right of access to medical care. (From Llewellyn Davies, M. (ed.), 1915,* Maternity: Letters from Working Women collected by the Women's Co-operative Guild*, G. Bell & Sons, London; reprinted in 1978 by Virago, London)*

Despite the emphasis on *maternal inefficiency*, few of the welfare benefits introduced at this time were available to individual working-class women. The aim of the welfare reforms was primarily economic; and women, even though more of them were at work, had little power in the market place.

This emphasis on motherhood did not lead to a rise in family size at any level of society. Exactly the opposite was the case. Middle-class women had been using *birth control* to limit the size of their families since the 1860s and, as you have seen, the birth rate was falling in the last quarter of the century. Immediately after World War I there was a brief increase in the birth rate, but the long-term trend was downward throughout Western Europe. This trend was assisted by the wider use of contraception which was spreading among working-class women by the turn of the century. The burden of unwanted births (see Figure 4.7) gradually began to lift.

Lady visitors

Increased *outside* intervention in working-class homes and important shifts between lay and formal sectors of care both took place. Areas of lay care were taken out of the home by the institutional route—the removal of large numbers of elderly women into lunatic asylums is one example. *Volunteer visiting* of the poor had a long history, but this tendency also became more marked from the 1860s onwards. In 1862, the Ladies' Section of the Manchester and Salford Sanitary Association undertook to spread health information among the poor of the community. Visiting nurses moved rapidly to other areas, promoting the care and welfare of young children at home. In London, the work of the Charity Organisation Society from the 1870s was focused on 'close personal surveillance'.

The main development at the end of the nineteenth century was that these 'visitors' were more likely to have a professional, or at least a trained background. Formal health visiting schemes expanded in the early years of the twentieth century and came ultimately under the control of Medical Officers of Health. By 1918, **health visitor** numbers had reached 1 000 and by 1919 uniform training requirements had been laid down. Their position was ambiguous in that they were expected to befriend and gently influence, but also to monitor and report. Ultimately the focus of their work did not address the real needs of mothers and infants.

Evidence collected by the Women's Co-operative Guild (published in *Maternity,* 1915; see Figure 4.7) and other surveys, showed the impact of poor diet in pregnancy and the stretching of inadequate wages. Problems arising from living conditions and economic situation were on a far greater scale than any individual inadequacies. But the magnified role for health visiting also demonstrated how lay networks of care were increasingly giving way to outside intervention, initially on a voluntary basis and subsequently trained and professionalised.

Sanitarianism in action

The sanitarian movement reflected the best and the worst features of Victorian society. Against a neglect of the root causes of poverty must be set the energy and dedication which led to the transformation of the urban environment. The unbridled industrial activity which blighted the lives and health of a large proportion of the working population also produced the waterworks, embankments, and pumping stations which stand as monuments today (see Figure 4.8). Parsimony and obliviousness to the sufferings of others were matched by passionate concern and a strong sense of public duty.

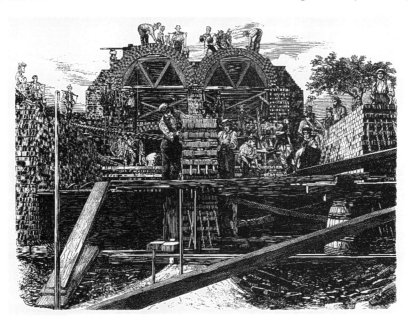

Figure 4.8 *6 000 men, directed by Sir Joseph Bazalgette, built London's main sewer system between 1858 and 1865: eighty miles of tunnel running north and south of the Thames with outfalls into the river at Barking and Crossness. '[T]he opening ceremonies at the southern outfall down the Thames were attended by the Prince of Wales, Prince Edward Saxe-Weimar, the Lord Mayor, the Archbishop of Canterbury, the Archbishop of York, and 500 guests, who dined on salmon while the city's excreta gushed forth into the Thames beneath them' (Wohl, 1983, p. 107). (Source:* Illustrated London News)

The classic period of public-health reform is represented by four very different charismatic figures: Edwin Chadwick, the Benthamite lawyer, whom you met in Chapter 3; William Farr of the Registrar-General's Office, the son of a Shropshire farm labourer; Florence Nightingale, the sickly upper-class spinster, who spearheaded sanitary reform of the army and of hospitals; and John Simon, a surgeon of Huguenot descent, and creator, after the dismantling of Chadwick's General Board of Health, of a medical department of government which prefigured the Ministry of Health. These figures had in common the ability to deploy information to devastating effect, using the characteristic Victorian weapons of personal influence, 'bluebooks' (official government reports), the press, and the pulpit. All were long-lived, and their influence extended until the turn of the century.

The successes of propaganda

The sanitary movement was very much a matter of effective propaganda and the creation of a responsive climate of opinion. Early sanitary legislation, from 1848 onwards, mainly facilitated the granting of powers to local agencies, and laid down administrative measures which had to be adopted only if local mortality rose to exceed a defined 'average' of 23 per thousand. Where powers did exist, the problems of enforcement were usually considerable. For the most part, early public-health administration consisted of talented and courageous use of duties to 'inquire and report'. The creation of *inspectorates* was central to sanitary campaigns. Much effort had to be devoted to the extraction and presentation of up-to-date data on changes in the level of mortality, since these constituted the basis on which action could be taken.

Victorian élites came to believe in quantification as a mode of reasoning, and *statistics* were central to the sanitary movement. However, medical certification of death was not compulsory until 1874; the notification of cases of certain infectious diseases, compulsory once adopted and providing information on morbidity, was not introduced nationally until 1889. In the meantime, William Farr, as Compiler of Abstracts, provided a running commentary on the broad generalisations issued in the Registrar-General's Reports, and constructed equations from the unpublished material which suggested natural laws of disease involving such factors as population density and height above sea-level. This was matched by independent inquiries conducted by individuals and local societies, like the Manchester Statistical Society (founded 1833) and the Epidemiological Society of London (founded 1850). The use of statistics by sanitarians is of course only one reflection of the development of the 'social sciences'—the

sense that not only the natural world, but also human society, could be studied scientifically.

Early sanitarianism was dominated by water supply and drainage, along with a successful campaign to halt burials in crowded urban graveyards. Chadwick was chiefly responsible for the introduction of the smallbore sewer pipe, an innovation which his successor Simon could hardly praise sufficiently:

> The adaptation of glazed earthenware pipes to serve as domestic and urban drains was the most valuable sanitary contrivance which had been introduced since Roman times. (Simon, 1897, p. 226)

Chadwick envisaged, but could not implement, a perfect, cyclic system in which flowing water scoured the sewers and the sewage was transported to enrich agricultural land. This system presupposed central, single-authority control. Chadwick's Board was axed by government in 1854 (a cholera year), and health responsibilities were transferred to the Privy Council. Simon, having attracted much attention as Medical Officer to the City of London, moved to become 'Medical Officer of the Committee of Council on Health'.

Simon initially avoided the Benthamite emphasis on direct central administration, and was only gradually converted because of the unreformed structure of local government. From the outset, however, he advocated a Ministry of Health, and defined areas requiring legislative intervention, including:

> The uncontrolled letting of houses unfit for human habitation; the unregulated industries of sorts endangering the health of persons employed in them; the unregulated nuisance-making businesses; the unchecked adulterations of food [see Figure 4.9]; the unchecked falsification of drugs; the unregulated promiscuous sale of poisons; and the absence of legal distinction between qualified and unqualified medical practitioners. (Simon, 1897, p. 255)

These were not new issues, but ones in which sanitarianism reasserted the moral duty of interference between buyer and seller.

Medical Officers of Health

Simon did however represent a shift of emphasis in sanitarianism which occurred as medical involvement increased. **Medical Officers of Health** (MOHs), at first attached to temporary Boards of Health in periods of epidemic crisis, became compulsory in London districts in 1855, and in all local government areas in the 1870s.

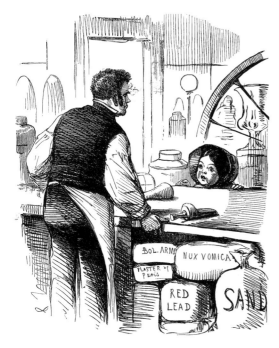

Figure 4.9 *Urbanisation and industrialisation increased the scale and severity of food and drug adulteration. In spite of spirited press campaigns, and legislation from 1860 onwards, effective and widespread testing was not established before the twentieth century. The little girl says: 'If you please, sir, Mother says, will you let her have a quarter of a pound of your best tea to kill the rats with, and a ounce of chocolate as would get rid of the black beadles!' (Source:* Punch *4 August 1855)*

For some practitioners, a Medical Officership was a routine part-time local appointment, somewhat better paid and higher in status than a Poor Law surgeoncy. Some MOHs were able and dedicated innovators with well-developed research interests. However, the reforming MOH was often unpopular, as in Darlington in 1851:

> The indiscriminate publication at length of the report...of the Officer of Health having been considered by the Board, it is resolved that indiscriminate publication is calculated to be injurious to the town. (Quoted by Brockington, 1965, p. 159)

□ The origin of the MOH can be traced to Chadwick, who had stressed the need for health officers to be full-time, salaried public employees. Can you suggest reasons for this requirement?

■ Conscientious MOHs were very often in difficulties because the insecure, low-paid, part-time nature of their employment left them dependent on continuing in private practice among the very people whose local interests they were seen as attacking.

The basic sanitary truths about filth and disease became enshrined in the public mind, and were reiterated for the whole of the period. Reiteration was often necessary, as the Rev. Joseph Dare of Leicester found in 1852:

> The completion of the Water Works will be a great blessing to the town...From the far villas on the London-road, to the extremities of 'the North' and the Belgrave-gate, fever and diarrhoea have spread their desolating blight. From these and other causes vast numbers of the poor are always in a low state of health. This is no doubt the reason why they are perpetually seeking after the nostrums of quackery. Of course, I have heard of the 'Wise Woman of Wing'. The London Board, by its dilatoriness and needless objections to the proposed Drainage Scheme, has been the best patron she has had in this neighbourhood. (Quoted in Haynes, 1991, pp. 43–4)

Moreover, it was not only the poor whose habits had to be changed, as Simon later recalled about his successes as MOH for the City of London:

> The abomination of cesspools had come to an end. At a time when cesspools were still almost universal in the metropolis, and while, in the mansions of the west-end, they were regarded as equally sacred with the wine-cellars, they had been abolished, for rich and poor, throughout all the square mile of the City. (Simon, 1897, p. 252)

'Scientific' sanitarianism

Little legislation on public health was added to the statute book after the great legal codifications of the 1870s: this also reflects the gap between legislation and its effective implementation (see Figure 4.10 *overleaf*).

By the 1920s, public-health agencies had built up a formidable system of controls, expanding into food production, workplaces, shops, housing, schools, hospitals and clinics (see Figure 4.11 *overleaf*).

However, the 'scientising' of public health from about 1860 meant a shift *away* from focusing on the environment *towards* the control of particular diseases and their causes—a move away from the 'filth diseases' like cholera, typhoid and dysentery, towards more directly infectious diseases and the behaviour of the infected individual.

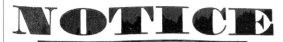

NOTICE
NEW CLOSET REGULATIONS.

The MIDDLETON LOCAL BOARD finding it impracticable, owing to the tidal action, to keep the drains in working order, have passed a resolution that the drain connected with the Hartlepool Engine Works be cut off. It has therefore been necessary to adopt a Closet on the Dry-earth System adjoining the Gatehouse. There is, however, so much trouble and difficulty in keeping such Closets in a proper sanitary condition, that whilst providing such a convenience, it is strongly recommended to the workmen to use instead their own conveniences at home; and as a premium towards encouraging the adoption of this recommendation, six tokens for admission to the Closet will be issued weekly, free of charge to each workman, of the value of Threepence, and if these tokens are not used, he will receive weekly that sum in addition to his pay on the following pay day.

The New Closet shall be open on and after Monday the 8th November, 1880, and shall henceforth be the only convenience of the kind, in these Works, for those employed in the PATTERN SHOP, FORGE, FITTING, ERECTING, and LATHE SHOPS, BOILER YARD, and SMITHS' SHOP.

Anyone in these departments using any other part of the Works, excepting this New Closet, shall be dismissed.

Everyone in these departments shall be allowed tokens to permit of his entering the Closet once a day, where he may remain not more than eight minutes.

Anyone remaining from his work longer than eight minutes, shall be liable to dismissal.

Everyone who enters the Closet, shall pay a token at the Gatehouse, previous to entering.

Six tokens shall be supplied free of charge, in the pay boxes, to every employee in the above departments, on Saturday the 6th November, 1880, and as many tokens every following pay-day, as the number of week-days he has been at work the previous week.

Should anyone use all his tokens before the end of the week, he will be required to pay a Halfpenny at the Gatehouse in lieu of a token previous to entering.

As soon as any workman has saved six tokens he should put them in his pay box and place same on a tray provided for the purpose, immediately after receiving his pay. Those not having six tokens to return shall place their empty boxes in the basket as usual.

BY ORDER.

N.B. For the present those employed in the BRASS and IRON FOUNDRIES, and COPPER SHOP, shall continue the use of the Closet at the top of Foundry Yard, and those employed in the LOW BOILER YARD shall also continue the use of their present Closet. These will not of course receive any tokens.

Hartlepool Engine Works.
4th November, 1880.

Figure 4.10 *As well as illustrating conditions at work in 1880, these regulations give examples of the impediments to effective sanitary reform. A system could be physically in place and yet not working. (Source: Shellard, P., 1970,* Factory Life 1774–1885, *Evans Bros., now HarperCollins Publishers Ltd, London)*

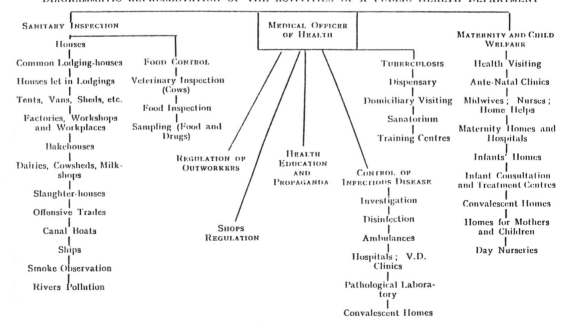

Figure 4.11 *This textbook diagram outlines the pyramid of responsibilities which had accumulated under the Medical Officer of Health by the late 1920s (Bannington, B. G., 1929,* English Public Health Administration, *P. S. King & Son Ltd, London, frontispiece from 2nd edition). The chief difference noted by the author since the first edition of 1915 was the growth of maternity and child welfare.*

The more refined epidemiology of Simon and his department was partly a political strategy, and partly a reflection of Simon's awareness of scientific developments in mainland Europe. Simon was able to capitalise on his contemporaries' belief that science was ultimately the means ordained for ordering the chaos with which many Victorians felt themselves to be surrounded.

This is not to say that science in the public domain went unquestioned. The anti-vivisection agitation of the 1870s is the most obvious example of this.

Moreover, the scientifically informed campaign against the infected individual had a strong tendency to bear hardest upon the most disadvantaged. *Vaccination*, compulsory for infants since 1853, closely associated with the Poor Law, and often poorly administered, had bred popular resistance from its inception. The later phases of this resistance stored up opposition to subsequent immunisation programmes.

In the 1860s, inequity in public-health policy was taken to an extreme by the Contagious Diseases Acts, which sought to control sexually transmitted disease by allowing, in garrison towns, the *compulsory* medical treatment of those suspected of prostitution. Many sanitarians advocated the extension of this legislation to the civilian population; the controversy went on even after repeal of the Acts in the 1880s. All policies of disease notification, disinfection, and segregation were more readily evaded by the better-off than by the poor, who were also more disadvantaged by loss of earnings or property.

The complex role of bacteriology

Public-health medicine gained new scientific credibility from the rise of the germ theory which began in the 1860s.[8] However, bacteriology had wider implications. The speed with which Louis Pasteur's discovery of living micro-organisms was taken up by conservative politicians and the medical establishment reveals their reluctance to acknowledge social and material explanations for infectious diseases. For some, bacteriology encouraged a sense of fatalism, or of alienation; it appeared to suggest the impracticability of modern urban society—that God, or nature, had ordained that human beings could not live together without danger.

The undoubted successes of bacteriology instilled both a 'single-factor' style of explanation for disease, in which all the emphasis was placed on the invading organism, and an expectation of equally single-factor solutions—'magic bullets', like the drug salvarsan, the

specific remedy for syphilis discovered in 1907—which in practice were rarely forthcoming. Bacteriology gave medicine an almost unprecedented reputation for effectiveness; but, because it shifted the centre of gravity of medical legitimation *away* from the hospital and the private patient and *towards* the laboratory, bacteriology also drove a wedge—especially in Britain—between the clinician and the laboratory scientist.

However, the focus on *single-factor* explanations was never absolute. Public-health doctors continued to advocate *environmentalist* views in the early twentieth century, with an updated emphasis on persistent re-infection among crowded populations. The environmentalists also turned to collectivist social remedies against infectious disease, demanding improved housing and diet, and town planning, in order to promote bodily resistance to infection. Medicine in general was deeply reluctant to relinquish its emphasis on the *constitution* of the individual (which by now had been given eugenic connotations). Doctors favoured a multifactorial, rather than a single-factor, approach even to infectious disease. Thus, even in a post-bacteriological era, many who would otherwise be opponents, could agree on the virtues of therapies such as open air and sunlight.

Overall, however, the end of the period saw a gradual shift away from collective, environmental approaches, towards an emphasis on individual responsibility and individual liability to disease. Public health had also moved somewhat away from concern with the acute infectious diseases, to consider conditions like cancer, TB, sexually transmitted diseases, and alcoholism.

Different routes to professionalisation

Medical practice continued to professionalise in this period, both to meet middle-class demand and to answer the requirements of an increasingly bureaucratic society. Nonetheless, both training and the rewards of practice remained very far from uniform, and the search for recognised qualifications was in part a response to pressures within an 'overstocked' profession.

Medical men (not women as yet) were also struggling to remain at the top of pyramids of public administration which were growing in areas like public health and education. The supervision of other health workers, such as nurses and midwives, formed part of this struggle and, as in earlier periods, could lead to medical sponsorship of the professionalisation of these groups. It would be wrong, however, to see factors related to professionalisation as the only cause of these changes. *Nursing* is an excellent example of this.

[8] *Medical Knowledge: Doubt and Certainty,* Chapter 4.

Nursing: religion, gender and social class

Because of the dominance of the Nightingale story, and because nurses are easier to detect in hospitals than elsewhere, the myth by which the down-at-heel, drunken, middle-aged 'Sairey Gamp' (immortalised by Dickens in *Martin Chuzzlewit*) was transformed into the young, pure, vocational nurse (see Figure 4.12) has been placed firmly in the context of the *reform of hospitals*, military and civilian.

However, this is to overlook other important factors that shaped nursing. The historian Anne Summers has stressed the need to see nursing history as a subplot to the history of Victorian Christianity. Earlier in the century, the churches had seen the pressures of industrialisation undermine the traditional practice of visiting the sick poor to advise on the health of body and soul. 'District Visiting Societies' emerged, which were successful enough to preserve the term *district nurse* for later use. The 'sisterhoods' of domiciliary nurses trained by some of these religious societies attended the poor without charge, but were in increasing demand in better-off households and in hospitals. Summers argues that hospital patients benefited from the higher standards of care imported by these nurses from their upper-class employments.

These developments precede the well-known story of Florence Nightingale's experience in the Crimea, and the founding of the Nightingale Training Schools after 1860. They also look forward to the marked trend at the end of the century towards home visiting, which we discussed earlier. We should also note that, although nursing was being recognised as an occupation, this was in the context of nurses being supervised by, and accountable to, their social superiors, whether these were male medical practitioners, or women philanthropists.

This social division was of importance in the struggle to organise nursing more formally as an occupation. The actual social background of recruits had changed much less by 1918 than might have been imagined. A handful of well-born women had become matrons or lady superintendents, but the majority of nurses still came from relatively humble backgrounds.

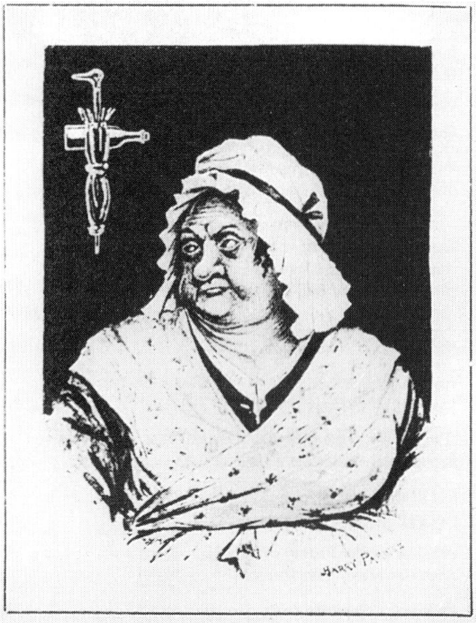

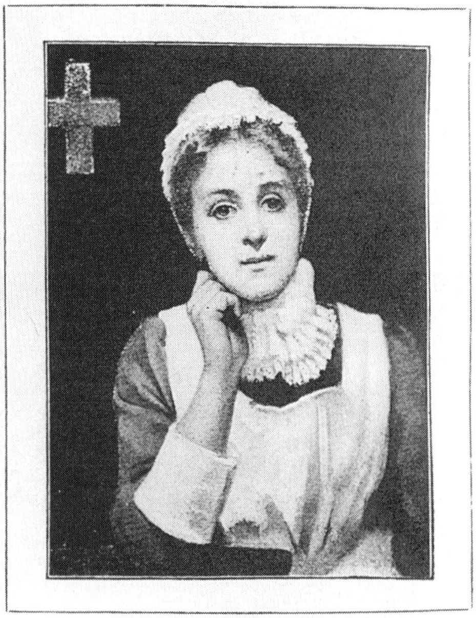

1838.   1888.

THEN.   NOW.

Figure 4.12 *These 'then and now' images should be seen as loaded with the biases of the later nineteenth-century campaigns for nursing 'sisterhoods'. Note the resemblance of the young nurse's uniform to a religious habit, and the cross behind her; the older nurse, on the other hand, has been given as her device a bottle of drink and an umbrella (or 'gamp'). Note too the element of prejudice against the mature woman, who is likely to have worked independently, on a self-employed basis. (Source: Supplement to the* Nursing Record, *20 December 1888)*

Table 4.1 Distribution of previous work experiences of recruits to nurse training, 1881–1921 (shown as percentages)

Previous work experience	Manchester Royal Infirmary (1881–1921)	The London Hospital (1881–1921)	Leeds Poor Law Infirmary (1895–1921)
actual number of recruits	1 696	4 454	370
	%	%	%
nil	28	28	28
nursing	39	26	35
domestic service	21	29	22
clerical and commercial	4	5	3
clothing and textiles	1	2	5
shop work	2	2	4
education	5	5	2
war work and miscellaneous	1	3	1

Data from Maggs, C. J. (1983) *The Origins of General Nursing*, Croom Helm, Beckenham, Table 2.2, p. 67.

□ What can you infer from Table 4.1 about the social background of nursing recruits and the social status of nursing?

■ Nurses were mostly from a working-class background and nursing shared a similar social status with domestic service and other manual occupations.

This division created tensions in establishing the status of nursing which have continued to the present day.[9] Was nursing to be a 'new profession for women'; or was it a form of refined domestic service, assigned a subordinate position in the hospital?

To this division was added that between the *general nurses* of the voluntary hospitals, and those engaged in *Poor Law nursing* which, despite its numerical significance, was seen as very much the poor relation. Following a professional pattern, general nurses stressed vocation, selflessness and dedication, and formed a College of Nursing in 1916. Asylum and Poor Law nurses, on the other hand, tended to join the trade union movement.

The principal arena for contests over the resolution of these complex divisions was the struggle for *nurse registration*, which began in the 1880s. For the next thirty years a 'nursing war' took place against a background of changed and widening employment opportunities for women of all classes. At the same time the number of hospitals increased and so did the demand for nurses.

The question of the *nursing shortage* (another parallel with present-day nursing issues) was an added and continuing complication in the debates around how nursing status could be established. During World War I the problem was dealt with by the introduction of Voluntary Aid Detachments (VADs) used in military nursing. These were women given a minimal introduction to nursing; their presence caused anxiety to the leaders of the trained nurses.

Registration was finally secured after the war in 1919 and established a standard system of accreditation; but it did not eliminate the tensions within nursing, between 'aristocratic' and 'democratic' conceptions of its role and status.

Midwives: marginalisation to rehabilitation

Issues of internal stratification and of gender also affected the status and development of *midwifery* in this period. As you will recall from Chapter 2, in the seventeenth century nearly all babies had been delivered by women. But in the eighteenth century more men had entered this area, aided by technological innovation. Soon the stereotype of 'ignorant midwives' was commonplace, much as the image of drunken old hags had tainted untrained nurses. By the middle of the nineteenth century, midwives had been virtually confined to attendance on the poor, combining help at childbirth with general work such as washing and cleaning.

But moves by women of 'professional' status to enter medicine had their impact on midwifery, as much as on medicine and nursing. The emergence of a class of highly educated and vocal midwives as a professionalising pressure group led to efforts over the last three decades of the nineteenth century to bring about training and control. The battle was between medical pressure groups seeking legislation to control midwives in their own interests, and the middle-class section of midwifery seeking independent professional status.

[9] For detailed discussion of present-day issues affecting the status of nursing, see another book in this series, *Dilemmas in Health Care* (Open University Press, 1993), Chapter 6.

The Midwives Act 1902 was to a great degree a compromise. It prohibited unqualified practice, but it placed midwifery in a disadvantaged professional position in the sexual division of health labour. The Central Midwives Board had a *medical* majority and local supervision was by the MOH. Moreover, the Act's immediate impact on unqualified practice was muted. By 1914 many such women continued to practise, for the Act allowed women in 'bona fide' practice to continue to work.

The proportion of trained women had risen considerably by the early 1920s (see Table 4.2).

Table 4.2 Percentage of trained midwives in three cities, 1911–35

	1911	1915	1920	1925	1930	1935
Birmingham	n.d.	31.5	53.3	76.4	90	97.6
Hull	30	43	38.9	83	91	96
Liverpool	88	86	100	100	100	100

n.d. = no data. Data from the annual reports of the Medical Officers of Health for Birmingham, Liverpool and Hull, cited in Lewis, J. (1980) *The Politics of Motherhood*, Croom Helm, Beckenham, p. 143.

The Medical Register: definition not prohibition

The modern definition of medicine as a *profession* is commonly dated to the Medical Act 1858, which created the General Medical Council and gave it responsibilities for medical education, registration and discipline. The qualifications it defined were valid throughout the British Empire.

Nonetheless, the Act was a limited achievement. It did not outlaw unqualified practice, but merely laid down what the law would recognise as a qualification. Homoeopaths and others were little hindered until *employment* was restricted to registered practitioners, as for example under National Health Insurance.

Moreover, the medical organisations were unable to agree on a 'single-portal' system involving only one set of national examinations. Consequently a wide range of qualifications were given legal status, and the numerous qualifying bodies could continue to set standards independently of each other. A *minimal* qualification was enough to ensure eligibility for the public service; and any *one* qualification legally entitled the practitioner to practise *all* parts of medicine, surgery and midwifery, even though his training may not have been of this general kind. As in earlier periods, the major call from patients was for general, not specialised practice.

□ You have seen that midwifery had low status; it was unremunerative and time-consuming. Yet many *male* GPs engaged in it. Can you suggest reasons for this?

■ Midwifery was in demand, and competition among practitioners meant that many could not pick and choose what services they offered. Practitioners offered midwifery services in the hope of securing the custom of the whole family.

Similarly, there was an incentive to sell drugs, however demeaning this was thought to be, because it was lucrative. Not surprisingly, medical practitioners pressed for regulation of their rivals in this area, the chemists and druggists.

Changing definitions? Some challenges to the medical hierarchy

Owing to the 'dreary and thankless task of learning the intricacies and jealousies of medico-professional politics' (Simon, 1897, p. 308), the necessary government interest in the defects of the 1858 Act was slow to develop. After a failure in the 1870s, effective action was delayed until 1886. By the 1870s the clinical ideal of *training by example*, on the basis of a gentlemanly background in natural philosophy, was being challenged by a stress on *scientific laboratory-based training* which derived from the research institutes developed in continental Europe.

Britain was here far behind developments in Germany and the USA. The medical academic scene in Germany had been an important influence on the Johns Hopkins School of Medicine in the USA, founded in 1889. In Germany, *research* became an essential component of medicine and a strong biomedical scientific influence was brought to bear on clinical medicine. The 1910 Flexner Report (produced by a layman, Abraham Flexner, working for the Carnegie Foundation) proposed that all American medical education be based on the German model. In Britain there was reluctance to embrace this emphasis on research, and full-time academic appointments, which could confer independence from private practice, did not develop in the London medical schools until after World War I.

Professional success continued to be closely linked to social status and family connections, partly because of the relevance of family circumstances to the kind of education which could be afforded. Social status underpinned the distinction between consultant and GP, which as yet had little to do with specialisation within medical practice (although specialties, for example in gynaecology, ophthalmology, neurology and psychological medicine, certainly existed).

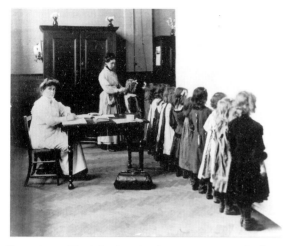

Figure 4.13 *The School Medical Service. Basic medical inspection (not treatment) of school children became the norm after the institution of this service in 1907 and served further to reveal social inequalities in health. (Source: Greater London Photographic Library)*

The different grades of medical practitioner earned very different levels of income. For most, profitable private practice with a prestigious hospital connection was a remote ideal. The reality consisted of competing for appointments in insurance companies, prisons, the army, the police, friendly societies, factories, mining companies, railway companies and Poor Law Unions.

You may have been wondering what part *women* doctors had in these events. Qualified medical practice remained a male preserve until the 1860s, and the first women entrants in Britain and the USA had to follow a policy of 'separate development', in separate medical schools and even hospitals. Integrated training did not necessarily prove advantageous: later, women practitioners tended to be concentrated in specialties relating to women and children, or in lower-status options such as the School Medical Service (see Figure 4.13).

Medical power versus lay control

The external power relationships of medicine were also fluid. Although much of medical practice remained under lay control at the end of the century, as for example in friendly society and 'sick club' practice, the balance of power was beginning to alter. The shifting pattern of authority within hospitals in this period shows a move from lay to medical control. Increasingly, lay trustees exercised control *indirectly* through bureaucratic channels symbolised by the appointment of house committees and senior lay administrators like hospital secretaries.

Doctors, on the other hand, formed themselves into medical committees to ensure that their interests were represented in management.

By the 1860s, a general pattern was for lay and medical committees to work in tandem, with responsibility for their own areas. In the latter part of the century, the balance of power shifted still further to the medical sector as the hospital moved towards becoming a more specialist scientific and research-based institution.

In the USA, doctors were less dominant in hospital management, and health managers and administrators were a more powerful group. In Britain, as you will see in Chapter 7, the development of *health management* as a challenge to medical power came only in the 1980s.[10] In some respects, this has echoes of the nineteenth century. This tension between, first, lay/voluntary and, subsequently, lay/bureaucratic forms of control, and medical dominance, is a theme which can be traced through from the eighteenth to the late twentieth centuries.

Institutions, insurances and the national interest

As you have seen earlier in this chapter, the latter half of the nineteenth century saw an expansion of institutional care; and, increasingly, in the first two decades of the twentieth century, publicly funded and centrally regulated health care developed as an outgrowth of the concern for national efficiency.

Asylums and hospitals

The asylum continued its inexorable growth.

☐ What does Table 4.3 (*overleaf*) show about changes in the institutional system for the treatment of insanity in the second half of the nineteenth century?

■ It demonstrates two developments: the increased number of institutional places available; and the rise in importance of the publicly funded County and Borough asylums. In fifteen years the numbers in these asylums had quadrupled. (Note also that large—perhaps greater—numbers of the 'insane' were kept in Poor Law institutions, notably the workhouses, *not* included in the table.)

[10] Shifts in the balance of power between health service managers, doctors and groups representing patients' interests in the 1990s, following the re-organisation of the National Health Service, are the subject of Chapter 2 in *Dilemmas in Health Care*.

Table 4.3 Mid-nineteenth-century asylum statistics

| | Patients in asylums in | | | | | |
| | 1844 | | 1860 | | 1870 | |
Institutions	No.	%	No.	%	No.	%
provincial licensed houses	3 346	30	2 356	10	2 204	6
metropolitan licensed houses	1 827	16	1 944	8	2 700	8
County and Borough asylums	4 489	40	17 432	73	27 890	79
others	1 610	14	1 985	8	2 369	7
total	**11 272**	**100**	**23 717**	**100**	**35 163**	**100**

Data (rounded to nearest whole number) based on Scull, A. (1979) *Museums of Madness: The Social Organisation of Insanity in 19th Century England*, Allen Lane, London, Tables 3 and 4, pp. 190 and 193.

☐ In the years between 1807 and 1890, the numbers of persons officially identified as insane (including those in workhouses and the community) in England and Wales rose from about 2 per 10 000 to almost 30 per 10 000. What different explanations can you think of for the steep rise?

■ There are three possible explanations:

1   that this represented a real growth in the extent of insanity in the population;

2   that it was an artefact (the collection of statistics was poor in the first half of the nineteenth century and medical diagnosis was less developed); and

3   that the increase represented a major reduction in the community's ability or willingness to contain and tolerate disturbed behaviour.

The American historical sociologist, Andrew Scull, has argued in favour of the last explanation. The growth of the asylum and the rise in the number of its inmates, in his view, were outgrowths of a rapidly urbanising society in which families were no longer able to support unproductive relatives. By the end of the nineteenth century, the pauper insane formed 90 per cent of the asylum population.

The *function* of the asylum also changed. The reformers who had supported its expansion had seen the asylum as a welcoming refuge, modelled on the pioneering Retreat at York. But the reality turned out to be very different.

It is a vast and straggling building, in which the characteristics of a prison, a self-advertising charitable institution, and some ambitious piece of Poor Law architecture struggle for prominence. The gates are kept by an official who is attired in a garb as nearly as possible like that of a gaoler. All the male attendants are made to display the same forbidding uniform. (Mortimer Granville on Hanwell Asylum, London, 1877, quoted in Scull, 1979, p. 195)

☐ What does this suggest to you about the function of the asylum?

■ By the end of the century the asylum was custodial, a prison for those classified as insane.

The *hospital system* also expanded in the late nineteenth century. This was not simply a matter of the growth of specialisms. To the voluntary hospitals were added the Poor Law infirmaries which expanded in London after a major onslaught on workhouse infirmary conditions by the *Lancet* and medical groups in the 1860s.

The Metropolitan Poor Act 1867 was a means by which finance could be raised for building large infirmaries. The Metropolitan Asylums Board, also established in 1867, developed one of the largest hospital systems in the world (note that the term 'asylum' was here being used in its general sense of 'place of refuge'). The Board's infectious diseases hospitals were originally intended only for use by paupers, but during epidemics they were used by all classes. In this way the principle of entitlement to free treatment was established. By 1908, over 18 per cent of all deaths in England and Wales occurred in public institutions, a figure which had doubled over thirty years.

☐ Table 4.4 shows some basic statistics about the growth of hospital provision in England from 1861 onward. What developments do you notice?

■ The numbers of beds in both voluntary and public hospitals had increased proportionately to population in this period. But the public hospital sector was far larger and continued to grow at a higher rate.

These developments brought changes in the role of patients and the relationship between doctors in and outside the hospital. One change was that out-patient numbers increased dramatically at the end of the century. Hospital out-patient departments, especially in London, provided primary health care for the entire local population (look ahead to Figure 6.2). Indeed, before the National Insurance Act 1911 (see below) 'going to the doctor' in his surgery was unusual for most of the British population.

Table 4.4 Growth of hospital provision (numbers of beds) in England after 1861

	Public hospitals		Voluntary hospitals		Total	
Year	Beds	Per 1 000 population	Beds	Per 1 000 population	Beds	Per 1 000 population
1861	50 000	2.6	11 000	0.6	61 000	3.2
1891	83 000	2.9	29 000	1.0	113 000	3.9
1911	154 000	4.3	43 000	1.2	197 000	5.5
1921	172 000	4.6	57 000	1.5	229 000	6.1
1938	176 000	4.3	87 000	2.1	263 000	6.4

Data (rounded to the nearest thousand) based on Abel-Smith, B. (1964) *The Hospitals, 1800–1948*, Heinemann, London, pp. 46, 152, 200, 353, 382–5.

You should now read the article by Rosemary Stevens in the Reader,[11] which compares the evolution of the health-care system in the USA with that in the United Kingdom in this period.

   □ According to Stevens, what effect did the expansion of the hospital system on both sides of the Atlantic have on the relationship between doctors inside and outside hospital medicine?

   ■ Stevens argues that in the USA the use of out-patient departments, and the rise of special hospitals in the last quarter of the nineteenth century, threatened the position of the GP; general practice was largely moribund by World War I. But in Britain, the relationship between the hospital specialist and the GP was settled to accommodate a continuing role for the GP (as you will see in the next three chapters).

Financing health care

This expansion in hospital usage brought particular problems for the *voluntary hospitals*. The proportion of beds they provided grew, but this led to financial crisis. The voluntary hospitals provided almost all the *acute* beds (i.e. those dedicated to short-stay patients in acute need of care); costs escalated owing to medical advances such as antiseptic and then aseptic surgery. Acute-care patients need more intensive nursing, and consequently running costs were also higher. Expanding services produced expanding costs.

   Money was raised through private charity and the introduction of *pay beds*. The charitable Hospital Sunday and Hospital Saturday Funds (which organised flag days and fund-raising) were established as sources of hospital finance in the 1870s. Hospitals, which had previously had a solely working-class clientele, began charging any

patients judged capable of paying, and also established private blocks, thus instituting first- and second-class forms of treatment.

Sickness insurance in Germany

There were moves to establish a broader entitlement to health care. The National Insurance Act 1911 was a significant step in this direction (see below), but Britain was slower to introduce a state insurance-based sickness system than many European countries. Compulsory sickness insurance was introduced by the German Chancellor, Otto von Bismarck, in 1883. This superseded earlier voluntary and co-operative sickness funds which had appealed to the better-educated workers in relatively stable occupations.

   That the sickness insurance funds *(Krankenkassen)* were initially limited to certain wage bands of urban workers who were the main supporters of socialism, explains Bismarck's political motives in the years following his anti-socialist legislation of 1878–91. Yet the insurance funds were autonomous, with worker and employer representation on a 2 : 1 basis. Ironically, from the 1890s, a number of leading socialists had careers in sickness insurance fund administration, and they were keen to extend benefits to family dependants, to emulate French schemes for maternity benefits (these were discretionary in Germany), and to include certain categories of disease (like sexually transmitted diseases), initially excluded from the scheme as attributable to personal moral failings.

   In the longer term, sickness insurance was extended by state legislation, so that by 1913 it covered 25 per cent of the German population (including, from 1911, such groups as domestic servants and agricultural workers), half of these having family dependants. In contrast to the British scheme, German workers contributed on a graduated scale in proportion to their earnings. The market for medical care was greatly extended, bringing new social sectors into regular contact with university-educated physicians. The prospect of a steady income

[11] 'The evolution of the health-care systems in the United States and the United Kingdom: similarities and differences' (1976), in *Health and Disease: A Reader.*

from insurance fees stimulated a doubling in numbers of the German medical profession between 1889 and 1898.

German socialist criticisms of unhealthy social conditions, and of the poor law as depriving recipients of civil rights, prompted the Prussian ruling elite in 1895 to launch an association for providing *sanatoria* for patients with TB. Once these were opened, patient costs could be covered by sickness insurance schemes, and by 1911 Germany had more public sanatoria (*Volksheilstätten*) than any other country.

As the cost of such sanatoria was high, welfare clinics and home-visiting schemes were devised, using pioneer French dispensary clinics as models. Whereas the French clinics provided treatment, pressure from the German medical profession limited the role of the German equivalents to diagnosis and the provision of welfare benefits. Dispensary clinics were organised for infant welfare, for alcoholism and, by 1914, for sexually transmitted diseases. Networks of urban 'policlinics' supplemented the French and German municipal hospital systems which were being extended and modernised from the 1880s. Improvements in hospital design and new therapies meant that by the turn of the century a broader social spectrum was making use of new children's hospitals.

Sickness insurance in Britain

The German system of social insurance became an influential international model. But the British system, although influenced by German example, was significantly different in several respects. The *1911 National Health Insurance scheme* limited benefits to the contributor alone, below a certain level of income, and did not include dependants (see Figure 4.14). However, a maternity benefit of 30 s. was available to insured working women and to the wives of working men.

Contributions were not graduated, but paid at a flat rate (4d for men and 3d for women per week), approximately half each by employee and employer; and the administration of the system was not centralised. Cash benefits for sickness, accident and disability were paid at a fixed amount regardless of severity, and continued to be distributed through familiar insurance companies, the so-called *approved societies*. Insured contributors had the right to free but limited care from a doctor on a local list or *panel* and the doctor received a capitation fee for each panel patient. Hospital treatment was available only to patients with TB.

The historian Bentley Gilbert has commented that:

> The aim of national insurance was to replace lost income, not to cure sickness. (Gilbert, 1966, p. 318)

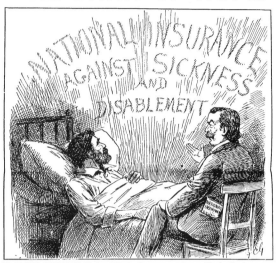

THE DAWN OF HOPE.

Mr. **LLOYD GEORGE'S** National Health Insurance Bill provides for the insurance of the Worker in case of Sickness.

Support the Liberal Government
in their policy of
SOCIAL REFORM.

Figure 4.14 *The National Insurance Act 1911 established for the first time in Britain the concept of benefits as a right, based on records of contributions. (Source: Hulton/Deutsch Picture Collection)*

The avoidance of pauperism was the main incentive: Lloyd George's intention was that sickness insurance, despite its limited coverage, should supersede the Poor Law. Yet even this limited scheme did not become law without a struggle. Doctors, via the BMA, fought hard to defend their right to private practice and to establish medical control over the activities of the approved societies. Many points were conceded, and the specialists and consultants who had been urging the BMA forward, found rank-and-file support waning. GPs clamoured to be admitted to the panels, which offered many a larger and steadier income than ever before. As a result of the panels, a GP service became available to manual workers, which resolved the conflict over hospital out-patients and brought clarification of the division between GP-primary and specialist-hospital care—a crucial development in British health policy.

One significant offshoot of the National Health Insurance system was the establishment of the Medical

Research Committee in 1913, funded from the proceeds of the National Insurance Act and originally intended to develop research into TB. Renamed the *Medical Research Council* after World War I, it financed a wide-ranging programme of medical research, focusing on the pre-clinical sciences.

Impact of World War I

In Germany, the war had a considerable impact on health services. The various state sickness insurance and voluntary medical measures were subject to increasing control by the central state (or *Reich*). The state began to acknowledge its responsibility to maintain the health of the population in the context of total war, and health innovations were accompanied by pronatalist propaganda in favour of 'child-rich' families. Legislation was introduced for maternity allowances, schemes were instituted to improve midwifery services on a domiciliary basis, district health and welfare centres were opened, and condoms as a barrier to sexually transmitted infections were officially sanctioned.

In Britain, developments were on a smaller scale. The pre-existing concerns for the health of mothers and babies rose to a new height during the war. The argument that it was more dangerous to be a baby than a soldier was well publicised. Infant mortality had, in fact, been in decline since the early years of the century and continued to fall during the war. The number of clinics and health visitors expanded, and the Maternity and Child Welfare Act 1918 imposed an obligation on local authorities to provide services in this area. However, the historian Jay Winter has concluded that rising incomes, and consequent better nutrition, had a more significant effect on the health of mothers and children than the patchy local provision of health services.

Somewhat surprisingly, civilian mortality rates also improved; even though 14 000 doctors were diverted to military service during the war, lack of medical attention did not prevent an overall increase in life expectancy.

Against this overall 'optimistic' picture must be set the increased death rate from *TB* (primarily a young person's disease), possibly because of cross-infection from troops and deteriorating housing; and higher death rates among the elderly, who were removed from hospitals and institutions to make way for the wounded. *Sexually transmitted diseases* (then known as 'venereal diseases' or VD) also spread rapidly in war-time conditions.

Government action was forthcoming in the cases of TB and sexually transmitted diseases. The government had made free treatment for TB (including sanatoria) available to insured workers and their dependants in 1911 under the National Insurance Act. An Act in 1921

extended local-authority responsibility for the treatment of TB. An Act of 1917 established a network of local-authority VD clinics where treatment was free and confidential. Arguments about condoning or encouraging immorality (paralleled by the arguments in the 1980s around the promotion of 'safe sex' and condom use against AIDS) prevented distribution to the troops of prophylactics against VD. The war had some impact on health-care provision, but little of the generalised effect of World War II; rather, there was a patchwork of services for special groups.

Mortality and medical progress

The latter half of the nineteenth century and the beginning of the twentieth was a time of *innovation* in hospital-based procedures and therapies in Britain and continental Europe.[12] Two crucial questions arising from these developments are: what *relevance* did they have for the general population; and what *impact* did they have on mortality and morbidity rates?

The debate about the impact of medical care is typified by two articles in the *Reader*, by Thomas McKeown and Simon Szreter.[13]

□ Can you recall the main thrust, first of McKeown's argument, and then of what Szreter has added to McKeown?

■ McKeown's interpretation has downgraded the role of medical care in favour of improved nutrition. Szreter's recent work has revised the McKeown account and has emphasised the role of public-health measures in improving health.

The general thrust of the McKeown argument still holds good. It makes the important point that scientific, high-technology medicine is often of limited impact by comparison with general improvements in living standards and the overall nutritional status of the population. These types of argument were important in later moves to

---

[12] Discussed in *Medical Knowledge: Doubt and Certainty* (revised edition 1994), particularly in Chapter 4 in relation to the treatment and prevention of tuberculosis.

[13] The articles in question are 'The medical contribution' by Thomas McKeown (1976) and 'The importance of social intervention in Britain's mortality decline, *c.*1850–1914' by Simon Szreter (1988), in *Health and Disease: A Reader* (second edition, 1995). Both were set reading for Open University students studying another book in this series: *World Health and Disease*.

reduce hospital dominance in the British health system and to upgrade the status of primary health care.

However, as you will see in Chapter 5, medicine's claims to effectiveness increase considerably after this period, on the basis of (for example) a wider range of immunisations, blood transfusion, vitamins, improved understanding of vector-borne diseases like malaria, and more potent drugs such as the sulphonamides.

Medicine and imperialism: the 'scramble for Africa'

The most important aspect of European expansion overseas in this period was the so-called 'scramble for Africa', beginning in the 1880s, in which Britain, France, Germany, and other European countries began to carve up the continent into colonies and 'protectorates' (see Figures 4.15 and 4.16). No single theory can explain why this development occurred, but behind imperial rivalry was increasing political and economic competition between Britain, France and the new German state. As you saw earlier in this chapter, these changes were bound up with the rise of industrial capitalism, the social consequences of which led to new forms of medical intervention, particularly in the field of public health. In much the same way, imperial expansion created or exacerbated

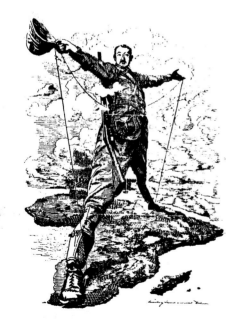

Figure 4.15 *British-born South African statesman Cecil Rhodes, shown by* Punch *as a colossus straddling the continent of Africa, was instrumental in expanding British territories.*

a whole range of medical and social problems in the colonies, which posed a threat not only to the health of indigenous peoples, but also to the durability and profitability of the colonial enterprise.

Problems of imperial efficiency had a profound effect on the development of medicine in Europe, particularly on the new sciences of bacteriology and parasitology, which formed the basis of a new discipline—**tropical medicine**. But the indigenous inhabitants of Africa benefited little from these advances in medical knowledge, or from the sanitary reforms which were transforming the urban environment in Europe. More often than not, if they encountered Western medicine, it was in the form of a coercive power, or was conditional upon the acceptance of European norms and values.

Tropical medicine

As you saw in Chapters 2 and 3, Europeans had begun to acquire a knowledge of the diseases of 'warm climates', based on a mixture of European and indigenous medical knowledge, and observations of the tropical disease environment. With few exceptions, however, this specialised knowledge had not been institutionalised; but from the 1880s, with the rise of a popular and political culture of imperialism, this began to change.

As well as being transformed internally by the specialisms of bacteriology and parasitology, tropical medicine was being shaped externally by a growing concern over economic and military efficiency in the colonies. The Liverpool School of Tropical Medicine founded in 1898, and the London School of Tropical Medicine founded in 1899, owed their existence to financial contributions from colonial merchants and the Colonial Office respectively.

However, the Liverpool and London schools embodied the professional aspirations of medical men as much as the economic objectives of European businessmen and politicians. In the last two decades of the nineteenth century, medical men in the colonies had made a number of discoveries that would eventually revolutionise the prevention and treatment of disease in the tropics. The micro-organisms causing malaria, cholera, brucellosis, sleeping sickness, bubonic plague and leishmaniasis were all discovered in the years between 1880 and 1918.

But until 1900, at least, those engaged in medical research in the colonies received little support from either their respective governments or their professional colleagues in Europe, many of whom were suspicious or ignorant of bacteriology and microscopical research. In the 1890s, professional journals, such as the *Journal of Tropical Medicine*, began to appear with the object of uniting those working in the field, and medical men

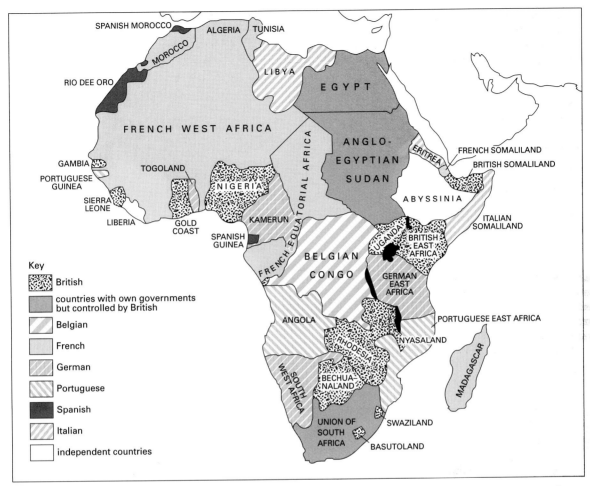

Figure 4.16 *The European partition of Africa, 1914. Medical provision varied considerably in the territories annexed by the European powers. Generally, medical services were focused on the needs of Europeans themselves, although in some colonies public-health measures were coercive. In Portuguese Angola and the Belgian Congo, for instance, colonial medicine was a powerful instrument of social control, constraining the movement of the indigenous population, or providing a pretext for their forcible relocation.*

began to lobby governments in the colonies and in Europe to make better provisions for laboratory research.

Those engaged in medical research in the tropics frequently presented themselves as heroic individuals, striving against official indifference and indigenous ignorance. For 'crusading' colonial medical officers like Ronald Ross, who became the first Director of the Liverpool School of Tropical Medicine, European imperialism was first and foremost a civilising force, capable of bestowing immense benefits upon indigenous peoples. According to Ross, Europeans were:

> …superior to subject peoples in natural ability, integrity and science…. They [had] introduced honesty, law, justice, order, roads, posts,

railways, irrigation, hospitals…and what was necessary for civilization, a final superior authority. (Ross, 1923, p. 17)

This paternalistic, if not racist, rationalisation of European domination was to set the tone for much of the propaganda surrounding tropical medicine until after World War II.

In reality, it was far from clear, at least before 1918, that tropical medicine had bestowed any substantial benefits upon the populations of European colonies. Research institutions established in the colonies before 1918, such as the French Pasteur Institutes and the Central Research Institute which opened in India in 1907, were little more than icons of Western scientific progress, whose research had direct benefit for only a small proportion of the indigenous population. The majority of medical research conducted in the colonies in this period was directed at health problems impairing military and economic efficiency.

This was clearly the case with the early work of the Liverpool School of Tropical Medicine in Africa. Its research and disease-prevention programmes were, in the words of the historian Michael Worboys, 'entrepreneurial activities', funded by subscriptions from among Liverpool merchants, which had the ultimate aim of improving labour efficiency in the colonies.

Most prominent among the school's early activities were *anti-malarial programmes* which attempted to control the disease by the eradication of its vector, the *Anopheles* mosquito[14] (identified by the school's director, Ronald Ross). These early, isolated, attempts at mosquito eradication in Africa appear to have met with little success—not surprisingly, since they were rarely followed up by colonial governments.

'The sick continent'

Disease in African society was a social metaphor as well as a biological fact. For Europeans, 'African' diseases came to symbolise everything they considered degenerate or threatening about African society. *Sleeping sickness* became a metaphor for the 'laziness' of the black African, while *plague*, which was introduced into Africa in the late 1890s, came to represent all that was considered unclean or dangerous about the indigenous population. In the French North African port of Dakar, as in many other cities throughout the European colonies, plague provided a medical rationalisation for racial segregation. The Dakar Sanitary Commission demanded:

> ...the transfer of the native population which takes pleasure in a deep-rooted and incurable filthiness, to a place far from the city, and the destruction or demolition of all shacks and huts, as the only measure able to stop the spread of the current epidemic. (Quoted by Headrick, 1988, p. 163)

☐ Are there any similarities between this statement and the extract from Sir Ronald Ross's memoirs, cited above?

■ Ross stresses Europe's 'civilising mission' whereas the Commission seeks only to protect Europeans, but both view native peoples as culturally inferior to Europeans, and both are extremely authoritarian.

[14] The life cycle of the malarial parasite and its transmission by mosquitoes are described in *World Health and Disease*, Chapter 3.

The high incidence of *malarial infection* among African children also led to attempts to segregate Europeans from native peoples. In Cameroon, in 1910, German administrators began a scheme to relocate the entire black population of the harbour city Duala to a fenced-off area inland. Although not fully completed before Germany lost the colony after World War I, the legacy of segregated housing and poor sanitation was upheld by the colony's new masters, the French.

Missionary zeal

In most areas of colonial Africa before 1918, and in many cases until the 1930s, indigenous peoples were most likely to experience Western health care in the form of **medical missions**. It was the medical missions which first introduced rural health care in Africa and which began to train Africans in midwifery and rural health work.

But while mission medicine employed the same medical technologies as the secular colonial state, its mode of operation was substantially different. An emphasis on spiritual salvation and on the Christian tradition of healing frequently obscured the humanitarian objectives of medical missions. Indeed, medical work was generally subordinated to the more urgent task of saving souls. Long-term care of the sick in leper asylums and mission hospitals presented missionaries with the best opportunities for evangelisation (see Figure 4.17), and *leprosy*, with its biblical connotations, became their *cause célèbre*.

The extent to which indigenous peoples availed themselves of the opportunities provided by the missions is far from clear, yet it seems that mission

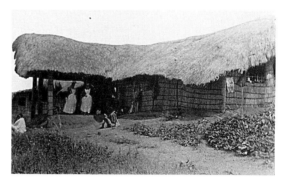

Figure 4.17 *Mengo missionary hospital, Uganda, 1898, from Foster, W. D. (1978) Sir Albert Cook: A Missionary Doctor in Uganda, Newhaven Press, Newhaven, Sussex. (Source: Church Missionary Society) Elsewhere in a missionary journal Cook commented: 'It is not our job, nor have we the power, to convert the souls of men, yet we do see again and again death beds irradiated by the smile of hope and peace given from on high'. (Mercy and Truth, 1904, 95, p. 338)*

dispensaries offering Western therapies and vaccination against smallpox had become quite popular in some areas of Africa by 1918. Certain forms of surgery such as the removal of cataracts also quickly gained the confidence of Africans. The results of cataract operations were fairly immediate and often impressive, and not unlike the biblical miracles preached by the missionaries.

Indeed, in Africa especially, the missions did succeed in converting a substantial number of their patients, many of whom went on to train as nurses and midwives. Generally, though, Africans were selective and incorporated only certain aspects of Western medicine and Christianity into their traditional systems. Missionaries viewed this tendency with some alarm, since African society was seen by them not only as heathen but as, itself, fundamentally sick.

☐ What does Figure 4.18 suggest to you concerning the way in which Africans were portrayed by African missionaries?

■ The appeal depicts Africans as sick, vulnerable, and unable to survive without Western medical aid.

The peoples of colonial Africa, like the inhabitants of India considered in Chapter 3, benefited little from the advances made in tropical medicine or from other 'fruits' of Western civilisation. Tropical medicine was not developed for the benefit of colonial peoples, but to improve colonial *productivity* and to safeguard the health of Europeans in the 'white man's grave'. Further, when Africans encountered Western medicine, it was often in the form of coercive public-health measures or missionary medicine, in which the task of healing the sick was perceived as less important than the saving of souls.

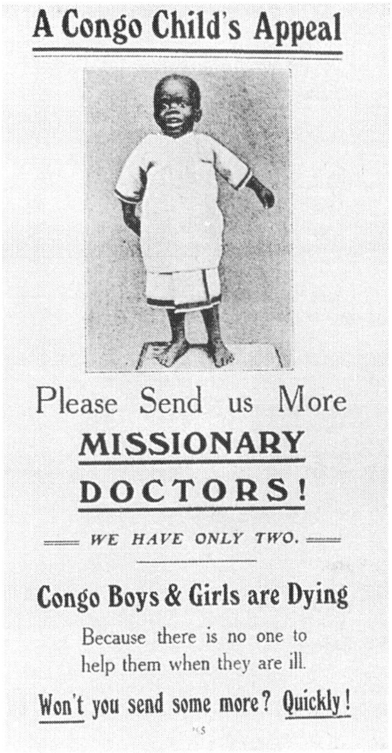

A Congo Child's Appeal

Please Send us More **MISSIONARY DOCTORS!**

=== WE HAVE ONLY TWO. ===

Congo Boys & Girls are Dying

Because there is no one to help them when they are ill.

Won't you send some more? Quickly!

Figure 4.18 *'A Congo Child's Appeal', 1909 (Source: Medical Missionary, 8(9), 1909 (Bodleian Library, Oxford))*

More generally, by representing African society as diseased, Western medicine was instrumental in creating a negative image of black Africans which has persisted in Western culture even to the present, reinforced by AIDS, which is considered in Chapter 8.

OBJECTIVES FOR CHAPTER 4

After studying this chapter, you should be able to:

4.1 Explain the shift from the ascendancy of the sanitarian movement and its representative, the MOH, to the deepening crisis of confidence over the state of health and health care, culminating in the concern over threats to 'national efficiency'.

4.2 Describe the ways in which the role of the family and the community in health care was eroded by professional, institutional and commercial developments.

4.3 Describe the moves towards professionalisation of nursing and other health-care occupations, noting the trend in control from lay to medical authorities.

4.4 Outline the moves in Europe towards social welfare systems providing health insurance and the way in which this trend was manifested in Britain.

4.5 Explain the ways in which European medicine was affected by colonial expansion and how European priorities dominated the provision of health care in colonial Africa.

QUESTIONS FOR CHAPTER 4

Question 1 (*Objective 4.1*)

The Rev. Joseph Dare of Leicester, long an ardent sanitarian, reported in 1875:

> In view of the excessive mortality of the 'little ones' that has so long distressed the town, and which must show that its causes are not yet well understood, a medical gentleman recently inquired of me, 'whether married female labour had not lately much increased?' I have made many inquiries amongst different branches of labour, and the general impression seems to be that it has much increased of late years. (Quoted in Haynes, 1991, p. 49)

What changes of view about the causes of major health problems does Dare (and the 'medical gentleman') represent?

Question 2 (*Objective 4.2*)

Read the following extract from an article published in 1906 in the *British Medical Journal*:

> The health visitors…must carry with them the carbolic powder, explain its use, and leave it where it is accepted; direct the attention of those they visit to the evils of bad smells, want of fresh air, impurities of all kinds; give hints to mothers on feeding and clothing their children—where they find sickness assist in promoting the comfort of the invalid by personal help, and report such cases…they must urge the importance of cleanliness, thrift, and temperance on all possible occasions. They are desired to get as many as possible to join the mothers' meetings of their districts, to use all their influence to induce those they visit to attend regularly at their respective places of worship, and to send their children to school. ('A Model Ladies Health Society' (1906), *British Medical Journal*, **i**, p. 152, quoted in Davies, 1988, p. 43)

What changes in patterns of family care does this advice to health visitors represent?

Question 3 (*Objective 4.3*)

In 1898, just before the (second) Boer war, a Miss Phipps wrote to a well-placed friend to ask:

> …how I, an amateur nurse, can get into the Red Cross Society—tell him [Lord Wantage, head of the National Aid Society] that I have done good work under St John Ambulance for which I got a Jubilee Medal and have worked as a nurse in a surgery in Rome—and all my life practised on our farm people—how brutal that sounds!…I *would* like to have the chance of being a R.C. [sic] nurse in case of war. (Quoted in Summers, 1988, p. 194)

How typical was this eager volunteer? And what does her background tell us about the state of nurse training at this time?

Question 4 (*Objective 4.4*)

To what extent did the sickness insurance scheme introduced by Lloyd George improve upon defects in German sickness insurance provision and what were its limitations?

Question 5 (*Objective 4.5*)

What does the pattern of health care in colonial Africa tell us about the nature and objectives of colonial medicine in this period?

5

The impact of war and depression, 1918 to 1948

The social welfare system which emerged in Britain during this period included a focus on the effects on health of poor housing and nutrition (especially among mothers and children). Data on the epidemiological associations of certain diseases with housing quality and nutrition were discussed in World Health and Disease, *Chapters 10 and 11. You may find it useful to look at the Reader article by Ramesh and Hyma[1] when studying the final section of this chapter. (This is optional reading for this chapter since it is set reading for Chapter 9.)*

Europe between the wars

The period covered by this chapter begins and ends with a world war. War, and in particular 'total war' of the type experienced in 1914–18 and 1939–45, has been said by historians to lead to significant social change. This was more the case for World War II than for World War I (although in the rest of Europe, the first war did lead to the establishment of welfare systems for the civilian population). World War II led to the establishment of the National Health Service in Britain, the first comprehensive state-funded system of health care in the West. The impact of World War I on health care has been more controversial, as we noted in the last chapter. The aftermath of World War I did not lead to the sort of reconstruction associated with World War II. There was no mood for radical change among the ruling elite; that section of society instead believed that the war had been fought to restore the world as they knew it before 1914.

[1]Ramesh, A. and Hyma, B. (1981) 'Traditional Indian medicine in practice in an Indian metropolitan city', in *Health and Disease: A Reader.*

The period following World War I remained one of ebbs and flows in entitlement to health care in its widest sense, including social welfare. Post-war reconstruction was more limited than that after World War II, but did point towards greater collectivism. Bureaucracies were now assuming that they could intervene in complex socio-economic affairs. Ministries of Health were established all over Europe and elaborate insurance-based health-care systems were enacted. In Britain, the Ministry of Health was established in 1919, as a partial realisation of the earlier aims of John Simon and other public-health reformers (as described in Chapter 4).

The war also led to the beginnings of *international standard-setting*, not only for medicines but also for health care. The newly established League of Nations set optimal standards for *nutrition* which made it possible to begin to evaluate deficiencies at a national level. The Rockefeller Foundation's global policies promoted medicine on a collectivist and scientific basis, policies which were controversial because of their stress on training new elite specialists in public health.

The inter-war years are, nevertheless, with good reason generally portrayed as a time of depression. In Britain, the period was dominated by rising unemployment, which never fell below a million, and rose at its peak to more than three million. (This represented a far graver recession than the 'slumps' of the early 1980s and early 1990s because a larger proportion of the 'working' population was unemployed.) The collapse of the Western economies in 1929 meant that developments in health care must be seen against a background of national crisis.

There were also continuing *crises of subsistence* and of *disease*. The 1919 'flu pandemic brought a huge number of deaths in its train (perhaps 200 000 in Britain alone). There were epidemics of typhus and of cholera associated with a severe famine in Eastern Europe in 1920–2, causing the deaths of many millions.

In Britain, the inter-war years were also a time of *financial conservatism*. The Treasury fulfilled its traditional role of cutting short any reform involving significant public expenditure. The coverage of compulsory health and unemployment insurance was widened from a quarter to a half of the adult population. But there was no attempt at a wide-ranging reorganisation of health services or any attempt to bring order into the funding of them.

There were a number of possible options facing policy makers in the inter-war years. These included the extension of the National Health Insurance (NHI) system (Figure 5.1), or basing health services firmly on the local authorities. The National Insurance Act 1911 and its subsequent revisions, as we have noted in Chapter 4, made only *lower* wage-earners eligible for state-subsidised insurance, and it excluded their families. But there were also other fundamental shortcomings in the insurance system. The system gave imperfect access to specialist services and many of those services, as you will see in the next section, were in a state of crisis—the voluntary hospitals in particular.

Other aspects of health administration were mostly left to local authorities, but here again there were problems, especially as the system of local taxation (rates) tended to result in the poorest services in the poorest areas. The downward trend of infant mortality and the decline in the major infectious diseases encouraged complacency and government economy. Exchequer contributions to the health insurance fund fell in the 1920s and the government refused to finance any extra burden of access to health care out of taxation. Government was determined to retrench and refused to extend health insurance further.

Social welfare systems were established in all Western European countries in this period, in spite of their contrasting political systems. Totalitarian regimes established in Italy and Germany produced their own solutions. Fascism, like its socialist antitheses, stressed the nation's health as was shown by Italian innovations in setting up a single (but inadequately financed) authority for maternal and child welfare, promulgating pronatalism geared to Mussolini's schemes for military conquest. At the same time, as part of the racial machinery of the Nazi state, there were efforts to promote a centralised welfare state by coordinating the hitherto autonomous sickness insurance funds, ending municipal autonomy by unifying state and municipal public health, and taking control of the Red Cross and other hitherto voluntary agencies.

Social welfare systems involving health care were also established elsewhere. The *New Deal* introduced

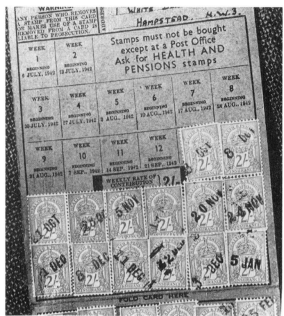

Figure 5.1 *The basis of National Health Insurance—a stamped up card for 1942. (Source: G. A. Paddon/The Pilot Press)*

under F. D. Roosevelt's Presidency in the 1930s included maternity and child health and child welfare services, all of them restricted to lower-income groups. The 'New Deal' was a kind of 'half-way house'; and when production began to recover in 1937, all government spending was cut back. Social democracies in Europe, most notably Sweden in the 1930s, introduced major programmes of social insurance and social reform—although health was not included in the minimum universal provision made in the decade after World War II for eradicating most of the major causes of poverty.

New directions for health care were apparent also in the post-revolutionary Soviet system. By the 1930s the Soviets could claim that the 1917 October Revolution had produced a radical change in the health position in the country and that they had successfully built the first mass national health service in the world. Western social and health reformers of the time were enthusiastic but often naive in their reports of Soviet achievements.

Various models of health care developed in Europe in the inter-war years, and in the colonies, as you will see later in this chapter, a paternalistic model of health care prevailed.

It was not until after World War II in Britain that comprehensive reconstruction of health services was attempted. The election of a Labour government in 1945 was partly in reaction to the financial stringency of the National government in the 1930s. Radical reconstruction was achieved, as it had not been after World War I. The Labour government succeeded in establishing a system of comprehensive health care for the first time in Britain but, as you will see shortly, its organisation and funding was rather different to what might have been expected from looking at the inter-war health services. Neither of the apparent options facing policy makers after World War I—extension of national health insurance or increasing access to local-authority-based services—were in the event adopted.

The health-care system: chaos and change

Two questions concern us in this section: what was the state of the health-care system in Britain between the wars? and what led to the establishment of the post-war National Health Service?

Health-care provision after World War I was a patchwork of ramshackle and uncoordinated services. The health-care system in Britain proved increasingly chaotic in its funding, operation and with respect to access: the *voluntary hospitals* often limited their admissions to specialised cases; the *workhouse infirmaries* coped with the mentally handicapped, senile, 'venereal' and chronic and elderly patients; *local-authority ante-natal clinics* and *GP panel services* under the NHI Commission catered for a minority of the population. There was poor coordination between services and relations were often openly hostile, leading to criticism of clinical standards. Any attempts at wide-ranging rationalisation or reform of the system were prevented by the stance of post-war governments towards economic problems, which were concerned with financial retrenchment rather than investment.

The *Dawson Report* of 1920 provided an ambitious blueprint for the integration and coordination of preventive and curative services. Its recommendation of a two-tier network of GP and specialist **health centres**, in which services would be concentrated and coordinated, stressed planning of local GP-based services and the accessibility of specialist care. But, as Sir George Godber, later the Chief Medical Officer in the Department of Health, subsequently pointed out in the 1980s:

> The British did not really believe in the capacity of government at any level to run such human services in 1920. (Godber, 1983, p. 4)

The Dawson Committee's recommendations remained unimplemented in the inter-war years. As you will see in Chapter 6, health centres only became a reality in the 1960s and then in rather a different form. Models of health-care provision were discussed in the 1920s, but little was achieved in the inter-war years to rationalise a hotch-potch provision of overlapping and 'special interest' services, dealing with conditions such as tuberculosis or sexually transmitted disease.

More was achieved in other Western European countries. During the 1920s, socialist municipalities in cities like Berlin and Vienna promoted innovative schemes in social medicine with health centres and model housing schemes. *Preventive* health care became linked with the promotion of *positive health*. There were innovative experiments with birth-control clinics, child guidance clinics (incorporating psychoanalysis) and cosmetic services for sufferers from facial cancers and other disfiguring illnesses. Soviet social medicine placed a high priority on preventive medicine, and medical services were shaped by theories that diseases were socially caused. Feminists praised the liberality of Soviet abortion legislation (overlooking the fact that abortion was subject to medical decisions by a physician).

In Britain, the recommendations of other committees of enquiry—for example, the 1918 Maclean Committee, or the 1926 Royal Commission on National Health Insurance, which attacked the hotch-potch of benefits and provision offered by the existing NHI scheme—all foundered in the face of government economy measures. The Economy Act 1926 incorporated a wide range of cuts, including the government contribution to the health insurance scheme which was reduced from two-ninths to one-seventh. Further cuts followed the world financial crisis of 1931; cuts in benefit to married women were made in 1932.

Hospitals in crisis

A significant omission from the NHI scheme (in addition to the exclusion of dependants from medical treatment) was the *lack of hospital treatment*. But the hospital services were a chaotic mixture: hospital services were unevenly distributed and especially limited in rural areas. The voluntary hospitals were in a state of crisis: they provided 25 per cent of all beds and had increasing financial problems. In 1921, a Committee headed by Viscount Cave pointed out that they were suffering from rising costs and recommended a £1m subvention from the state. The government provided only half the amount and refused any permanent commitment.

The voluntary hospitals' problems arose from a number of factors. First, the steadily improving capacities of medicine created a demand for better-equipped hospitals. Technical standards began to fall behind those in the USA. In the best American medical schools, *research* became an essential component of clinical medicine and hospital teaching after World War I; in Britain, such developments were slower to materialise.

Second, in British voluntary hospitals, the increased *salaries* of resident medical and nursing staff outstripped the growth in income from voluntary sources. The hospitals increasingly became dependent upon means-tested payment by patients, and upon payment from local authorities for treatment undertaken on their behalf. Hospital contributory systems were set up, but were expensive to operate. The Hospital Saturday and Sunday Funds (charities mentioned in Chapter 4) continued to supplement income. To meet increasing demand from would-be patients who earned above the £6 per week income limit, many hospitals expanded their wards for fee-paying patients. Even given these financial expedients, by the end of the 1930s, many of the voluntary hospitals were in financial difficulties, and the major teaching hospitals faced the worst of these problems.

Table 5.1 Sources of income of London voluntary hospitals, 1938 and 1947 (percentages)

Source of income	Percentage of income in	
	1938	1947
voluntary gifts	34	16
investments	16	8
public authority payments	8	46
other payments (patient fees, etc.)	42	30
total	**100**	**100**

Data from Eckstein, H. (1958) *The English Health Service*, Oxford University Press, Oxford, p. 75.

□ Look at Table 5.1. What changes strike you in the voluntary hospitals' sources of income between 1938 and 1947?

■ The proportion of income derived from donations declined and support from public authorities increased. The proportion derived from patient fees also declined, but remained a significant section of income.

The local-authority-based health service developed in a piecemeal way. The Local Government Act 1929 empowered local authorities to take over Poor Law infirmaries as *municipal hospitals*, but, outside London, the local authorities were slow to take up the opportunities offered by the 1929 Act.

Health care finance in crisis

Finance was also a problem in the general operation of health services before World War II. The NHI scheme, based on the *approved societies* (which collected contributions and distributed cash benefits to claimants; see Chapter 4), faced increasing financial difficulties. The inter-war recession took a heavy toll on approved society finances, and by 1930, the huge profits revealed in 1925 at the second valuation had dwindled to virtually nothing. New support systems introduced in the early 1930s to help members who could not afford to keep up with contributions cost the societies huge sums. Even so, by 1934, over four million policies were in arrears.

The commercial approved societies were a powerful lobby and were not willing to 'pool' resources as the 1926 Royal Commission had proposed. Even if this had been done, there would not have been sufficient funds to meet the needs of the working population. By the end of the inter-war period less than a dozen societies catered for nine-tenths of the insured population.

In addition, the number of friendly societies (to which workers might make 'sick club' contributions) fell sharply between 1918 and 1936 as almost one-third went out of existence. The health insurance system could do little other than survive; it failed to expand as its founders had hoped, mainly because of the political and economic climate within which it operated.

Although the operation of NHI has attracted much comment from historians (in part because of the debates about health insurance in the 1980s), the bulk of income for medical services in the inter-war period did not emanate from insurance funds, but from public authorities. Table 5.2 shows the major sources of revenue for health services in 1938–9.

□ What strikes you about the patterns of funding revealed by the data in Table 5.2?

Table 5.2 Funding sources for health services, 1938–9

Source of funding	£m	Percentage of total
Exchequer	3.0	4.6
rates (local property taxation)	40.3	61.1
NHI	11.2	17.0
voluntary sources	11.5	17.4

Data (rounded to the nearest decimal place) from C. Webster, previously unpublished, based on Treasury data.

■ The bulk of funding for health services was provided from the rates at the outbreak of war. Other contributions, including NHI, were roughly equal. (Note that the inter-war 'free market' system, often alluded to in policy debates around health service funding in the 1980s, was in fact largely funded from public sources.)

By the outbreak of war in 1939, a growing chorus of influential opinion demanded change to the chaotic and uncoordinated nature of health services. The *Socialist Medical Association* called for a free national health service administered by local authorities; and, as you will see shortly, the *BMA* also began to demand change.

Far more influential in terms of public opinion was a report published in 1937, by *Political and Economic Planning* (PEP), an independent and non-party group, on *The British Health Services*. The report attracted considerable attention, being welcomed on publication day by leading articles in eleven national and provincial dailies. It also received a welcome from most of the specialist medical journals; and was subsequently republished in abridged form as a 6d Pelican paperback. The report concluded:

> The health services suffer greatly from confusion and overlapping, and in order to minimise this we propose their reorientation around the general practitioner, who should be enabled to bring the resources of the health services on the one hand into contact with the needs and peculiarities of the individual patient on the other.... The general practitioner, however, cannot function satisfactorily unless he has behind him a range of better coordinated and less fragmentary health facilities of a specialised nature, to which cases can be readily referred where necessary...perhaps the most fundamental defect in the existing system is that it is overwhelmingly preoccupied with manifest and advanced diseases or disabilities and is more interested in enabling the sufferers to go on functioning in society somehow than in studying the nature of health and the means of producing and maintaining it. From this it naturally follows that millions of pounds are spent in looking after and trying to cure the victims of accidents and illnesses which need never have occurred if a fraction of this amount of intelligence and money had been devoted to tracing the social and economic causes of the trouble and making the necessary readjustments. (PEP, 1939, p. 205)

□ The PEP report identified the fragmentary and chaotic nature of the inter-war health system. What did it propose as solutions?

■ It placed emphasis on the role of the GP; on a coordinated specialist system backing up primary care; and on preventive as well as curative medicine.

The proposals in the report were in fact based on an extension of NHI; a completely free service was rejected on the grounds of cost.

The birth of the NHS

Change was in the air before 1939; but two crucial questions remain for us to consider: how much would have been achieved but for the impact of war? and what would have been achieved without the election of a Labour government in 1945?

The impact of war was certainly considerable. It led directly to the establishment of an *Emergency Medical Service*, planned before the war (and fully in operation by 1941) in order to cater for the large numbers of expected civilian bombing casualties. Hospitals were run by existing authorities, but within a regional framework and with the Ministry of Health deciding what role each should play.

A further strong impetus to comprehensive proposals came with the publication of the Beveridge Report in 1942 on *Social Insurance and Allied Services* with its recommendations for a comprehensive health service. With the publication of the White Paper, *A National Health Service* (February 1944), the political temperature began to rise. The White Paper indicated the progress made since the outbreak of war. Whereas in 1941 the government had spoken only in terms of a *hospital* service, by 1944 a *comprehensive* service was planned, with free treatment financed from taxation.

> To ensure that everybody in the country—irrespective of means, age, sex and occupation—shall have equal opportunity to benefit from the best and most up-to-date medical and allied services available. To provide, therefore, for all who want it, a comprehensive service covering every branch of medical and allied activity.
>
> To divorce the case of health from questions of personal means or other factors irrelevant to it; to provide the service free of charge (apart from certain possible charges in respect of appliances) and to encourage a new attitude to health—the easier obtaining of advice early, the promotion of good health rather than only the treatment of bad. (Ministry of Health, 1944, p. 47)

However, it was becoming clear that one of the major planks of opposition to a national health service was the medical profession itself, and in particular the BMA. The latter resolutely opposed any move to a salaried service and local-authority control of services for two reasons: first, the threat this offered to valued 'clinical freedom', and second, the echoes of nineteenth-century systems of lay control through the friendly societies and the Poor Law. The BMA also wanted an enhanced role for the voluntary hospitals and their consultants.

The BMA had won substantial concessions on the 1944 White Paper by 1945. But the election of a Labour government and the arrival of Aneurin Bevan as Minister of Health changed the situation. Bevan espoused the *nationalisation* of the hospitals (under appointed local bodies) rather than local-authority control, which was until then Labour Party policy. By doing so, he exploited already existing divisions within the medical profession between consultants and GPs, and, within the BMA, between the wealthier and the majority of poorly remunerated GPs. Although struggles between Bevan and sections of the medical profession continued even after the 'Appointed Day' for the inception of the **National Health Service (NHS)** on 5 July 1948, he had effectively won over both the influential consultants and the majority of GPs, neither of whom would have countenanced local-authority control.

The *National Health Service Act 1946* established a nationally directed and financed **tripartite system** of hospitals; GPs, pharmacists, opticians and others; and local-authority teams. Both the voluntary and local hospitals were nationalised and placed under the control of regional boards consisting of local-authority and voluntary hospital representatives. GP, dental and pharmacy services were to be administered by Executive Councils, half professional and half lay. GPs remained 'independent contractors' under the NHS in continuity with NHI; proposals for a salaried service were dropped. Counties and county boroughs retained responsibility for health centres, clinics and other services such as health visiting and ambulances.

The original intention was that health centres, provided by local authorities, would be the key coordinating agency between the three services. But, as shown in Chapter 6, this proposal was abandoned.

Bevan's achievement was a considerable one. It is easy enough to think of the NHS as a 'natural' development from the pre-war discussions, but historical research has shown that the much trumpeted mood of 'war-time consensus' was largely illusory. Under the Labour Minister of Health, supported by key civil servants in the Ministry of Health, reform proceeded further and faster than it would have done under the 1944 White Paper.

The following memory of the arrival of the new service gives some indication of what it meant for poor families.

> I well remember our Brian being born. He was delivered by a doctor up at Oldham, a Scotsman, he got called up and killed in the war, so we never paid for Brian. The doctors were very good. You'd go to the doctor. He had your name and address. And after, you got a bill, and if you couldn't pay it, which very few people could, each doctor had his own collector. The collectors used to come round each week and you'd pay sixpence. My wife's father and mother used to say they'd never be straight in their lifetime. When the National Health came in all them doctors' bills were written off. The collectors always used to be the same type who were park keepers in them days—they'd be no use today, kids'd throw them in pond—but they were always little wizened fellers. (Gray, 1986, p. 88)

Some historians have argued that the establishment of the NHS was not unique, and that the principle of *regionalisation* (the regional planning and organisation of health services) was being established as a basic form of service organisation in many countries at this time. Certainly, in the period in which the NHS was being set up in Britain, parallel schemes were in operation or preparation elsewhere in Europe, Australia and the USA. But there were numerous differences of detail of funding and of access.

The European insurance-based systems were founded on non-governmental, non-profit-making public bodies, while in the USA insurance was provided by commercial companies. The British system was *unique* in its free and open access to all. All of the systems were dominated by hospital-based medicine. The unusual *nationalised* hospital system in Britain possessed certain advantages, but among its disadvantages were the fragmentation of the health system, an escalation of hospital costs, and a lack of democratic accountability. These drawbacks became increasingly apparent as time passed, as you will see in Chapter 6.

Lay care and boundaries with formal care: tipping the balance

You have seen how welfare systems were established in the inter-war period in a number of European countries. But the role of domestic, family and neighbourhood networks in providing health care remained central, in particular for poor families. The historian Elizabeth Roberts has collected memories of people living in Lancashire in the 1920s and 1930s. Here is one reminiscence. Mrs A. as a child, was part of a very large extended family in Preston. Her aunt, her mother's oldest sister, lived next door and was regarded as the family's expert:

> She was the one who, if we were ill, my mother always wanted guidance from. If anything was wrong with us it would be 'go and bring aunt Martha'.

The grandmother of the family had a stroke:

> She wasn't quite 71 and she was 77 when she died. She was in bed all the time. It paralysed her all down one side and she could get out of bed...but couldn't get back. So my auntie next door took her and she had her in the front room in the bed downstairs and my mother looked to her in the daytime and auntie looked to her at night. (Roberts, 1984, p. 51)

☐ Compare this description with the role of family members in health care today—what differences strike you?

■ Most obviously that there is no mention of any professional medical intervention in the home or any perceived role for institutional care. The old lady does not go to hospital or to a home; care is confined within the extended family.

☐ In Chapter 2 you read criticisms of the idea of a 'golden age' when every family looked after its own relations. How would you assess this quotation as historical evidence?

■ You should be aware of the limitation of oral evidence. This situation of informal care from the family was undoubtedly the case here, but may not have been universally the rule. It also ignores the contribution of lay care *outside* kinship networks, for example by friends and neighbours.

Establishing the boundaries

Traditions of lay care persisted, in part because of the limitations of existing formal services (see, for example, Figure 5.2 (a)). The rudimentary statutory services were piecemeal, and the lack of service provision especially affected women and children. Only in a minority of cases would children's health problems be detected and treated under the school medical service (see Figure 5.2 (b)).

☐ Can you recall why health care before the NHS was particularly inadequate for women and children?

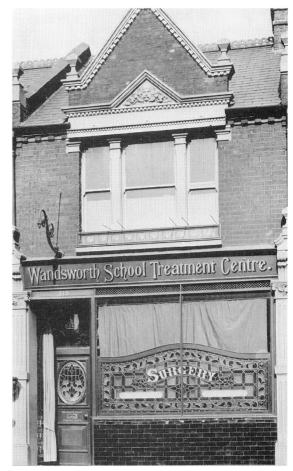

(a)

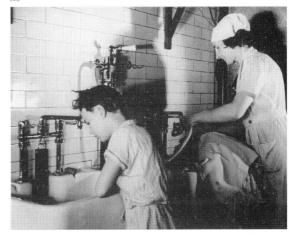

(b)

Figure 5.2 *(a) Wandsworth School Treatment Centre operating room, photographed in 1911. (Source: Age Exchange/Alec Schweitzer) (b) Hair disinfestation in the 1930s; one function of the school medical service. (Source: Age Exchange/Alec Schweitzer)*

■ The NHI scheme did not cover dependants, so women and children had no formal entitlement to 'panel' GP care.

It was customary in some working-class families to belong to the local hospital scheme, but this only covered emergencies and did not provide regular medical care. Maternity and child welfare clinics were established under local-authority control especially after the *Maternal and Child Welfare Act 1918*, but provision of these was patchy and often encountered opposition from local GPs, who feared the competition emanating from the clinics.

There was also, at least in the period immediately after the war, a current of popular disbelief in the *efficacy* of formal health-care provision. Health visitors established their status and role in the inter-war period, but friction between mother and visitor was common. One former health visitor described how she was resented as an authority figure and referred to by many of the women she visited in the East End of London as 'the Town 'all'.

Unqualified midwives also continued to be widely used: they were cheaper than qualified ones, they were generally thought friendlier and less 'starchy' and there was hardly any popular criticism of their competence. The *Midwives Act 1902* had made the training of new midwives and the registration of established ones compulsory, but untrained women continued to practise throughout the inter-war years. A coordinated midwifery service involving trained practitioners (see Figure 5.3) was not widely available until after World War II.

There was also a different working-class health 'culture'; and health beliefs were not the same as those in other sections of society. For example, there was a concern for death as well as for health. Almost all families would attempt to contribute to some form of death insurance. Elizabeth Roberts comments that:

> …the strengths of working-class mores, and the demands of working class respectability, were such that the little surplus income there was, went, not towards health care for the living, but towards ensuring a decent funeral for the dead. (Quoted in Pickstone, 1980, p. 40)

Self-medication was still the norm, as in the nineteenth century. Boots the Chemist continued its nineteenth-century expansion (see Figure 5.4) and Woolworths became the major supplier of spectacles in the United Kingdom.

There was also a widespread reliance on well-established popular remedies. Robert Roberts, who was brought up in a Salford slum, remembers what was used:

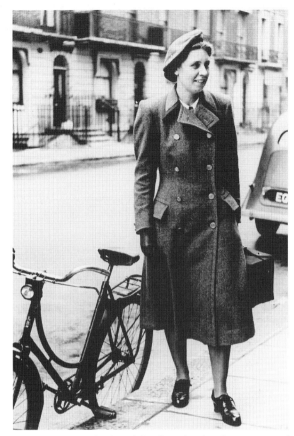

Figure 5.3 *A midwife with her bicycle, the classic image of the new trained and professionalised service. (Source: Age Exchange/Alec Schweitzer)*

At weekends people purged themselves with great doses of black draught, senna pods, cascara sagrada, and their young with Gregory powder, licorice powder and California syrup of figs…the working class had an awful fear of constipation…. Pills sold at a penny a box, any doubts as to their potency being quieted by the venerable image of their maker smiling from the lid. He had cause for amusement. Nearly all the pills appeared to possess a dual purpose: they 'attacked' at one and the same the ills of two intestines 'Head and Stomach', 'Blood and Stomach', 'Back and Kidney', 'Back and Bladder' and indeed almost any pair of organs that could in decency be named. (Roberts, 1971, pp. 124–5)

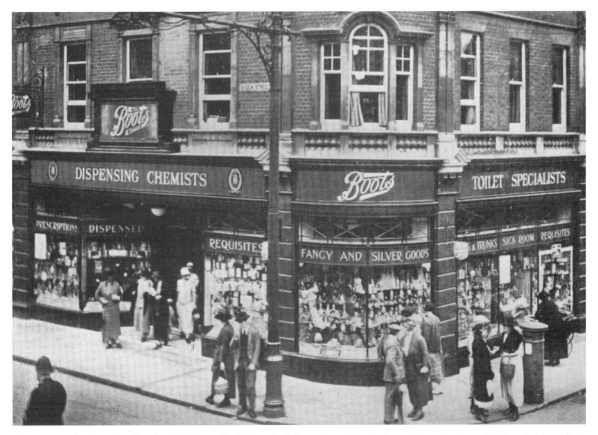

Figure 5.4 *The imposing facade of this branch of Boots in Pelham Street, Nottingham, in 1935 reflects the size of the market for self-medication and toiletries in the inter-war years. (Source: The Boots Company, plc, Nottingham)*

□ How could you investigate the extent of self-medication in the 1920s and 1930s?

■ You could draw on your own or local experiences of self-medication now. You could talk to a sample of older people about the remedies which were most commonly used and how they were obtained. (You could also look at books listed in the References such as *Can We Afford the Doctor?* for reminiscences of self-medication.)

The role of local pharmacists in lay medical care was considerable. They frequently provided diagnosis and advice. One remembered in an interview:

We were the first filter as it were…we had to do a bit of diagnosing in our own way and be responsible for it. 'Would they for example bring children in and say "What is the matter?" ' Oh my goodness yes. 'What sort of things would

be the matter with them?' It might be just nettle rash, it might be measles—very often it was measles and teething trouble, a little feverish, constipation or something like that, the usual childish ailments but we had to be very, very careful in case there was little yellow spots behind the throat and then write to the doctor…. 'You didn't charge for this advice?' Oh dear no. Anything had to be inexpensive… (Roberts, quoted in Pickstone, 1980, p. 45)

□ What strikes you about the role of the pharmacist here by comparison with the occupation's present position?

■ In some respects, the current role of the pharmacist is not that different. (It is interesting that policy documents on pharmacy in the 1990s have emphasised the role of the pharmacist as a first-line practitioner.)

Changing aspirations

These patterns of lay care were in many respects little different from those we have described in the nineteenth century. But change was detectable in the inter-war period, in particular in *aspirations to health*. Higher standards of living and shorter hours of work, together with the extension of paid holidays to wider groups of workers, provided an impetus for an increase in almost every type of leisure activity. The widespread popularity of the cinema (a survey of Liverpool in 1937 found that 40 per cent of the population went at least once a week), radio and commercial magazines, served to raise social expectations and made information about health more widely available.

Active participation became the norm: sport, hiking, holiday camps (which had accommodation for more than half a million people by 1939), all found increasing popularity. Physical recreation and fitness was an aspiration for large numbers of working- and lower-middle-class people, although Britain was in general backward in providing state facilities for recreation, especially where they were needed most. Physical fitness was also an important part of preventive medicine in Germany and other central European states, for example Czechoslovakia. However, outside observers were suspicious of it as militaristic in intention.

In this period, family health and hygiene was promoted as a special part of a woman's 'role'. Under-population rather than over-population was seen as a threat, but reformers were also concerned about the *differential* birth rate. The fear was that the 'wrong' people (the poor and the unfit) would breed and might overwhelm the educated and upper classes of society. These 'eugenic' ideas have been a continuing theme in the birth-control movement; in addition to humanitarian concerns for women dragged down by endless pregnancies.

Organisations such as Women's Institutes and the Women's Co-operative Guild promoted birth control, hygiene and responsibility for family health among the working classes. The most important advocate of birth control and a more open attitude to sexual matters was Dr Marie Stopes. The popularity of her writings reflected a massive public demand for birth-control advice. In 1921, she opened her first clinic in Holloway Road, North London. In 1930, Stopes and others formed the National Birth Control Council, which in 1939 became the *Family Planning Association*.

Experiments in improving the diet of mothers were undertaken in the 1930s in South Wales and in the North East by the National Birthday Trust Fund and the People's League of Health. These had an indeterminate effect on the maternal mortality rate, which continued to rise across the classes in the inter-war years, largely unaffected by improvements in maternity services. By 1939, however, sulphonamides were a more important means of reducing the death rate among women in childbirth.

☐ What does Figure 5.5 indicate about changes in the level of maternal mortality?

■ From 1900 to the mid-1930s there was little change in the rate. A steep and sustained decline followed. This, so it is argued, was associated both with effective drug therapies and with the increase in trained midwifery.

Changes in attitudes towards childbirth reflected wider changes in lay attitudes towards formal health services. The trend was towards medicalised childbirth; in 1927 only 15 per cent of births took place in hospital, but by 1946, this had risen to 54 per cent. This trend gave obstetrics a new status; it was also supported by women who recognised the need for more aseptic procedures. It thus reflected both medical and consumer demand and also developments taking place in the USA and across Europe (although not in the Netherlands, where home births remained the norm).

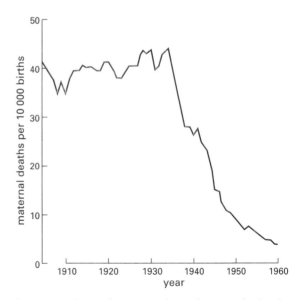

Figure 5.5 *The trend in maternal mortality in England and Wales, 1905–60 (data from MacFarlane, A. and Mugford, M., 1984,* Birth Counts: Statistics of Pregnancy and Childbirth, *HMSO, London; graph from Loudon, I., 1991, On maternal and infant mortality, 1900–1960, Social History of Medicine,* **4**(1), p. 38)

In itself, hospitalised childbirth was not an essential component of maternal and infant health. In the inter-war period in the United Kingdom, most births still took place at home, but here, too, there was a less fatalistic attitude to childbirth and a lessening of women's role in assisting at the event. The help and advice of outside trained experts—the doctor, health visitor and clinic—were increasingly referred to instead of relatives and neighbours. The final tipping of the balance towards professional help came only after the establishment of the NHS in the late 1940s.

Public-health services: in search of an identity

The reluctance of the laity to seek professional help may have been prolonged by a significant mismatch between the issues that working people saw as affecting their own and their family's health—low pay, unemployment, poor housing and nutritional standards—and the concerns of public-health doctors and the services they controlled.

In the nineteenth century, environmental issues were central to public health, and were the responsibility of the emergent **public-health profession** advising governments or local authorities. In the twentieth century such environmental issues did not disappear, as you will see from the following discussion of housing, incomes and nutrition. But they became less central to the *work* of the MOH and other public-health doctors employed in local government, and to the *ideology* of public health to which these doctors adhered. The inter-war years were, in one sense, a 'golden age' of public health, when public-health doctors had more responsibility at the local level than before or since. In another sense, they were a period of crisis when the profession and the ideas of public health failed to adapt themselves to the realities of poverty and unemployment in the Depression.

Despite a dramatic growth in the statutory powers of public-health departments in local authorities, the nineteenth-century concern to deal with all aspects of the environment and housing as a means of promoting health and cleanliness gradually disappeared. Increasingly, public-health departments focused on what the *individual* should do to ensure personal hygiene; for example, the instruction of women in family hygiene at the infant welfare clinics which we mentioned earlier. Public health justified its emphasis on clinic work with mothers and children as 'applied physiology', a kind of preventive clinical medicine. Both before and after the transition to the NHS, this brought MOHs into competition with GPs, who also claimed control over this work.

Public health established itself substantially at the local level in the inter-war years. Between 1918 and 1939, some twenty pieces of legislation extending the remit of *local-authority health services* were passed. By 1939, local authorities were providing maternal and child welfare services; the school medical service; TB clinics and treatment; infectious disease, ear, nose and throat and VD services; and *health centres*—the most elaborate being that built by Finsbury Borough Council in 1938. In addition, the *Local Government Act 1929* allowed local authorities to take over the Poor Law hospitals. Finally the *Cancer Act 1939* placed responsibility for the development of local regional cancer schemes on the local authorities.

This was a substantial increase in power and influence, but, as the historian Jane Lewis has argued, it also meant that public-health practice had no clear guiding philosophy during the inter-war years. The *aims* of public health were formulated according to the functions *actually being carried out*. Public-health departments added to their responsibilities without questioning what was distinctive about public health.

Looking back in 1939, R. M. F. Picken, Professor of Preventive Medicine at the Welsh School of Medicine, felt that the profession of MOH had gone down the wrong path:

> Public health might have developed on very different lines. It might well have remained purely preventive, grown out of sanitation to be concerned mainly with the problems of the nutrition of the people, their physical fitness, and public education generally, and kept away from any sort of medical advice and treatment of the individual… (Quoted in Lewis, 1986, p. 29)

☐ Picken thought that public health should have kept away from individual medical advice and treatment. What was his suggestion for public health?

■ His view, although broader than questions of medical treatment, is still focused on prevention of disease at the *personal* level and *individual responsibility* for health rather than the environmentalism of nineteenth-century public health.

The neglect of social causes of ill-health

One result of public health's 'administrative focus' during this period was its relative neglect of sources of danger to the people's health. Public-health doctors were on the whole little involved in the debates on the effects of *unemployment* on health. They did not bring to public notice the large number of cases of *malnutrition* in the

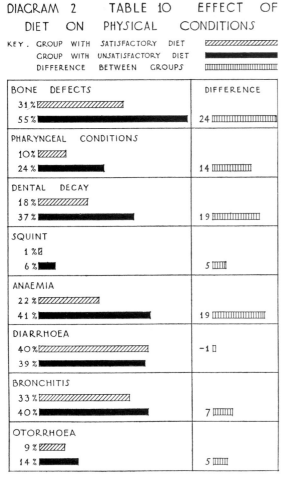

DIAGRAM 2   TABLE 10   EFFECT OF DIET ON PHYSICAL CONDITIONS

KEY. GROUP WITH SATISFACTORY DIET
GROUP WITH UNSATISFACTORY DIET
DIFFERENCE BETWEEN GROUPS

BONE DEFECTS	DIFFERENCE
31%	
55%	24
PHARYNGEAL CONDITIONS	
10%	
24%	14
DENTAL DECAY	
18%	
37%	19
SQUINT	
1%	
6%	5
ANAEMIA	
22%	
41%	19
DIARRHOEA	
40%	−1
39%	
BRONCHITIS	
33%	
40%	7
OTORRHOEA	
9%	
14%	5

Figure 5.6 *Dr M'Gonigle's tabulation of the relationship between diet and poor physical condition. (Reproduced from M'Gonigle, G. and Kirby, J., 1936,* Poverty and Public Health, *Victor Gollancz, London, p. 98)*

depressed areas, or the widespread sickness among *childbearing* women.

British people during the 1920s and 1930s did experience some overall improvement in living standards. Average life expectancy was up and mortality down; and inter-war surveys found poverty levels lower than in the late Victorian investigations. But social class and regional disparities persisted and in some cases worsened. This was demonstrated through surveys of *diet and nutrition*. Sir John Boyd Orr's study, *Food, Health and Income*, published in 1936, showed that a tenth of the population, including a fifth of all children, were chronically ill-nourished. Dr George M'Gonigle, the MOH for Stockton-on-Tees, found that in 1936 the death rate

among the poorer section of the local population (families with an income of 25–35s per week)—who spent only 3s a head per week on food—was twice that of the more affluent (families with an income of 70–80s per week), who spent 6s a head.

☐ Figure 5.6 is taken from M'Gonigle's report. What general point does it illustrate? And what cautionary note should we bear in mind when interpreting these data?

■ M'Gonigle's data make a strong connection between poor diet and poor physical condition. He relates 'unsatisfactory' diet to the incidence of a large range of physical defects (he discounted diarrhoea, which was the result of infection, but is in fact exacerbated by under-nutrition). However, he has used his own definition of satisfactory and unsatisfactory diets, and has neglected the effects of repeated illness on general health.[2]

The association between *unemployment*, poverty, under-nutrition and health during this period is also controversial, as it remains today[3] (see Figure 5.7). In the 1930s, a general overall improvement in health disguised a tremendous regional diversity. As always, ill-health and malnutrition had the greatest effect on women and children.

Regional diversity was also evident in the attempts to improve *housing conditions*—part of the public-health mandate in the nineteenth century. Slum clearance got under way to a significant extent after World War I, although progress was patchy. Rents were controlled and subsidies offered for private house-building.

Between 1931 and 1939, local authorities built over 700 000 houses, supposedly rehousing four-fifths of existing slum dwellers (the numbers in the slums were actually underestimated). In Leeds, the Quarry Hill Scheme saw 2 000 slum houses demolished and 938 new flats built at a cost of £1.5 million. New standards for space and design were laid down. But the most dramatic developments took place in private house building, and poor housing remained one of the most pressing social issues.

[2]Problems associated with defining an 'adequate' diet and distinguishing the health-damaging effects of under-nutrition from those of repeated infections, particularly in childhood, are discussed in World Health and Disease, Chapter 11.

[3]See World Health and Disease, Chapter 10 for a full discussion.

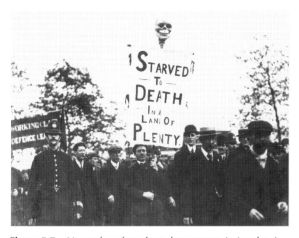

Figure 5.7 *Unemployed workers demonstrate in London in October 1908. (Source: Hulton/Deutsch Picture Collection)*

New council estates (see Figure 5.8) tended to be occupied by skilled and white collar workers, leaving behind the poor in rapidly deteriorating housing stock. London had one of the worst problems: a survey in 1933 revealed that almost half a million people in the capital were suffering from overcrowding.

The lead in raising the questions about the complex relationship between housing, unemployment, low pay and nutrition in the 1930s came from political lobby groups such as the Children's Minimum Council, not from within the public-health profession. In the 1940s, moves were made to reorientate public-health practice round the new academic discipline of **social medicine**. This aimed to link the *planning* of health and social services to the *needs* of the population. Social medicine became an academic specialty, its flagship the Oxford Institute of Social Medicine, with the philosopher clinician, John Ryle, as Professor.

However, this initiative failed to influence the medical schools and medical education, and was alienated from the practice of public health. Ryle's chair at Oxford

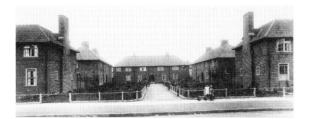

Figure 5.8 *This London County Council estate at Dagenham provided a good standard of new housing in the inter-war period, typical of the house-building programme of the time. (Source: Greater London Photograph Library)*

was not filled when he died in 1950, by which date social medicine was seen as a failed experiment, a telling indication of the declining importance of environmental issues and public health. As you will see in the next section, this was just one of many boundary disputes among health-care occupations.

Formal health-care occupations: disputed boundaries

Health-care occupations in general underwent considerable development in the inter-war years and there was increasing professionalisation among what (by the 1960s) had become known as the **professions supplementary to medicine**[4]: opticians, dentists, radiographers, chiropodists and physiotherapists. Whatever their many differences, health-care occupations were, and remain, similar in their quests for occupational monopolies. Some of the supplementary professions attracted medical patronage, but their ambitions soon began to clash with those of groups of physicians and surgeons also intent on shaping their own specialist fields.

These clashes mounted, particularly after the 1914–18 war. The new Ministry of Health and the medical professional bodies were forced through several stages of response. The sociologist, Gerald Larkin, has characterised these as follows:

> …the initial stage was an often contemptuous dismissal of 'auxiliary' ambitions by the Ministry and medical profession; this was followed by the offer of a compromise by the Ministry and the doctors, usually involving lower status alternatives to an occupational monopoly; and finally came the eventual collapse of this alliance of medical and Ministry interests and the concession of the case for further forms of state registration. (Larkin, 1987, pp. 51–2)

The first two stages took place in the 1920s, 1930s and 1940s; final establishment of registration and monopolies took place in the 1950s and will be discussed in Chapter 6. The first stage began after the success of nurses (1919) and dentists (1921) in securing state registration (see Figure 5.9, *overleaf*).

[4]This term came into use in 1960 with the *Professions Supplementary to Medicine Act*. By the 1980s the term had been replaced in common usage by 'professions allied to medicine' (PAMs).

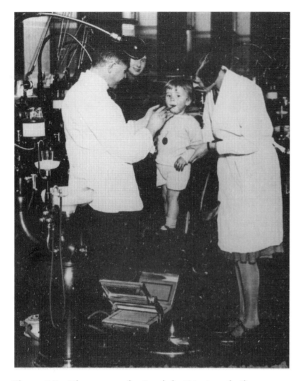

Figure 5.9 *The new professional dentist at work: the Eastman Dental clinic at the Royal Free Hospital in 1930. (Source: Age Exchange/Alec Schweitzer)*

This encouraged smaller groups such as the *opticians* to emulate these achievements. But the Ministry and medical officials worked together to frustrate claims which, in their view, meant licensing inferior alternatives to medical practice. Ophthalmic opticians, for example, expressed their aspirations for professional status through the 1920s, but their claims to share the sight-testing market were sidetracked into a Ministry of Health Committee of Enquiry, dominated by medical interests.

Similarly, a 1928 *chiropody* bill was opposed. Limited recognition was achieved in the 1920s by *radiographers* who were allowed 'to describe the appearances of X-ray plates' to doctors, but not to attempt diagnosis. *Physiotherapists* were also advanced via a royal charter, granted in 1920 through the aristocratic connections of early masseuses; but this also expressly forbade treatment without medical referral.

By 1928, the BMA council had decided on a policy of shaping, rather than automatically rejecting, auxiliary ambitions in order to establish the doctors' authority over the other groups. In the 1930s, the BMA worked for a *Board of Registration of Medical Auxiliaries,* which was set up in 1936 under BMA control. Its constitution had two features: a permanent medical voting majority; and a

duty for all affiliated to it to work *exclusively* under medical direction and supervision. But the Board failed and was unable to reconcile a number of dilemmas. Expansion of its remit was opposed by existing affiliates because this diluted the scarcity value of medical expertise. There were, in fact, few requests for affiliation because the entry terms required a thorough subordination to BMA interests in order to satisfy demands for medical control.

After World War II, as the inception of the NHS came closer, the BMA pressed for the Board's inclusion as an instrument of management under its own control. But there was considerable government opposition to this course of action. In the ten years after the NHS was established (as you will see in Chapter 6), the BMA failed to secure its policy, while the state was pushed into a more immediate managerial responsibility for qualified health-care workers within the NHS.

The BMA, as you can see from this brief history of its relationship with the 'para-medical' professions, was growing in power as the trades union representing doctors. The BMA also aspired to influence national health policy and developed its views on the evolution of the health services. It aimed to put the *National Health Insurance panel* at the centre of health-care organisation. The BMA joined the debate on the health service when it issued its proposals for *A General Medical Service for the Nation* in 1930. This suggested a system of health insurance for virtually all adults and their dependants. By 1938, when a revised version was issued, it had almost been overtaken by events. But its basic principle was a faithful reflection of the more idealistic approach to health care which was gaining acceptance at this time:

> That the system of medical science should be directed to the achievement of positive health and the prevention of disease no less than to the relief of sickness. (BMA, 1938, p. 8)

The role of the general practitioner

The BMA's version of a national health service put the GP centre stage. The NHI panel scheme suited GPs well. By 1938, 90 per cent of all GPs were participating; and 42 per cent of the population were covered on the basis of the £250 per annum income limit (only those earning below this sum were part of the scheme). This upper limit was not raised (to £420 per annum) until 1942.

A striking feature of the BMA's 'trades-union' activities in the run-up to the NHS was its defence of GP panel practice. Doctors had come to appreciate the NHI scheme because it provided a firm basic income for those practitioners who could expect to earn least from private practice (see Figure 5.10), but without the lack of incentive implied by a salaried service. Moreover, it did not jeopardise the prizes to be won from private practice.

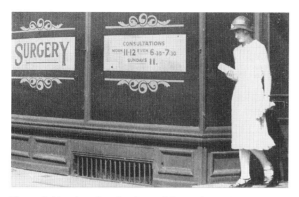

Figure 5.10 *A patient leaving a GP panel practice surgery in the 1930s. Panel practices were generally in less well-to-do districts. When a panel doctor sold his practice to another GP, the patients usually remained on the panel of the purchaser. (Source: Dorien Leigh/The Pilot Press)*

Table 5.3 shows the pattern of GP earnings in the inter-war period.

☐ What strikes you about the trends shown in Table 5.3?

■ GPs were showing a substantial increase in earnings, which was proportionately higher than that for most other groups, particularly in the period of the Depression in the 1930s.

The pay structure of GPs at this time is well illustrated by Dr G. L. Pierce, who practised in a mining valley in South Wales and gave evidence to the Spens committee on GP pay in 1946. He varied his private fee according to the patient: a more prosperous person might be charged half or even 1 guinea for a service while a poorer person would pay 3s 6d or 5s for the same service. This system was sometimes referred to as 'climbing over the backs of the poor into the pockets of the rich'. It was an argument used later to justify the existence of pay beds in NHS hospitals; these were said to subsidise access by non-paying patients.

The GP panel system, although it suited doctors well in some respects, also led to a sense of poverty and insecurity among many GPs and demanded long working hours (in England one half day off during the week and an early finish on Sunday was common practice).

The relationship between general practice and the hospital system had its difficulties. The growth of hospital contributory schemes (already discussed earlier in this chapter) worried GPs. By admitting patients directly to hospital, it threatened to short-circuit the referral system they had established at the turn of the century. Many GPs resorted to establishing *cottage hospitals*, the numbers of which expanded from fewer than 200 at the turn of the century to over 600 by 1935.

This ensured that GPs continued to be involved in surgery; in fact, we still call their premises the 'surgery'. In 1938–9 it was estimated that 2.5 million surgical operations were performed by GPs—an average of three per doctor per week. (This tendency may be revived in the 1990s since the NHS contract for fund-holding GPs carries inducements for them to carry out 'day surgery'.)

Table 5.3 GP earnings in the inter-war period, compared with average earnings in selected professions and occupations

	1913–14 £	1922–4 £	1936–8 £	Change 1913–14 to 1922–4 %	Change 1922–4 to 1936–8 %
higher professionals					
GPs	395	756	1 030	91	36
barristers	478	1 124	(1 090)[1]	135	−3
solicitors	568	1 096	(1 238)	93	13
dentists	368	601	676	63	12
clergy	206	332	370	61	11
army officers	170	390	205	129	−47
engineers	292	468	–	60	–
chemists	314	556	512	77	−8
higher professionals[2]	328	582	634	77	9
lower professionals[2]	155	320	308	106	−4
all men (including manual workers)	94	180	186	91	4

[1]Figures in brackets are more uncertain. [2]Average weighted by the constituent numbers employed in corresponding years. (Data from Digby, A. and Bosanquet, N., 1988, 'Doctors and patients in an era of National Health Insurance and private practice, 1913–39', *Economic History Review*, **XLI**, p. 77, Table 3)

In Europe, the relationship between general practice and hospitals developed differently. Sickness insurance schemes meant that patients had direct access to specialists rather than being referred by their GP as in Britain. Specialists often developed their own elaborate private clinic facilities rather than being hospital-based. Specialism thus developed further in the rest of Europe during this period. For example, families would consult a paediatric specialist about their children's ailments—the 'family doctor' in the British sense, caring for all family members, was less common in Europe except in rural areas. In the USA also, specialisation of doctors persisted, as you should recall from the Reader article by Rosemary Stevens,[5] which you read when studying Chapter 4.

The crisis in nursing

The NHI system had greatly enhanced the prestige of the medical profession, but the status of other health-care professions was more indeterminate. This is emphasised by the deepening crisis which beset *nursing* in this period.

Registration of nurses—achieved in 1919—was not the hoped-for solution in terms of occupational monopoly and status. Many practising nurses failed to meet the requirements for registration and yet still regarded themselves as nurses. The state had become a substantial employer of nurses and so had an interest in the matter. It did not want to grant **registered nurses** a monopoly when it was possible to keep the ranks of nursing more open and costs down. The issue of who should and should not be on the register continued to be an area of contention in this period and one in which the Ministry of Health played an important role. It is clear that the advance of the public sector led to improvement in the status of nurses because of the imposition of standardisation of conditions and terms of employment. Nurses came to enjoy the benefits of other local government employees. Certification was helpful for grading nurses on the local government wage scales.

During the 1920s and 1930s, as hospitals expanded, the *nursing shortage* dominated the period. Unregistered nurses were hired in increasing numbers and trade union militancy spread among them for better conditions and pay. On the eve of World War II, the *Athlone Committee* recommended that a second level of nurse, the **enrolled nurse**, be trained and recognised. This marked a step towards the emergence of a formal hierarchy of nursing grades (see Figure 5.11). The struggle between the Ministry of Health and the College of Nursing over the status

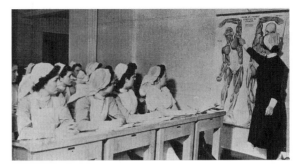

Figure 5.11 *A class for nurses aged 17 and over at Beckenham Hospital in the 1930s, part of the drive to recruit and train more nurses in the inter-war period. (Source: Sport & General/The Pilot Press)*

and grading of nursing continued in the post-war years and indeed the debate continues to the present day.[6]

We conclude this analysis of the period between the World Wars by looking beyond the parochial concerns of health care in Britain, to health care in the colonial territories governed by Britain and other European powers.

Empires and exchanges: the limits of paternalism

The years 1918–48 witnessed crucial changes in Europe's relations with its overseas colonies. Prior to World War I, former settler colonies like Australia had been granted the status of self-governing *Dominions*, and in India nationalist politics had reached a new pitch, with an intensification of violent protest against British rule.

The 1914–18 war did much to accelerate these trends. Troops drawn from the colonies to fight in Europe returned with new aspirations, including expectations of democratic reform and better social provisions such as health care. But in only a few cases did indigenous peoples benefit from collective health provisions such as those described earlier in this chapter. Even where more extensive provisions were made in the colonies, they were, as in Europe, severely constrained by the prevailing mood of financial conservatism in the late 1920s and 1930s. Health care in the colonies also remained paternalistic, although in India and some other colonies indigenous peoples began to play a greater role in the health services established by the colonial state.

India: devolution and diversity

In India, political reforms in 1919 devolved responsibility for certain areas of administration—including health

---

[5]'The evolution of the health-care systems in the United States and the United Kingdom: similarities and differences', in *Health and Disease: A Reader.*

[6]See *Dilemmas in Health Care* (revised edition 1993), Chapter 6.

care—upon provincial governments which had by then become responsible to a majority of elected representatives. For the first time, Indians began to play a major role in decision-making in medical policy and matters of public health.

At first sight, the 1919 reforms appear to have provided a stimulus to the provision of health care in India, with provincial government expenditure on health rising substantially between 1919 and 1939, and more rapidly than other areas of revenue expenditure. However, provincial governments continued to operate within strict financial limits, particularly during the economic depression of the early 1930s. The Indian economic historian V. R. Muraleedharan has argued that the Government of Madras was 'far more concerned about reducing its financial commitments' than providing adequate health care, and that it showed a 'lack of concern for the efficiency and effectiveness of the measures taken' (Muraleedharan, 1987, pp. 333–4).

Retrenchment also adversely affected medical research in India, its budget being cut drastically in the 1920s and 1930s (see Figure 5.12).

One other feature of health care in India between the wars, which it had in common with other colonial countries, was the durability of *indigenous medical systems* (you might like to refer to the Reader article by Ramesh and Hyma at this point).[7]

It is difficult to assess the precise impact of colonial rule on indigenous medicine, although it is certain that traditional systems like *ayurveda* and *unani* (which you encountered in Chapter 2) enjoyed something of a renaissance around the turn of the century, as a result of attempts by some nationalists to revive Indian culture, and with the expansion of the middle-class market for medical services. Many new colleges were established to train practitioners in both Islamic and Hindu medicine, gradually replacing the old system of training by apprenticeship.

However, much of the funding for these institutions came from private sources, with the provincial governments, including many Indian representatives, ambivalent or even hostile to traditional Indian medicine. Many 'modernising' nationalists, who drew their inspiration from the West, denounced Indian medicine as 'unscientific', creating a debate on the relative merits of the two systems which persisted beyond political independence in 1947.

The fate of *folk medicine* under British rule is harder to gauge and appears to have fluctuated greatly according

[7]Ramesh, A. and Hyma, B., 'Traditional Indian medicine in practice in an Indian metropolitan city', in *Health and Disease: A Reader*. This is set reading for Chapter 9.

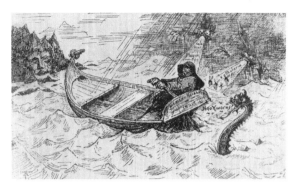

Figure 5.12 *A cartoon from the* Indian Medical Gazette *of June 1923, showing the risk that 'Medical Research in India' ran of being wrecked by the policy of the Inchcape Commission. The Commission recommended drastic reductions in research personnel and in the amount of money allocated to medical research. The sea monsters are labelled 'plague', 'malaria' and 'hookworm'. (From Balfour, A. and Scott, H. H., 1924,* Health Problems of the Empire, *Collins, Glasgow, p. 134)*

to local economic conditions. In general, it seems that specialist remedies such as bone-setting were in many areas displaced by Western medicine, but that non-specialist traditions, such as the use of local plants for medicinal purposes, continued to thrive. Health care in the colonies, as in Britain, remained essentially pluralistic.

☐ Why might indigenous medical systems continue to thrive at a time when Western medical intervention was also increasing?

■ Western medical provisions were still limited and often unacceptable because of their links with an alien regime. Indigenous systems were more widespread, were not hindered by cultural obstacles, and, in many cases, were equally effective.

Africa: the 'great campaigns'

The Indian experience of health care between the wars was, however, untypical. Western forms of health care in Africa and other colonies usually remained in the hands of the European authorities, in conjunction with non-governmental organisations (such as the Rockefeller Foundation) sponsoring medical research and the prevention of disease. Such programmes were geared not so much to the health needs of Africans—they usually ignored diseases associated with poverty—but to the economic and medical requirements of the colonial state. According to the historian of Africa, Megan Vaughan:

In the first half of the twentieth century, any contact which the majority of Africans had with colonial medicine was likely to have been in the

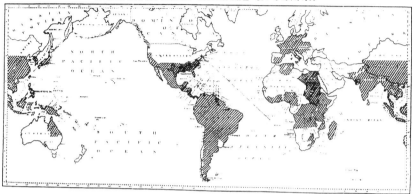

MORE THAN
900,000,000
PEOPLE
Live in hookworm infested areas

THE FIELD OF OPERATION✶
OF THE
ROCKEFELLER FOUNDATION
INTERNATIONAL ✶ HEALTH ✶ COMMISSION

SEVERAL·HUNDRED
MILLION·PEOPLE
Are to day suffering from hookworm disease.

Follow the RED lines to the dark areas in the Tropical Zone belting the Globe
WHERE HOOKWORM DISEASE IS FOUND.

Figure 5.13 *Field of operations of the International Health Commission in 1916. (Courtesy of the Rockefeller Archive Center)*

form of a 'great campaign'. [In these campaigns] Africans were conceived of as an undifferentiated mass, part of a dangerous environment which needed to be controlled and contained. (Vaughan, 1991, pp. 39–40)

Attempts to eradicate diseases such as sleeping sickness could, however, be promoted as acts of imperial beneficence, and used to justify or rationalise European domination. This was particularly true of those regimes, like that of the Belgian Congo, which had been heavily criticised in the British press earlier in the 1900s for its treatment of indigenous peoples.

Similar motivating forces propelled the work of non-governmental organisations such as the *Rockefeller Foundation*. Having begun its work in the United States, the Foundation became increasingly involved, between the wars, in funding overseas medical programmes against so-called *tropical diseases* like hookworm and bilharzia. Figure 5.13 illustrates the vast geographical range of the Rockefeller Foundation's 'medical empire'. The trustees of the Rockefeller Foundation saw Western medicine as a vehicle for American commercial expansion as much as for humanitarian endeavour. It was hoped that medical campaigns in the colonies would present Western culture and capitalism in a good light.

Yet it cannot be denied that these military-style campaigns had some beneficial effect. In her study of sleeping

sickness in the Belgian Congo, Maryinez Lyons records that by 1930 the state medical service had examined 3 million people and had treated 104 000 for sleeping sickness. By 1940, 5 million had been examined, and by 1955 the number had risen to 6.6 million. Since the population of the colony in 1951 was only 11.7 million, Lyons concludes that, from the point of view of organisation at least, the sleeping-sickness campaigns were impressive.

However, like the majority of recent writers on disease in colonial Africa, Lyons maintains that these campaigns were little more than 'justification after the fact' (Lyons, 1988, p. 253), since the problem of epidemic sleeping sickness had itself been created by upheavals caused by colonisation.

Colonial medicine in transition

The great campaigns typified the paternalistic approach which had, until this time, dominated the provision of health care in the majority of European colonies. But, by the 1930s, and in some cases even earlier, there was increasing recognition that health programmes could be made more effective by encouraging the active participation of indigenous peoples.

In the Cook Islands, for instance, the New Zealand government began nurse training programmes for the islanders in 1917, and after World War I, a more ambitious scheme for the training of rural health workers was inaugurated by an American, S. M. Lambert, who was director of the Rockefeller Foundation's health programme in the Pacific. At the same time, in Africa, the colonial state began to employ village headmen as vaccinators and 'sanitary police'. By the 1930s, Africans were far more likely to encounter Western medicine via indigenous personnel than through the 'white doctors' of the Colonial Medical Service. This trend gradually gained pace and underpinned the primary health-care revolution in Third World countries in the 1970s, which will be considered in Chapter 8.

Although the chief objective of medical education in the colonies was to supply subordinate medical staff for missions or government service, there were also limited opportunities to study for a medical degree. In India, indigenous peoples had had access to Western medical education since the 1830s, and a medical career was an attraction second only to law among the new Western-educated elite. After World War I, medical education in India expanded rapidly, and the number of medical graduates per annum rose from 800 in 1905 to over 2 000 by 1934.

However, in British eyes, education in the Indian medical schools was inferior, particularly in midwifery, and in 1924 the *General Medical Council* refused to recognise medical degrees from Indian universities, agreeing to do so only in 1930, after certain reforms had taken place. At the same time, medical education in Britain became an increasingly attractive option for those Indians who could afford it.

Another major development of the inter-war years was the establishment of health programmes focusing specifically on women and children, who had so far benefited little from the health policies of colonial governments. In the years after World War I, in the light of concern over child welfare in Britain, the spotlight came to rest on high levels of maternal and infant mortality in the colonies: a source of growing embarrassment to colonial apologists and a barrier to colonial development.

Initiatives to reach women and children began in India in the mid-1880s, with the establishment of the *Dufferin Fund*, which sought to provide female medical personnel for the treatment of women. As late as the 1930s, according to the *Indian Medical Service* officer Henry Holland, the seclusion of women was still so widely practised that:

> ...rather than allow a man doctor to attend the women of the household, the family would often let a patient die. (Holland, 1958, p. 178)

Treatment usually centred on the dispensary, where women and children were treated as out-patients for eye-diseases, dysentery and diarrhoea, and other ailments that were endemic in many parts of India. But

dispensaries were educational as much as therapeutic institutions, and were the main conduit for Western notions of hygiene, diet and child-care. Where they succeeded in reaching indigenous peoples, such measures undoubtedly had beneficial consequences for the health of women and children, but the underlying causes of ill-health—poverty and malnutrition—were, in this period, seldom addressed.

Malnutrition in the colonies

Research into the physiological effects of malnutrition began in India before World War I by an Indian Medical Service officer, Robert MacCarrison, who first published his research on goitre and *deficiency diseases* in 1921. By the mid-1920s, more general nutritional surveys were being conducted in Africa, first among livestock and then among indigenous peoples.

These investigations, which were primarily concerned with the effects of malnourishment on labour efficiency, eventually led to international recognition of the problem. In 1933, the full Assembly of the *League of Nations* considered a *Report on Nutrition and Public Health* drafted by its Health Organisation, which argued that nutrition ought to be made an integral part of public-health policy. As the historian Michael Worboys has noted, these claims signalled the impending emergence of nutrition as a discipline in its own right.

Many of those associated with this emerging discipline held radical political views, critical of imperialism, and attributed malnutrition to economic inequalities created by colonialism itself. But, as Worboys points out:

> ...the technical dimensions of this problem allowed for this radicalism to be lost as the definition changed from one of inappropriate structures to one of inadequate knowledge.... Colonial malnutrition was rapidly reconstructed from...an epidemic problem to an endemic one, for which colonialism had little responsibility and over which it could exercise little control. (Worboys, 1988a, p. 222–3)

The political dimensions of colonial and post-colonial malnutrition remained submerged until after World War II, when they were again exposed through the efforts of organisations such as OXFAM.

The 1918–48 period, then, brought significant changes in the nature and extent of health-care provision in the colonies, with the increasing participation of indigenous peoples in Western systems of health care, and the growing involvement of philanthropic organisations such as the Rockefeller Foundation. But the intervention of these bodies, and of the colonial state, continued to be motivated largely by self-interest, which meant that many important areas of health remained untouched.

This was particularly the case in relation to malnutrition, where European governments and medical practitioners chose to ignore the economic causes of ill-health. You will recall from earlier in this chapter that in Britain too, the effects of the Depression were underplayed in favour of an emphasis on individual responsibility for health. All this was to change after World War II, as Britain mobilised for total welfare.

OBJECTIVES FOR CHAPTER 5

After studying this chapter, you should be able to:

5.1   Use examples to illustrate the chaotic nature of health services in Britain and their funding in the inter-war years.

5.2   Assess the variety of forms in which lay medical care manifested itself; and the shifts which took place between lay and formal care in this period.

5.3   Describe the changing emphasis of public health in the inter-war years.

5.4   Analyse the tensions and conflicts in the moves towards greater professionalisation among health-care occupations prior to and during World War II.

5.5   Describe the new developments in colonial health care in this period and explain why many fundamental medical problems had still not been addressed.

QUESTIONS FOR CHAPTER 5

Question 1 (*Objective 5.1*)

In 1920, the Central Council on Medical and Administrative Services, chaired by Sir Bertrand Dawson, recommended the 'close coordination' of preventive and curative services and spoke of:

> …the increasing conviction that the best means of maintaining health and curing disease should be made available to all citizens. (Dawson, 1920, p. 3)

What in fact happened to health services and their funding in the inter-war years?

Question 2 (*Objective 5.2*)

Read the following extract from an interview conducted in 1979 with an elderly Englishwoman, Mrs Cooper:

> My father you know, he worked for a licensed vet…he learned a lot…all about these medicines…. He used to send me…to the chemist in Golborne Road, N. Kensington and buy three penn'orth of laudanum, three penn'orth of red lavender and three penn'orth essence of peppermint. Well that was for dysentery, diarrhoea and all that. The neighbours used to come to him for that. (Mrs Cooper, quoted in Berridge, 1979, p. 51)

What does this quotation tell you about lay care and self-medication in the inter-war years? What was happening in general to lay care?

Question 3 (*Objective 5.3*)

How did public health differ in practice and in theory in this period from nineteenth-century public health and what criticisms have been made of the inter-war approach?

Question 4 (*Objective 5.4*)

What problems affected the moves towards greater professionalisation of nursing during this period?

Question 5 (*Objective 5.5*)

In India, wrote R. Palme Dutt, a Marxist critic of British rule:

> …provision for the most elementary needs of public hygiene, sanitation or health is so low, in respect of the working masses in the towns or in the villages, as to be practically non-existent. (Dutt, 1940, p. 79)

From what you have read in this chapter, how justified do you think Dutt was in making this claim, and to what extent might his remarks apply to other colonies between 1918 and 1948?

6

Mobilisation for total welfare, 1948 to 1974

This is the first of the chapters discussing health care in the period since World War II. The first sections of the chapter are much concerned with the British National Health Service. The parts of this chapter describing this vast and complex organisation, eventually employing about 1 million persons, require careful reading. You will need to pay particular attention to the terminology introduced to describe the modern health service. Look ahead to Box 7.1, where the differences in administration between the parts of the United Kingdom are briefly explained. For reasons of simplicity the description of the health service in the present chapter largely refers to England and Wales. This chapter provides the historical background to subjects treated in **Dilemmas in Health Care**. It will also be helpful for you to read again the Reader article by Rosemary Stevens, 'The evolution of the health-care systems in the United States and the United Kingdom: similarities and differences' (first published in 1976).

Welfare capitalism

The return of peace to Western Europe, the inception of political stability, and prolonged and exceptional economic growth, created a contrast with the dismal events that followed World War I. This new expansionist climate was conducive to demands from the underprivileged classes for a more egalitarian social order, and for concessions from the elite. Whether arising from altruism or necessity, wide consensus was achieved for decisive measures to secure economic stability and social harmony. There was broad agreement on basic means to prevent a renewed slide into economic depression and the rebirth of Fascism.

In Britain, the new spirit was epitomised by adoption of the economic principles of John Maynard Keynes and the social programme of William Beveridge, which implied:

- commitment to full employment;

- economic planning; and

- active state investment in industry and welfare.

The world order after World War II was of course strikingly different from the pre-war system. The Soviet bloc adopted its own path to social progress. Western Europe entered into the closest economic, political and military integration with the USA. Paradoxically, owing to more favourable indigenous traditions and appropriateness of existing institutions, welfare regimes developed on a more ambitious scale in Europe than proved practicable in the USA, despite the latter's incomparably greater intrinsic wealth.

As indicated in Chapter 5, the groundwork for more systematic state provision for welfare was laid before World War II, but the final construction was a product of the post-war settlement. Western states varied enormously in the mechanisms employed, but all participated in what Abram de Swaan called 'mobilisation for total welfare'. The period between 1948 and 1974 seemed to witness exponential growth on all fronts. De Swaan concludes that 'after 1945, democratic society everywhere seemed to imply a welfare state' (De Swaan, 1988, pp. 223–4).

The era of the **welfare state** involved action across a wide front, including income protection, housing, economic and urban planning, education and social services. Formal health-care provision constituted one of the prime areas of commitment. Although the services developed took on a vast diversity of forms, they shared certain common features. De Swaan describes the welfare state as a:

> …vast conglomerate of nationwide, compulsory and collective arrangements to remedy and control the external effects of adversity and deficiency. (De Swaan, 1988, p. 218)

Although it would be a mistake to see this development as an expression of unmitigated altruism, the arrival of the welfare state conveyed undoubted benefits to the working classes, as a result of which they became protected from the vagaries of the capitalist system better than ever before. In the rest of this chapter you will see that the positive gains and the dysfunctions of the welfare mechanism are well illustrated by the health services. Although modest in their scale at the outset, the Western health services gradually emerged as one of the most dominant, expensive and indispensable elements in the modern welfare regime.

Health services for all

Between 1945 and 1964, all sixteen countries in Western Europe greatly extended collective responsibility for health care. Most of the services were components of compulsory insurance-based schemes for social security, developed in linear descent from the Prussian social security reforms instigated under Bismarck. Consequently they generally involved connection between payments and benefits, and organisation on a decentralised and highly bureaucratic basis. Of the European schemes, that in Sweden approximated most closely to the United Kingdom model, but its universal scheme was not established until 1955. Even then the range of services was less comprehensive and it involved a higher level of direct payments from patients.

It is notoriously difficult to draw definitive conclusions about the performance of the rival systems of health care in Europe. However, it is safe to say that the British system was one of the most generous in its basic design. On the other hand, the NHS possessed intrinsic weaknesses that have never been effectively corrected and which, when combined with relative resource starvation, have prevented the British health service from fulfilling the high ambitions of its architects.

The NHS introduced in Britain by the post-war Labour government was an ambitious conception. However, the initiators of the NHS were only dimly aware of the nature of the commitments into which they were entering. Speculations concerning the likely *cost* of the health service expressed at the outset represented a spectrum of opinions which find their modern counterparts. The Labour Cabinet and the civil servants thought that the new service would involve *cosmetic* adjustments of the inherited system. Beveridge subscribed to the somewhat naive, but widespread fallacy, that the health service

might constitute a *diminishing* drain on public funds as the service progressively cleared up avoidable problems of ill-health within the workforce.

However, Aneurin Bevan, as the Minister responsible for the new health service in England and Wales, was in no doubt that the nation was embarking on an expensive venture, on account of previous underfunding, a great backlog of untreated conditions, and massive prospective liabilities associated with rising expectations, an ageing population, and the high cost of medical innovation. Taking Bevan's argument to an absurd extreme, critics of the NHS argued that the government had unleashed uncontrollable demand for health care, which would result in escalation in costs, economic ruin and political dislocation. Such polemicists as Dr Frangcon Roberts argued that the 'Welfare State will surely end in the Totalitarian State' (Roberts, 1952, p. 193).

With respect to its formal commitments, the new health service decisively turned its back on the multitude of limitations and discriminations inherent in the previous system. From the outset it was determined that the service should be universal and comprehensive:

> The proposed service must be 'comprehensive' in two senses—first that it is available to all people and second, that it covers all necessary forms of health care. (Ministry of Health, 1944, p. 9)

☐ In what ways was the NHS improving on NHI in its coverage and range of services?

■ The NHS was universal, whereas NHI was effectively confined to manual wage earners and provided no coverage for dependants. NHI provided for GP care but not for specialist or hospital services.

The NHS made available for the first time—to the whole population—treatment for defects of teeth, eyes and hearing. Indeed the most publicised aspect of the early NHS was the massive supply of dentures, spectacles and hearing aids. By this means the NHS contributed significantly to transforming the quality of life of elderly people.

Aneurin Bevan was committed to making a decisive break with the ethos of services associated with charity, means-testing and the Poor Law. The new service was therefore completely free of *direct charges* to patients, and designed to provide the highest quality of care, what he called 'universalising the best'. He was conscious that the nation was embarking on 'the biggest single experiment in social service that the world has ever seen undertaken' (quoted in Webster, 1991, p. 140). The enlightened ethos of the new health service is indicated by the text of the introductory leaflet shown in Figure 6.1.

The New
NATIONAL
HEALTH
SERVICE

•

Your new National Health Service begins on 5th July. What is it? How do you get it?

It will provide you with all medical, dental, and nursing care. Everyone—rich or poor, man, woman or child—can use it or any part of it. There are no charges, except for a few special items. There are no insurance qualifications. But it is not a "charity." You are all paying for it, mainly as taxpayers, and it will relieve your money worries in time of illness.

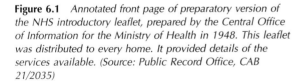

Figure 6.1 *Annotated front page of preparatory version of the NHS introductory leaflet, prepared by the Central Office of Information for the Ministry of Health in 1948. This leaflet was distributed to every home. It provided details of the services available. (Source: Public Record Office, CAB 21/2035)*

Containing the cost of services

In the event, even in the expansionist atmosphere of the post-war decades, it proved impossible to summon the political will to commit resources on anything like the scale required to fulfil Bevan's remit for the NHS. After a

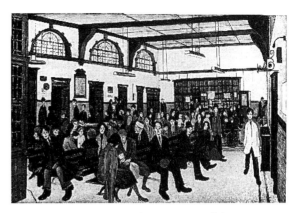

Figure 6.2 Ancoats Hospital Out-Patient Hall *by L. S. Lowry (1952). Situated in north-west Manchester, the Ancoats Hospital was built in the 1870s with money raised by voluntary donations and bequests. Nationalised in 1948, it continued as a general hospital in the NHS until 1982, when it was converted for use as a specialised orthopaedic unit. (Source: Whitworth Art Gallery, University of Manchester)*

hesitant start, the Labour government pegged down NHS expenditure, imposed direct charges for spectacles and dentures, and prepared the ground for the prescription charge. Thereafter, both Conservative and Labour governments gradually expanded these charges.[1] Until 1960, NHS expenditure was rigidly contained, to the extent that its share of GNP actually *fell*—so contradicting the apocalyptic forecasts of critics like Roberts. The low cost of the NHS was independently confirmed by an interdepartmental committee established by the Conservative government (HMSO, 1956; the 'Guillebaud Report').

Eventually the imposition of a severe regime of economy on the NHS proved untenable. By 1960, political embarrassment was being caused by such factors as long waiting lists, the slow pace of improvement of services, and the antiquated state of hospital buildings. The backwardness of the health service was also evident in the light of obvious comparisons with the rapidly expanding educational sector, or against health services in other Western states. The dreary, overcrowded atmosphere of the typical out-patient department (Figure 6.2) shows that in reality the NHS was slow to adjust to the best modern practices and rising expectations.

[1]The proportion of total cost of the NHS raised by charges to patients between 1950 and 1990, under successive governments, is discussed in *Dilemmas in Health Care*, Chapter 3.

The evident shortcomings of the NHS led to unavoidable pressures for increased expenditure, as a result of which the NHS share of GNP rose from 3.8 per cent to 5.7 per cent between 1960 and 1975. This boost reflected sporadic responses to crises by both Conservative and Labour governments. Modest increments in expenditure allowed the launching of urgently-needed initiatives, the most expensive being the *Hospital Plan*, the large hospital rebuilding programme launched in 1962.

From the outset, the main priority was establishing a comprehensive specialist service, and the resources of the NHS were heavily concentrated on this task. The scale of this undertaking is described by Sir George Godber, one of the chief planners of the system:

The result...was an immediate and large increase in the amount of specialist time available, especially in hospital centres outside the large cities. By the end of 1949 there had been a substantial increase and the equivalent of the whole-time three and a half thousand consultants was provided by the five and a half thousand individuals available in England and Wales. This process was to continue and by the end of 1970 there was two and a half times as much consultant time and double the number of medical staff in all grades. In the same period the number of nursing staff including the number of trained nurses doubled; the hospital professional and technical staff, other than doctors and nurses, increased more than two and a half times and included many new technologies and skills.

General medicine and general surgery were the largest medical specialties in 1948 but increased little after the first few years while other specialties were established and grew rapidly. Neurosurgery, thoracic surgery, and plastic surgery which had been established in a few centres were quickly provided by the Health Service in every region. Regional radio-therapy services separate from diagnostic radiology were established. The deficiencies in pathology and diagnostic radiology had been exposed by wartime needs and partly remedied, but needed expansion and re-equipment. Anaesthesiology developed rapidly into the largest specialty followed by pathology and psychiatry. The increase in consultants was

thus not only in numbers, but much more importantly in range of expertise. Geriatrics and child psychiatry developed from almost nothing; urological and cardiological units were established at least in main centres, pathology became subdivided; orthopaedic surgery became predominantly concerned with repair of trauma and defects at birth or of ageing. But rheumatology and rehabilitation were often neglected. (Godber, 1975, pp. 27–8)

It was a massive and genuine achievement to make available the most advanced diagnostic and treatment facilities for the entire population. However, because of the shortage of resources the **acute hospital sector** (i.e. catering for short-stay patients suitable for immediate treatment, including maternity care) was developed at the expense of everything else.

Given the revolution in the capacities of high-technology medicine from the mid-century onwards, it is understandable that the new health service should place the first emphasis on specialist and acute hospital services. There was an urgent need to bring Britain's old-fashioned and under-resourced hospitals up to the standards existing elsewhere in the advanced economies, modernise the conditions of employment of hospital doctors, and remove obstacles of access to patients.

The aim was to provide such basic functions as safer and effective accident and emergency services, properly equipped operating theatres, X-ray and pathological laboratory diagnostic facilities, and a comprehensive blood transfusion service. There was also increasing demand for hospital childbirth. The acute services were also politically the easier priority because hospitals were under direct state control. This also met the expectations of the public, who were inundated with media publicity about advances in hospital medicine.

The acute services absorbed the increasing resources made available to the NHS in the 1960s. Also they took up an increasing slice of the total expenditure, as Table 6.1 shows.

□ Examine Table 6.1 for evidence of gains and losses in the competition for NHS resources between 1949–50 and 1964–5.

■ The hospitals enjoyed a 13 per cent increase at the expense of general medical, dental and ophthalmic services. The great majority of the increased spending was on current expenditure, i.e. the cost of running the hospitals.

Table 6.1 Comparison of the percentage expenditure on parts of the NHS financed by central government in 1949–50 and 1964–5

	1949–50	1964–5
Hospitals		
current	49.6	58.5
capital	2.3	6.7
(subtotal)	(51.9)	(65.2)
Executive Council Services		
general medical	10.6	8.5
pharmaceutical	7.8	12.0
general dental	10.9	6.2
general ophthalmic	5.6	1.8
(subtotal)	(34.9)	(28.5)
other	13.2	6.3
total	**100.0**	**100.0**

Data from C. Webster, previously unpublished, based on Treasury data.

You will notice from Table 6.1 that spending on new buildings and refurbishment of hospitals (capital expenditure) was always at a low level in the first fifteen years of the NHS, but this Table indicates a small increase in 1964–5, which marks the beginning of implementation of the Hospital Plan. Between 1965 and 1975, the gathering pace of hospital development was responsible for further reducing the share of NHS resources devoted to the family practitioner services administered by Executive Councils, which today we would refer to collectively as *primary health care*. You will find in Chapter 7 that the above trend was reversed in the 1980s.

The pattern of expenditure recorded in Table 6.1 contributes to the view that primary health care, community, preventive and health promotion services were cut off from the mainstream of advance concentrated in the acute hospital sector of the NHS. From the outset the NHS failed to capitalise on the potentialities of preventive and primary care, a defect which has never subsequently been completely corrected.

Barriers to coordinated services

In principle, under the NHS, GPs treated all members of the family on an equal basis and gave access to modern drugs. However, the majority of patients were seen by over-stretched and doubtfully competent GPs, working from poorly equipped and inadequate accommodation, a situation little different from pre-NHS practice described in Chapter 5.

During the first two decades of the NHS there was no specific training for general practice in medical schools and no systematic post-graduate education. Older GPs were therefore increasingly out of touch with developments in chemotherapy and diagnosis, and they were not likely to be informed about new approaches to such problems as psychosomatic illness, alcohol and drug abuse or tobacco addiction.

An expert on health administration, Gordon Forsyth, noted the static character of general practice:

> In terms of organisation, there has been undoubtedly no change as a result of the NHS. Admittedly, partnerships have been encouraged by financial incentives; but many partnerships are financial fictions, not operational realities.... We still talk about coordinating the family doctor with the district nurse, the health visitor and the social worker, but we have failed to provide the institutional framework within which these services might be coordinated. The Health Centres never materialised. The family doctor is still the independent self-employed entrepreneur that he was in the 19th century. (Forsyth, 1963, p. 10)

☐ Examine Figure 6.3 (*overleaf*) and consider ways in which the *actual* organisation of the NHS provided the barriers to coordination mentioned by Gordon Forsyth.

■ You will notice especially that *health centres* were supposed to provide the coordinating link between services administered by Executive Councils and those provided by the local authorities. Abandonment of the health-centre plan severed the vital connection between the GP and community services.

Later in this chapter, you will find out more about changes within general practice. First we consider the hospitals inherited by the NHS. Not all the hospitals shared in the advances experienced in the acute sector. The worst defects of the NHS were hidden from sight in the vast conglomeration of asylums, mental deficiency institutions, and workhouse infirmaries taken over by the NHS and converted into mental hospitals, mental handicap[2] hospitals, and geriatric hospitals (all parts of the

[2]The term 'mental handicap' was commonly used during the period covered by this chapter. It has since been replaced in literature from more enlightened sources by less-pejorative terms such as 'learning difficulties' or 'learning disabilities'.

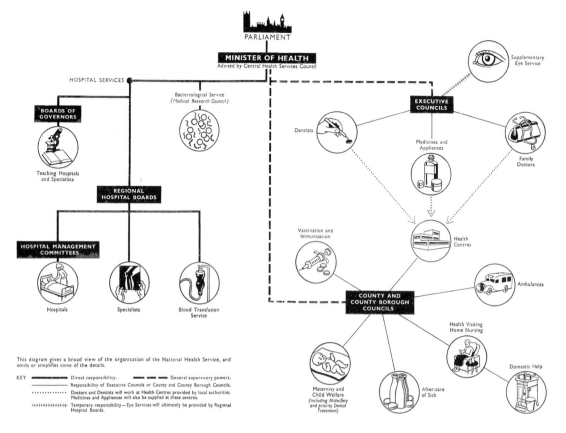

Figure 6.3 *Diagram of the intended inter-relationship of services in the NHS in 1948, taken from a pamphlet,* The National Health Service, *published by the Central Office of Information at the time. (Source: Ministry of Health and Central Office of Information)*

chronic sector). In 1948, these institutions housed about 300 000 patients and constituted more than half of the bed capacity of the NHS. With good reason these services became known as the *Cinderella* of the health service.[3]

This massive sector lapsed into a neglected backwater until a series of public scandals erupted in the 1960s. An extract from one of the more restrained reviews of the problem gives an insight into the true horror of the situation.

> A very great number of elderly people sit waiting for death in mental hospitals where they have no business to be. They are there because the mental hospitals are being used as a

dumping ground for the elderly, whose mental problems are caused by untreated physical illness. The mental hospital staff cannot possibly give them proper care, let alone rehabilitate them. There are not enough staff, not enough money, no facilities. The buildings in which they are expected to work are shameful. We cannot dodge the accusation that we, as an advanced and civilized country are treating a very great number of our old people in a manner that is far worse than merely barbarous. (Editorial in the *Nursing Times,* 10 June 1966)

Pressure for reorganisation

It was increasingly realised that the problems of the NHS could not be entirely solved by higher expenditure. The structure of its administration came under increasingly

[3]Plans to redistribute funds to the 'Cinderella' services in the 1970s are discussed in *Dilemmas in Health Care,* Chapter 3.

critical scrutiny. No sooner was the ink dry on the 1946 NHS legislation than the question of *reorganisation* of the health services emerged, and it soon joined expenditure as the major policy obsession. Reorganisation was expected to bring about greater harmony, unity and cooperation, thereby unlocking gains in efficiency.

Although presented as the result of deliberate planning, the original administrative structure adopted for the NHS was an untidy compromise (for reasons indicated in Chapter 5), designed to reconcile a wide variety of conflicting groups. These demands forced the government to abandon its scheme for a *unified* service. Instead a divided service was adopted, involving three entirely different forms of administration:

- that dealing with hospitals (the Regional Hospital Boards and Boards of Governors);

- local government services, administered by County and County Borough Councils; and

- family practitioner services, administered by Executive Councils.

This came to be called the **tripartite system**, based on the accidental parallel with the post-war tripartite system of secondary education. The system was further complicated by lack of uniformity between the parts of the United Kingdom (which are signified in Box 7.1 in the next chapter). You have already examined the contemporary representation of the complex 1948 structure given in Figure 6.3. Apart from changes in terminology, local government and family practitioner services represented continuations of pre-NHS administration, except that local government was stripped of its hospital responsibilities.

The real innovation in the Labour government's scheme was the *nationalisation* of all hospitals, and the creation of a new form of *regional* hospital administration with Hospital Management Committees at the periphery. However, although *teaching* hospitals in England and Wales were nationalised along with the rest, they each retained independent management, outside the regional structure. This represented a concession to the voluntary hospital tradition and it anticipated the formation of self-governing NHS Trusts in the 1990s.

The new system was therefore a failure as an exercise in unification, simplification and rationalisation. In England and Wales alone there were more than 400 hospital authorities and a total of about 700 (and in Scotland 170) administrative authorities involved in the health service. Arrangements for cooperation worked badly, even within the hospital service. In certain respects the NHS constituted a step back from the degree of coordination obtaining in the larger local authorities before 1948. Coordination and efficiency were impaired and there was no mechanism for decisively improving the situation.

Although the existing system was universally accepted as detrimental to the best interest of patients, there was a reticence to displace the delicate balance achieved by the 1948 compromise arrangements. However, the many illogicalities and inefficiencies of the system suggested that reorganisation was unavoidable.

☐ Again examine Figure 6.3. Indicate the separate authorities responsible for providing care in an imaginary provincial town in England and Wales possessing a medical school.

■ The Hospital Management Committee of the Regional Hospital Board would provide general hospital services; the Board of Governors would supply more specialist teaching-hospital services; the Executive Council would superintend the family practitioners (the GPs, pharmacists, dentists and opticians); and finally the County Borough Council would provide a miscellaneous range of preventive and community services.

Planners were faced with two alternatives for improving the organisation of services. One idea was unification of the health services under local government, a possibility enhanced by the imminence of local government reform. However, this arrangement was unacceptable to the medical profession, and was against the trend of events. The alternative was unification under expanded hospital authorities, continuing the trend begun in 1948.

During the 1960s, pressures from all sides mounted for reform and the prospect emerged of a radical simplification of the existing service—perhaps unifying all health and personal social services under as few as 40 new area health authorities in England and Wales. A Green Paper making this suggestion was issued by the Labour government in July 1968, shortly before the Ministry of Health was amalgamated with the Ministry of Social Security to form the *Department of Health and Social Security* (DHSS). There was then a delay before the second Green Paper of February 1970. Further delay was occasioned by a change in government. The Conservative consultative process then began in May 1971 and was concluded with the reorganisation which took effect in 1973 in Northern Ireland and in April 1974 in the rest of the United Kingdom.

As you will see in Chapter 7, any expectation that this reorganisation would bring about unification, simplification, efficiency or economy was rapidly dispelled.

Lay care and the welfare state

The coming of the NHS in 1948 and increased access to formal medical services for women could have dispensed with the role of lay care. But the situation in the post-war years, which is discussed in this chapter and in Chapter 7, turned out to be rather different.

Community care with health service support

Lay care, defined as care by *informal family networks*, became entwined with the concept of **community care**. This concept became a prominent policy goal of governments of both the main political parties after World War II. But despite widespread agreement about the necessity for 'community' rather than institutional care, no consistent meaning has been applied to the term. The social policy analyst, Alan Walker, has commented that the attractiveness of the term 'community care' owes much to its manipulation to encompass the widest possible range of constructions—it is all things to all politicians and policy makers.[4]

Community care, so far as it can be defined, developed a number of broad and interrelated strands, some of which have implications for lay care. Care in the community could be provided formally or informally. It is thus possible to distinguish between formally-organised care given primarily by health and personal social services, formal and quasi-formal care by voluntary organisations; and informal care by neighbours, friends and kinship networks. The concept has also been taken to mean different things at different times and in relation to different groups in need. Many of the terms used in this chapter (and Chapter 7) for people who provide community care, are euphemisms for 'women'. As you will see, the development of community-care provision has taken for granted women's role as 'natural carers'.

Behind the development of community-care policies lay a post-war change in the age-structure of the population. On the one hand, the birth rate was lower and the children that were born were healthier. But there was also a huge growth in the proportion of elderly

people in the population.[5] The numbers of elderly people had been growing rapidly between the wars as well, but the potential scale of their demand on the contemporary welfare system had been disguised by the crisis over unemployment during the Depression.

When Seebohm Rowntree conducted his first survey of York, published in 1901, the proportion of the British population aged 65 and over stood at 4.7 per cent. In his 80s, he returned to the town in 1951 to make a last survey. The proportion of the population over 65 was then 11 per cent and rising. Rowntree found that the elderly population dominated his tables: old age accounted for 68 per cent of the causes of poverty, with sickness the next largest category at 21 per cent; unemployment failed to register at all (Vincent, 1991, p. 135).

The initial concern of government was with questions of labour shortage, in particular the shortage of skilled labour. From the mid-1950s, in an attempt to maximise the available workforce, the Ministry of Labour launched a vigorous and unprecedented campaign to create a positive image of the older person (those in their later 60s). But the campaign was an entire failure. Since the late nineteenth century, the proportion of the workforce who retired in their mid-60s had been gradually increasing, and in the post-war period this trend accelerated.

The age-structure of the elderly population had implications for patterns of care. The rising numbers of elderly people—and in particular those in their 70s and 80s—added to the build-up of pressure in the **chronic hospital sector** (the long-stay wards and institutions). Proposals for community care of the elderly population were developed: in 1958, the Minister of Health stated that:

> ...the underlying principle of our services for the old should be this: that the best place for old people is in their own homes, with help from the home services if need be. (Quoted in Townsend, 1962, p. 196)

The same policy was also developed in the field of mental health and the *Royal Commission on Mental Illness* in 1957 recommended a shift in emphasis from hospital to community care for people diagnosed as mentally ill and mentally handicapped. This was also one of the first uses of the term 'community care' in the official literature.

---

[4]Community care in the 1990s, particularly for elderly people, is discussed further in *Dilemmas in Health Care*, Chapter 8.

[5]Demographic trends in the age of the population of the United Kingdom are described in *World Health and Disease*, Chapter 2 and the effects of an ageing population on disease patterns are discussed in Chapter 6.

The principles of community care in policy statements in the immediate post-war period can be summarised as:

- ensuring individuals remained integrated with their families and neighbours;

- a pattern of non-institutional care; and

- the provision of support in the home from a wide range of services.

In theory, the structure of health services at the local level and in particular the local-authority-based *domiciliary services*, was sufficient to achieve this aim. But, as you saw earlier, coordination within the fragmented tripartite structure of the NHS was poor.

The idea of *domiciliary teams* comprising a range of health-related occupations was widely discussed in the 1950s. The work of home nurses, home helps, health visitors (who were beginning to work to an increasing extent with elderly people) and social workers, as well as the 'meals-on-wheels' service undertaken largely by voluntary agencies, were seen as important in maintaining elderly people in their homes. But these services were generally inadequate and their extension insufficient to meet the needs of the ageing population. The home-help service, for example, which was recommended but not obligatory under the 1946 NHS Act, remained small in relation to the size of its client groups. Inevitably, lay carers (usually women) filled the gap.

In the 1950s and 1960s, 'community care' was also redefined to encompass **residential care** in the community. Local authorities developed the more traditional alternative of building residential homes for elderly people. By 1960, such residential accommodation housed a total of 84 000 persons, including 39 000 in homes opened since 1948. Residential homes were provided mostly for elderly people, but a small number of homes were given over to handicapped people and other groups. Residential homes of the model type containing places for about 60 residents received much publicity. Community care became what the sociologist Philip Abrams called *community treatment*.

Peter Townsend, a sociologist, questioned the whole philosophy of this development in his book *The Last Refuge: A Survey of Residential Institutions and Homes for the Aged*, which was published in 1962. In his view, the expansion of residential homes was an illustration of the absence of clear policy and detailed planning around the concept of community care.

Coordination between separate services quickly became a dominant policy theme and this, rather than the expansion of domiciliary services and the closure of institutions, became the primary goal of community-care policy. Policy was, however, ambiguous. In the White Paper, *Better Services for the Mentally Handicapped* (DHSS, 1971) it was argued that the services in need of greatest expansion included residential homes for children and adults, and a target increase of 15 per cent was set for the number of mentally handicapped persons in residential care. But planning forecasts for domiciliary services were completely omitted.

It was only in relation to elderly people that the need to support families caring for dependants, and for shared responsibility between the family and domiciliary services, was recognised. Initially, in this period, lay care was not given the dominant role in community care which it came to occupy later.

Lay care and family life

The tendency in other areas of health care, most obviously childbirth, was for the formal health service to exclude the lay carer. The pre-war trend towards the increased *hospitalisation of childbirth* continued and accelerated in the 1950s and 1960s. In 1927, 85 per cent of births were at home; in 1961, this had fallen to 32 per cent; and in 1980, only 1.3 per cent of confinements took place there. And within the hospital, the extent to which women gave birth without intervention from a doctor or midwife also changed, as Table 6.2 (*overleaf*) shows.

☐ Looking at Table 6.2, what developments do you notice in childbirth in the immediate post-war period, and in the 1960s and 1970s?

■ In the 1950s, the number of medical interventions in the process of birth increased only slightly, but in the 1960s and 1970s they rose much more quickly: overall, the rate of Caesarean sections and instrumental deliveries more than trebled, and two new interventions (induction and episiotomy) became commonplace.

However, family support and advice on health matters continued to play a major role in working-class lives. In the mid-1950s, two sociologists, Michael Young and Peter Willmott of the Institute of Community Studies, spent three years on 'field work', observing working-class family life in Bethnal Green and a new housing estate, Greenleigh, where many of the families were rehoused during this period. In what has become a classic study, they demonstrated the continuing role of family involvement in childbirth and child health. Mrs Banton, for example:

Table 6.2 Trends in obstetric intervention, England and Wales, 1953–78

| Year | Estimated percentage of all deliveries in England and Wales[1] | | | |
	Induction of labour or artificial rupture of membranes	Caesarean section	Instrumental delivery[2]	Episiotomy[3]
1953	–	2.2	3.7	–
1958	–	2.3	4.4	–
1963	8.9	3.1	5.3	–
1968	18.0	4.0	7.9	–
1973	34.9	5.0	11.0	44.0
1978	36.3	7.3	13.3	53.4

[1]Includes women resident outside England and Wales. [2]Forceps or vacuum extraction. [3]A small cut made to enlarge the vaginal opening. (Data from MacFarlane, A. and Mugford, M., 1984, *Birth Counts: Statistics of Pregnancy and Childbirth*, HMSO, London, p. 575, Table A7.32(a))

I take more notice of my mum than I do of the welfare. She's had eight and we're alright. Experience speaks for itself, more or less, doesn't it? If you're living near your mother, you don't really need that advice. You've got more confidence in your mother than you would have in the advice they'd give you.... (Young and Willmott, 1962, pp. 53–4)

Lay diagnosis and treatment outside the professional medical sector remained important throughout this period. A 1950s study of a working-class housing estate found two-thirds of the people interviewed were taking some self-prescribed medication, often in addition to a prescribed drug. Laxatives and aspirins were most commonly self-prescribed (quoted in Helman, 1990, pp. 72–3). At the end of the 1960s, the same pattern was evident. A major study was undertaken in 1969 by two sociologists, Karen Dunnell and Ann Cartwright, who found that 80 per cent of a large sample of the population drawn from across the country said that they had taken some medicine in the two weeks prior to the interview. Self-prescribed medicines—aspirin again and tonics, skin preparations and antacids—outnumbered those prescribed by doctors by two to one.

At the end of the 1960s, then, lay care both in terms of informal care and assistance and in terms of non-professional advice and self-medication, was thriving. This was despite the advent of a formal welfare state which, at least in theory, could have superseded it. In the 1970s and 1980s, however (see Chapter 7), lay care assumed a new and growing importance as the foundation of government community-care policies.

The changing division of work in health care

Bevan's nationalisation of the hospitals in 1948 had been facilitated by the support of the influential hospital consultants. The voluntary hospital consultants and the leaders of the medical profession were well pleased with the 1948 settlement, which gave them security, prestige and high remuneration, while also permitting the continuation of private practice. In the post-war period, the process of incorporation of the profession as a whole in the structure of decision-making by the state continued and expanded. But there were also changes within the medical profession.

The division of labour, relative role and status of hospital doctors and GPs changed; there were boundary shifts between doctors and nurses, and between nursing and ancillary workers within hospitals. The 1980s have been associated with the rise of 'managerialism' in health administration but, as you will see, this is a tendency that had its origins in the 1960s. Management, so it has been argued, has replaced the power of doctors in the health service and health policy-making. Whether that is the case still remains to be seen.

Working in hospitals

The status and areas of competence of the hospital-based occupations underwent significant change. As you will see in Chapter 7, the successive reorganisations of the NHS and management changes between 1974 and the present have altered relations between categories of workers, and nowhere more so than in the hospital service.

Initially, as the sociologist Margaret Stacey has commented, the NHS was composed of three occupational hierarchies; medical, nursing and administrative. Nursing served medicine and administration facilitated the services of both doctors and nurses. Hospital doctors were at the top of the power structure, but both nurses and administrators had some areas of control. The alternative power base of the matron in a hospital, in charge of all nursing services, was considerable.

The general tendency since the 1960s has been to seek *organisational* solutions to problems of health service costs and control. The application of the managerial ethos led to changes in the distribution of power between the three hierarchies. Nursing was the first to be affected.[6] The 1966 Salmon Report led to a new managerial structure for nursing, by which managerial grades were instituted above the ward sister and superseded the hospital matron. The work of nurses employed by local authorities was reorganised on similar lines. The Salmon Report greatly increased the hierarchy of management in nursing.

Moreover, the Salmon reorganisation effectively blocked career opportunities in *clinical* nursing; the only route to upward mobility for a nurse was to leave the bedside and take a management post. The new structure had the effect of further dividing nurse leaders from the great bulk of the nursing rank and file. At that level there was increasing militancy and unionisation from the 1960s onwards, as government efforts at cost containment focused on nursing salaries, the largest sector of the health-care budget.

At the same time, within hospitals, what was termed *functional management* was introduced (i.e. an appraisal of the functions that different occupational groups carried out, which led in some cases to reallocation of tasks and responsibilities). Nurses became more conscious of the distinction between direct *nursing* care of patients and other commonly undertaken duties which came to be seen as outside nursing; for example, domestic services were separated out from nursing, and laundry was organised on an area basis.

The progressive dilution of nursing by the development of lower-level staff to carry out less technical aspects of care continued with the unplanned growth of the *nursing auxiliary* in the 1950s and 1960s. By 1958, these unqualified nurses in general hospitals exceeded registered nurses by 50 per cent. The registered nurses'

[6]Strategies for increasing the status of nursing in the 1990s are discussed in *Dilemmas in Health Care*, Chapter 6.

hostility to their use was consistent. Nurses have been criticised for the elitism that this hostility invoked. For example, Robert Dingwall, a medical sociologist who has studied the nursing profession, complained that:

> The obstruction of more systematic training and a properly defined role for auxiliaries under the supervision of registered nurses merely denied patients such benefits as more skilful practical carers could have brought them. (Dingwall, *et al.*, 1988, p. 116)

Proliferation of occupations

The use of auxiliaries underlined a more general development in this period—the increased number of divisions in health labour. In general, the range of non-medical workers, scientists, technicians and workers in the para-medical professions expanded in the post-war period. By 1960, all the para-medical professions had achieved state registration (the opticians through a 1958 Act and the remainder through the Professions Supplementary to Medicine Act of 1960). Some commentators thought this marked an 'end to medical hegemony'. But there were also powerful arguments against this point of view. Not all changes went against doctors.

Changes in obstetric practice and the moves from home to hospital-based childbirth reduced the status of midwifery. Gender divisions between female midwives and (largely male) doctors complicated questions of division of labour. The sociologist Gerald Larkin, in his analysis of the relationship between medicine and para-medical occupations, argues that recognition of para-medical skills did not imply a dilution of medical hegemony; it was a matter of redrawing the boundaries without equalising all the parties. At the end of the 1960s little had yet effectively challenged overall medical dominance.

The general practitioner: decline and revival

Consultants may have been satisfied with the 1948 settlement, but for GPs the situation was much less clear cut. GPs had fought off the threat of a whole-time, salaried service and retained their status as 'independent contractors', i.e. each practitioner acted as an independent small contracting business. But the process of exclusion from hospitals continued.

GPs had been partially excluded from major hospitals in the inter-war years. The NHS made this process more absolute by forcing a choice between a general practice or a hospital career, and by placing what one commentator called an 'antiseptic barrier' between the two branches of the profession. Obstetrics remained a battleground where GPs retained some rights to hospital access and care of their patients; but, in general, few GPs found a role in hospitals in the post-war decades.

This was in sharp contrast to the American system of health care, where many GPs passed completely into the specialist category and the boundaries between hospital and general practice were much less clear-cut. Think back to the Reader article by Rosemary Stevens that you read during your study of Chapter 4.[7]

□ What reasons does Stevens give for the different patterns of development of the professions in health-care systems in Britain and the USA?

■ Stevens places emphasis on the systems of checks and balances which emerged from the pre-specialisation era in Britain. The old social division between branches of practice have continued in the separate functions of primary and secondary care. In the USA, in contrast, there were no medical guilds; no national focus for an elite; and, until the 1870s, relatively few hospitals.

In Britain, the status of the post-war GP was in decline and their image was fusty and old-fashioned (see Figure 6.4). Access to the new laboratory-based diagnostic techniques remained under the control of hospital specialists; GPs were not allowed to use them until the 1960s. Loss of hospital work had severely reduced the status of GPs, who had seen their exercise of surgical skills as conferring prestige. Above all, they were overwhelmed, so it seemed to them, by trivia. One GP interviewed by the sociologist Ann Cartwright in 1964, complained:

> We're swamped with trivialities. This isn't the sort of work one spent years at university preparing oneself for. There's the utter futility and humiliation of a professional man who feels his training is wasted. The GP has no status because he doesn't do medicine. (Quoted in Tudor Hart, 1988, p. 85)

Few medical students in the 1960s actively wanted to be GPs. In 1968, the Royal Commission on Medical Education found that only 23 per cent of final year medical students favoured a career in general practice, but 50 per cent ended up there, having failed as hospital trainees.

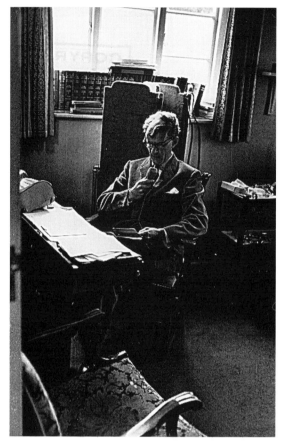

Figure 6.4 *The British GP of the 1950s typically worked alone from a private house, usually his (rarely her) own home. Secretarial help in record-keeping and booking house calls was often provided by the GP's wife. Contrast this with Figure 7.6. (Source: Jean Mohr)*

After a hesitant beginning, the GP has in fact gained new status and power under the NHS. How did this come about? Two factors need to be stressed. A new vision of general practice emerged from doctors themselves; and general practice became an important 'front-line' health service to governments who were increasingly conscious of the costs of a hospital-dominated service.

The internal rejuvenation of general practice was inspired by what Margot Jefferys and Hessie Sachs, in *Rethinking General Practice* (1983), have called the 're-habilitation of trivia'. The GP's importance as a friend, guide and counsellor began to be stressed. In 1950, the newly formed section of general practice of the Royal Society of Medicine held a discussion on 'what is general practice?' It concluded:

[7]Stevens, R. 'The evolution of the health-care systems in the United States and the United Kingdom: similarities and differences', in *Health and Disease: A Reader.*

The essence of general practice is to live amongst your patients as a definite cog in the whole machine, knowing them so well both in health and in sickness, and from birth until death. (Quoted in Armstrong, 1983, p. 80)

☐ This quotation describes the 'new conception' of the family doctor. Think back over the development of general practice described in Chapters 4–6; how have the GPs' functions changed over time?

■ In the nineteenth century, the GP could also have undertaken some salaried work, such as Medical Officer to a friendly society or Poor Law Medical Officer. In the inter-war period, some ran their own cottage hospitals. In the post-war period, they lost hospital access, but gained a wider role in the community.

The history of general practice was reconstructed to promote a vision of a distant era in which deep insight into the family life and character of patients was the very essence of good practice; the idea of the 'family doctor' was revived. The work of Michael Balint and his book *The Doctor, His Patient and the Illness* (1956) provided GPs with a holistic model of medical practice which refuted the mind/body dichotomy of much of hospital medicine. The influence of Balint, in particular among GPs active in the newly established *College of General Practitioners* (founded in 1952), was enormous.[8] John Horder, later its President, describing the work of Balint, claimed he had taught GPs that:

> …since every patient is unique, diagnosis must be like biography and is inseparable from treatment. (Quoted in Armstrong, 1983, p. 81)

To this internal rethinking of the role of the GP was added a concern for general practice in the government health departments in the late 1960s. The continued viability of general practice came to be seen as essential to contain mounting health-care costs, and strategies were instituted to revive it. The main elements were contained in the *Family Doctor's Charter* of 1966, agreed by the government and the General Medical Services Committee of the BMA, representing GPs.

Doctors were to work in common premises, and to employ support staff. They were encouraged to use hospital diagnostic services and to have opportunities to

refresh their professional expertise with funding from their postgraduate education allowance. The attachment of other health workers to general practices was encouraged; GPs were to be 'king pins in a hierarchy of dependent occupations' (Jefferys and Sachs, 1983, p. 326). The idea of *health centres*, dormant since their post-war failure, revived in the 1960s in response to enthusiasm from GPs.

Regular training posts for doctors entering general practice and a qualifying examination were instituted. The non-specialist role of the GP was then accordingly reconstituted as a form of specialism. The boundaries between hospital and general practice changed as a result; GPs clawed back some of the medical work from hospitals, in particular through the moves to community care discussed earlier and to which we return later in the chapter. The GP became an established and important part of the panoply of community health and welfare services.

Public-health doctors: loss of an empire

With the establishment of the NHS in 1948, the primary role of public-health doctors in hospital administration was abandoned. Although local-authority control of all health services had originally been Labour Party policy, Bevan secured the nationalisation of the hospitals as a condition for the acquiescence of consultants in the fledgling service. The voluntary hospital system became the dominant model for the rest of the hospital service. At a stroke, public-health doctors lost the hospital empires that they had built up in the inter-war decades.

Local authorities were left with substantially reduced responsibilities for a range of services—maternal and child welfare, midwifery, health visiting, home nursing, home helps and so on. Public-health doctors were gloomy and despondent about their role in the new service. But, as historian Jane Lewis has commented, they bore some responsibility for the outcome in 1948. Their vision of public health in the inter-war years had been too limited:

> …public health doctors were happy to extend their activities in whatever direction the Ministry permitted and anticipated that eventually this gap-filling exercise would be transformed into a fully-fledged state medical service in which they would play a dominant role. It was a dream doomed to disappointment, for neither the Ministry nor the medical profession shared it… (Lewis, 1986, p. 49).

The public-health profession could have been a unifying force in the tripartite fragmentation of the health service.

[8]Balint's work is discussed more fully in the revised edition of *Medical Knowledge: Doubt and Certainty* (Open University Press, 1994), Chapter 9.

But it was buffeted in this period between the rest of the medical profession and local government structures. The public-health empire in local government began to disintegrate and relationships with GPs remained difficult.

The Medical Officer of Health could have acted as the coordinator of community health services under the developing policies of community care. The role of health visitors as providing the link between general practice and public health was also an important one. But from the 1960s onward, cooperation was achieved by attaching health visitors to GPs. Health centres, which expanded from the late 1960s, operated not as the original intention had been, as a means of providing *integration* of the health services and community care, but as a focus for the establishment of *group general practices*. The volume of clinic work for local-authority doctors declined, as much of this work gradually passed to the GPs. There were tensions between the two groups of doctors as a result.

The position of public health as a specialty within the local authorities also caused problems. By the late 1960s, the idea of the MOH based in the local authority as the coordinator even of community services was no longer a practical possibility. Parts of the public-health empire were beginning to break away. Sanitary inspectors had begun to claim autonomy in the 1950s and had their own specialist training; they were renamed *public-health inspectors* in 1956. A major defection a decade later was that of the *social workers*. In 1968, the Seebohm Committee recommended the removal of social work from local-authority public-health departments and the setting up of separate social work departments.

A new definition of public health was beginning to emerge in the late 1960s. This was the concept of **community medicine** and of the *community physician*, replacing the role of the old MOH. These ideas were also developed in the late 1960s in a number of policy documents, in particular the *Todd Report* on medical education of 1968. The local-authority role of public-health doctors had gone, but a range of policy documents published in 1972 predicted an important new role for them as community physicians within the NHS. However, that role was poorly specified.

The twin components of community medicine were seen as *epidemiology* (the study of patterns of disease in populations)[9] and *medical administration*. But how these functions would operate in tandem—and how the community physician would operate within the NHS— remained unclear. Notice that, despite their title, community physicians were not involved in community care. As you will see in the next chapter, the fate of public health was closely bound up with the larger issue of NHS reform.

Campaigning for public health

☐ How did the ethos of public health change in the early part of the twentieth century (as described in Chapters 4 and 5)?

■ Public health concerned itself much more with questions of individual behaviour and lifestyle, rather than looking at the structural and economic issues involved in the health of the people. In the inter-war years public-health doctors took on the administration of hospital services, a role which gave them considerable powers, although at the expense of the possibility of playing a broader role in defining key issues in health care.

As you saw earlier, public health as a profession suffered by comparison with the rise of the GP in the post-war period and by the defection from the inter-war public-health 'empire' of both sanitary inspectors and social workers. This opened the way, at least in theory, for public-health doctors to take the lead in campaigns to improve public health on a broad range of issues. But this opportunity was not grasped. In the 1970s, the transition to community medicine saw public health redefined with a narrower, rather than a broader, focus.

'Single-issue' campaigns

In the 1950s and 1960s, environmental and public-health issues tended to be dealt with as **single-issue campaigns** for action against a particular cause of ill-health or for the introduction of a certain treatment or policy. Such campaigns were advanced by pressure groups, not by public-health doctors.

For example, the question of air pollution came to the fore in the 1950s. The 'great London smog' of 1952 brought matters to a head (see Figure 6.5). From 5 to 9 December, London was subjected to a dense smoke-polluted fog of catastrophic proportions, responsible for at least 4 000 deaths. Deaths on this scale had not been seen since the 'flu epidemic of 1918–19. The *Clean Air Act 1956* passed in part because of this and other 'smogs' established smokeless zones and controlled domestic smoke emissions for the first time.

---

[9]The methods and philosophy of epidemiology are taught in another book in this series, *Studying Health and Disease* (Open University Press, revised edition 1994), and further exemplified in *World Health and Disease*.

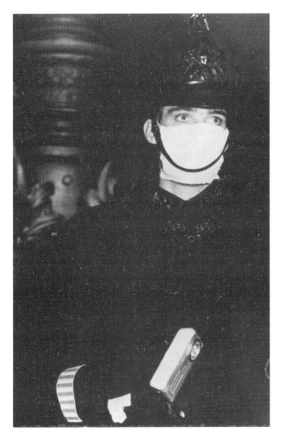

Figure 6.5 *A London smog in the 1950s. Police on duty were forced to wear smog masks. (Source: Hulton/Deutsch Picture Collection)*

But the passing of the Act was the result of pressure from the *National Society for Smoke Abatement*, a cross-party group of MPs—and a few committed MOHs. The Act played a substantial part in the reduction of air pollution. Two million tons of smoke were discharged into the atmosphere in 1954; by 1971 this had fallen to 700 000 tons, a reduction of 65 per cent. This was a successful environmental campaign, although not one in which the public-health profession had been prominent.

Another area of public health with which the public-health profession had little to do was the struggle to establish *birth control*. The post-war 'baby boom' and the reassertion of the importance of women's prime role as wife and mother in the home (via the writing of John Bowlby and others) led to services promoting contraception being given low priority. A breakthrough came in 1955 when the *Family Planning Association* celebrated its silver jubilee and received its first official recognition with a visit from Ian Macleod, then Minister of Health.

Between 1955 and 1960, despite opposition from some quarters, the battle for respectable contraception had been largely won (see Figure 6.6). At the Lambeth Conference in 1958, the Anglicans came out firmly in favour of birth control, which was accepted as a 'right and important factor in Christian family life'.

Another key development was the advent of the contraceptive pill, approved by the Medical Advisory Panel of the Family Planning Association in 1961. By 1964, there were about 480 000 women on the pill in Britain. The pill was 'scientific' and available only on prescription, and this put contraception for the first time firmly in the hands of the medical profession. As the historian, Barbara Brookes, has commented:

> …the pill and medical control ensured matters of fertility control became an integral part of medical practice rather than a separate moral issue. (Brookes, 1988, p. 128)

Mass publicity methods were used in the 1970s, for example the poster shown in Figure 6.7 (*overleaf*).

The same tendency was apparent in *abortion reform*, stimulated by public outrage at the thalidomide disaster (in which prescription of an anti-morning-sickness drug caused malformations in the fetus and large numbers of children were born with deformities), and at the lengths women had to go to obtain an abortion. The key pressure

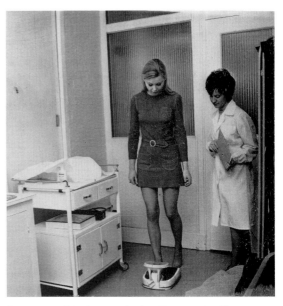

Figure 6.6 *This photograph of a client at a Family Planning Association (FPA) consultation in the 1960s was used to promote the 'modern' image of contraception among young women. (Source: Brook Advisory Centre)*

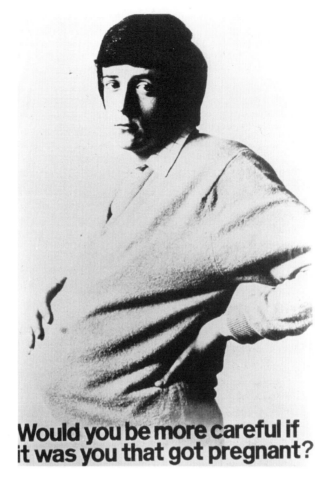

Would you be more careful if it was you that got pregnant?

Figure 6.7 *The Family Planning Association's 'pregnant man' poster attracted widespread publicity in 1974–5. (Source: Saatchi & Saatchi, London)*

group in this campaign was the Abortion Law Reform Association, which saw the *Abortion Act 1967* as a victory. But the Act also served to strengthen medical control and left women reliant on the profession's good will in sanctioning abortions.

Public health and housing policy

Birth control and abortion were 'single-issue' campaigns *par excellence*. Housing was a more politically divisive issue, although no less important from the health perspective. In the post-war period, the Labour Party consistently tried to increase the stock of council housing, while the Conservatives gave priority to expanding owner-occupation. Under the Conservatives, from 1954 to 1964 a greater proportion of private houses were built. This balance of construction also continued under Labour as a

result of the impact of the 1967 devaluation of the pound on public expenditure programmes.

By the mid-1970s, the overall standard of housing had considerably improved. But 'new slums' had been created in the high-rise council estates of the 1960s. In the medium term, these became the foci of deprivation and social degeneration, exacerbating instead of diminishing health inequalities.

The composition of the housing market also altered. The introduction of 'fair rents' and the protection of sitting tenants by the *Rent Act 1965* (following the abuses of 'Rachmanism', named after the scandals of rent extortion by a landlord, Peter Rachman) brought a drastic decline in private rented housing and new overcrowding problems. The housing market in the 1970s was divided between owner occupiers and an expanded council-house sector.

The erosion of welfare

The Conservative government of 1970–4 began to mount a reaction against the apparently inevitable extension of the interventionist state. Many of its measures had public-health implications. Increases in prescription charges and the price of school meals, and the abolition of cheap welfare milk were among the first assaults on the welfare state. In the 1980s, as you will see in Chapter 7, the erosion of welfare gathered momentum and had further implications for public health.

But before considering our own more recent past, we turn to health issues in the colonial, and former colonial territories held by Europe at the end of World War II. As you will see, a more nineteenth-century construction of public health was still in practice there.

'Scientific' medicine and the Third World

Up to the 1940s, international public health had been strongly influenced by the association made in colonial times between tropical medicine and the study and treatment of parasitic diseases. Expatriate civil servants, military personnel and managers were threatened by tropical diseases that were non-existent in Europe, or of limited importance. As a result, several important parasitic diseases including malaria and schistosomiasis (bilharzia) received considerable attention, and huge strides were made in understanding their causes and their natural history.

As you will recall from earlier chapters, schools of tropical medicine, established in Europe at the beginning of the century, took over from the predominantly military schools of medicine. As a more stable basis for research was needed, laboratories were established in colonial territories in what we now refer to collectively as the *Third World*: the Dutch specialised in Indonesia, the Belgians in Zaire, Rwanda and Burundi, the Germans in what was then Tanganyika. Britain and France's interests were more widespread because of their colonisation patterns. The American *Rockefeller Foundation* also played a dominant role in supporting research institutions in a number of Third World countries.

The early 1940s were characterised by great confidence in medical science and its ability to challenge disease. The advent of sulphonamides, penicillin and the wide-spectrum antibiotics between 1930 and 1950 gave Western medicine what were described as *magic bullets*, i.e. synthetic and naturally occurring drugs which could destroy infectious organisms without harming the living host.[10] In Africa, the use of penicillin injections to cure the infectious disease yaws and sexually transmitted diseases made such an indelible impression that injections continue to this day to be considered by many people the best medicine for any ill.

The synthesis of DDT and its application to control malaria-carrying mosquitoes seemed equally magical and, by the 1950s, vaccines which gave protection against many important infectious diseases gave added impetus to the triumph of medical science and its wonder drugs. Such pharmaceutical advances strengthened expatriate beliefs that indigenous systems of health were unscientific and potentially harmful, further undermining alternative traditional systems of care.

International initiatives

Medical confidence was paralleled by a social climate of reform in the wake of the 1930s recession and World War II. In the late 1940s, in a wave of idealism and wish for global peace, a number of new non-governmental organisations were set up within the United Nations system. The agency with a major responsibility for health was the *World Health Organisation* (WHO), with headquarters in Geneva, and six regional offices around the world. Its main aim was to promote international cooperation in the field of health. It evolved from an earlier agency of the League of Nations, established in 1923. Another UN agency closely involved with health was *UNICEF* (United Nations Children's Fund), its target group including both mothers and children.

Countries became members of WHO in order to gain from its expertise and influence policy on health. This exchange at the international level was important in terms of influencing thinking about health policy. For instance, one of the earliest programmes supported and initiated by WHO and a number of big donor agencies was against *malaria*. World War II had drawn attention to the powerful influence of this disease, which in Asia and the Pacific area caused far more illness and deaths among military forces, than occurred as casualties of war. Largely as a consequence of this world-wide sensitivity to an old problem, WHO launched a *malaria eradication programme* in 1955 (see Figure 6.8, *overleaf*).

[10]The mechanisms by which infectious organisms produce disease symptoms in people, and the effect of antibiotics on bacteria are discussed in another book in this series, *Human Biology and Health: An Evolutionary Approach* (Open University Press, 1994), Chapters 5 and 6.

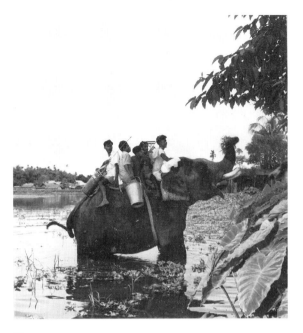

(a)

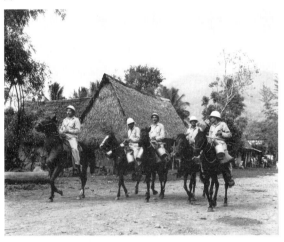

(b)

Figure 6.8 *Illustration of the WHO malaria eradication campaign, launched in 1955. (a) In India, a malaria team makes its way into the depths of the forest through marshes and across lakes. (b) In Mexico, the campaign was launched with the thoroughness of military organisation and spray teams were deployed as though they were combat troops. In this picture the 'malarial cavalry' set out from Jacaltepec to climb the bridle-paths into the High Sierras. (Sources: (a) WHO/photo by P. N. Sharma; (b) WHO/photo by Eric Schwab)*

This programme was a great success in parts of Europe and North America where malaria was endemic and in some parts of South America and the Western Pacific. By 1968, about 1.1 billion[11] people were protected from malaria as a result of environmental measures. But by then the momentum of the eradication programme was slowing down: DDT, the insecticide which had successfully killed off strains of mosquitoes in some areas, was increasingly seen to have environmentally negative effects, and resistant strains of mosquitoes evolved which were immune to spraying.

In the poorer tropical countries, the eradication campaign illustrates how difficult it is to sustain public-health measures when there is no basic rural infrastructure of health facilities to carry out essential activities (for example, spraying houses regularly; cutting down bush near homes; preventing stagnant pools of water in order to discourage mosquitoes breeding, and treating people with choloroquine when they were ill). The name of the programme changed from 'eradication' to 'control'. A successful eradication programme implies a significant measure of social reform.

Importing European health care

Social reform was also manifest in thinking about improving state provision of health services. Many of the ideas embodied in the Beveridge report in the United Kingdom were shared by others. The ex-colonies of South Africa and India set up Commissions in the British tradition, to explore how to organise health systems that would more effectively meet people's needs. The *Bhore Commission* in India explicitly looked towards a socialised system of health services in which public health predominated, and eventually replaced private medical practice.

The Bhore report was radical in its recognition that nutrition and general living standards were major determinants of health, and that 'it is the tiller of the soil on whom the economic structure of the country eventually depends' (quoted in Jeffrey, 1988, p. 113). The report therefore recommended, among other things, the establishment of a health system in India that emphasised

[11]Throughout this book, 1 billion is taken to equal 1 000 000 000 (one thousand million).

preventive measures and was based on salaried workers in a public-health service that linked villages to district health centres.

The *Gluckman Commission* in South Africa was asked to advise on an:

> ...organized national health service in conformity with the modern conception of 'health' which will ensure adequate mental, dental, nursing and hospital services for all sections of the people of South Africa. (Gluckman, quoted in Marks, 1988, p. 8)

However, only a few of the recommendations of the Bhore and Gluckman reports were implemented. This was partly due to the political and administrative structures of those countries, which gave considerable responsibility for health care to the states or provinces, with the central government retaining only minimal control over policy. But it was also due to political tensions, the resistance of the medical profession to radical change, and the beginning of the Cold War during which any ideas that seemed socialist or communist in origin were viewed with suspicion in the West.

Throughout the Third World, the medical establishment encouraged the founding of medical schools and training curricula modelled on those in the industrialised world. Universities and research institutions were set up, often in partnership with universities from the 'mother country'. There was a strong emphasis on comparability of standards and building up 'centres of excellence' which would equal the best of the medical schools and teaching hospitals of Britain, France, Italy and Germany. Curricula were imported from European schools, and medical students were taught about the chronic diseases of Europe rather than the infectious and other more relevant conditions (at the time) of their own countries.

Moreover, because of the emphasis on professional comparability, many Third World doctors and nurses left their own countries for further training in the industrialised world, and many never returned (a topic to which we come back in Chapter 9). The international ramifications of the 'brain drain' were analysed in the 1960s. The key findings were that it represented a huge donation from poor to rich countries. By 1982, the Philippines alone had lost a total of 14 000 doctors and 89 000 nurses—mostly to the USA. In the industrialised

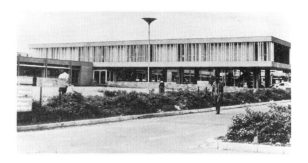

Figure 6.9 *The Kenyatta National Hospital in Nairobi (photographed in 1974) compared well with hospitals in the industrialised world, but absorbed a huge proportion of Kenya's total health budget. (Source: Diesfeld, H. J. and Hecklau, H. K., 1978,* Kenya: A Geomedical Monograph, *Springer-Verlag, Berlin)*

countries, these health workers filled important gaps in the less prestigious hospitals and specialties.[12]

In order to emulate the medical systems of the industrialised world, disproportionate amounts of health budgets went on teaching hospitals, importing diagnostic and therapeutic technology and medicines that were extremely costly (see Figure 6.9).

By the 1960s, it was clear that what the expert in tropical diseases among children, David Morley, has called the 'three-quarters rule' was true all over the developing world: three-quarters of spending on health care was for high-technology care in *urban*-based hospitals and staff (he called them 'disease palaces'), although three-quarters of the population lived in the *rural* areas, and three-quarters of all *deaths* were due to conditions that could be prevented by relatively *simple and inexpensive measures*.

By the 1970s, health policies that had encouraged the importation of Western or industrialised models of health care were increasingly criticised, and Third World countries themselves were experimenting with alternative systems of care. In Chapter 8 we look at how these changing ideas and experiences laid the basis for a revolutionary change in policy—the introduction of the *primary health-care* approach.

---

[12]The relative status of health-care workers in the United Kingdom who are of African or Asian origin or ethnic group is discussed further in *Dilemmas in Health Care*, Chapter 6.

OBJECTIVES FOR CHAPTER 6

After studying this chapter, you should be able to:

6.1 Describe the principal innovative features of the NHS.

6.2 Identify the intrinsic organisational weaknesses in the NHS as it was originally established.

6.3 Analyse the development of the concept of 'community care' in the period 1948–74, and its interaction with continuing patterns of lay care.

6.4 Describe the changes in the relative status and areas of competence of the medical profession in this period and the changes in the health-care division of labour.

6.5 Use examples to illustrate the changing nature of 'public-health issues' in this period and their relationship to the formal public-health profession.

6.6 Describe some of the ways in which Third World health systems mirrored those of the industrialised world, and how far such emulation undermined their own needs.

QUESTIONS FOR CHAPTER 6

Question 1 (*Objective 6.1*)

What factors led planners to concentrate their energies on building up the acute hospital services of the NHS? What effect did this policy have on the range of services available under the NHS?

Question 2 (*Objective 6.2*)

Aneurin Bevan argued that:

> ...the undertaking to provide all people with all kinds of health care...creates an entirely new situation and calls for something bolder than a mere extension and adoption of existing services. (Quoted in Webster, 1991, p. 41)

To what extent was the NHS in practice unable to break free from the inherited pattern of health care?

Question 3 (*Objective 6.3*)

What did community care mean in the period 1948–74? How did it relate to patterns of lay care?

Question 4 (*Objective 6.4*)

List the factors involved in the change in status of GPs in the period 1948–74.

Question 5 (*Objective 6.5*)

How did the function of public health change in the post-war decades? Cite examples of some public-health campaigns in this period and their relationship to the organised public-health profession.

Question 6 (*Objective 6.6*)

Describe the main influences on Third World health systems that stemmed directly from the industrialised world.

7

The crisis of welfare, 1974 to the 1990s

This chapter includes a detailed discussion of the complex changes to the organisation and structure of the NHS between 1974 and 1992. A more detailed analysis of specific areas of service provision in the 1990s and wider social policies to promote health in the United Kingdom, can be found in another book in this series.[1] We do not discuss the colonial dimension of Third World health care in this chapter in the way that we did in previous chapters in this book; this is the subject of Chapter 8. During your study of this chapter, you will be asked to read the article by Patricia Day and Rudolf Klein, entitled 'Britain's health care experiment' (1991), which you will find in the Reader.[2] This article is longer than most of the previously published articles you have been asked to read, but it is an essential source of information about the reorganisation of the NHS in the 1990s.

Feeling worse

Paradoxically, the massive expansion of the welfare state in Britain in the 1950s and 1960s served only to draw attention to the scale of unsatisfied demand. Every phase of the development tended to reveal fresh problems, expose the needs of further neglected groups, and stimulate public demand for further services. Public opinion, informed by radical critics among the social theorists (such as Ivan Illich, whose ideas are discussed in another book in this series[3]) increasingly called for dismantling of traditional structures and creation of alternatives more appropriate to the needs of such groups as women, racial minorities, disabled people, or the ever-expanding elderly and very elderly population. The 'urban masses' could no longer be relied upon to accept indignity with docility. Within the social and health services, personnel belonging to subordinate occupations were no longer willing to accept unquestioningly the dictates of bureaucrats or high-ranking professionals.

Although traditionally enjoying high esteem, the health sector in the 1970s and 1980s was not immune from critical scrutiny. The anti-psychiatry movement[4] demonstrated the strength of the case for the social construction of disease and underlined the evils of incarceration. Long-stay hospitals were vigorously criticised. High-technology medicine was no longer seen as an undisputed success or total panacea. The power of the medical profession was increasingly questioned; the unspoken philosophical assumptions of Western medicine were thrown into doubt; there were renewed calls for holistic medicine, and a passionate following developed for every form of alternative medicine. The medical profession declined in political authority. Thus, although the demand for health and welfare was voiced more actively than ever before, there was uncertainty about the way forward.

Dreams of an expanding and ever-more pluralistic welfare state were shattered in the autumn of 1973, when the price of oil was quadrupled by the producers, an action which abruptly plunged the Western economies into crisis. Western governments found themselves unable to sustain the unimpeded expansion of welfare services. The strains of the situation immediately disrupted the long-standing consensus surrounding welfare policy. Governments of the political Right pledged themselves to the maintenance and improvement of many individual welfare programmes. On the other hand, they

---

[1] *Dilemmas in Health Care* (Open University Press, revised edition 1993).

[2] *Health and Disease: A Reader* (revised edition 1995).

[3] *Medical Knowledge: Doubt and Certainty*, Chapter 8.

[4] Discussed further in another book in this series, *Experiencing and Explaining Disease* (Open University Press, revised edition 1996), Chapter 6.

attacked the basic philosophy of the welfare state, and were pledged to reduce taxes and public expenditure. Thereby the Right found itself committed to ever-more ambitious welfare objectives on the basis of ever-decreasing public expenditure.

In the event, although Left and Right diverged in political rhetoric, their record in office was not dissimilar. Governments of the Left failed to mobilise the resources to realise their ambitions, whereas the inertia of the system and political prudence inhibited governments of the Right from undertaking changes within the welfare system on the radical scale wanted by their more ardent ideologues.

Consequently the crisis affecting the welfare state has, in the decades since 1974, become increasingly more severe. Welfare provision, like foreign aid or environmental support, has tended to become a casualty of each recession, while its position has not been proportionately restored during economic upturns. This spiral of decline is serious for the poor of the West, but its impact inevitably spreads wider and, as you will see in Chapter 8, adds to the scale and severity of the enormously greater problems affecting the people of the Third World.

The health services: perpetual crisis and constant reorganisation

The malaise affecting the welfare state in this period carried particularly strong implications for the health services. In all Western nations, health care expanded in relative importance to become one of the largest and most expensive elements in the welfare system, to the extent of absorbing at least 10 per cent of the Gross Domestic Product (GDP)[5] in some of the leading Western economies. The Western nations became involved in a frantic search for economy in their health expenditure.

As you will see in more detail in Chapter 9, the British health service was considerably less expensive than most of its European and American counterparts. By the mid-1970s expenditure on it reached a peak of 6 per cent of GDP. Despite its relative economy, the NHS was one of the largest unified civil organisations in the Western world. The personnel engaged in the NHS doubled since its inception to reach almost one million by 1980. The oil crisis imposed a brake on a system which, at least

in the alarmist imagination, showed every sign of escalating out of control. Once applied, this brake was never again more than momentarily relaxed.

Expanding commitments

The economic downturn could not have come at a worse time for the health services. By 1974 there had emerged seemingly irresistible pressures for expenditure increases on all fronts. After a slow start, the hospital modernisation programme had reached its peak. Every sphere of the acute sector faced expenditure commitments brought about by the vastly increasing capacities of high-technology medicine.

After a long period of neglect there was demand for better services, in particular for elderly, disabled, mentally handicapped,[6] and mentally ill people. Although these groups to some extent required replacement of hospitals by community services, it was by no means obvious that the alternative was cheaper. The steady growth in the population of elderly and very elderly people imposed new demands on both the health and social services.

Finally, the *Family Doctors' Charter* of 1966 provided conditions for the development of *primary care*. As a result, after a period of almost total neglect, health centres were established at a hectic pace between 1966 and 1976. This was associated with an acceleration towards *group practice* of GPs and creation of *primary care teams* (both of which are discussed later), innovations which improved the quality of services, but inevitably involved additional expenditure.

Expectations were undoubtedly aroused that the most advanced treatment would be provided at all points within the health service. In every community, progress was anxiously monitored in provision of scanning devices, special care baby units, intensive care units, kidney dialysis units, cancer treatment (oncology) units, or hip replacement, transplantation and open-heart surgery facilities. Public appeals raised funds for modern equipment, especially connected with new imaging techniques.[7] Improved diagnostic facilities and introduction of screening for breast and cervical cancer, or for cardiovascular disorders, created a demand for treatment

[6]During the period covered by this chapter, 'mental handicap' was still the most commonly found term in documents arising from within the policy-making levels of central government, the NHS and sections of the social services.

[5]GDP is a measure of national wealth and is explained in Chapter 9 of this book.

[7]New medical technologies are discussed in *Dilemmas in Health Care*, Chapter 7.

which health authorities found difficult to meet.[8] This added to the already serious problem of waiting lists.

To meet the growing demands of the health services, governments since 1974 have become involved in a frantic process of policy reassessment and search for economies. There has been surprising lack of settled policy, even in major areas such as hospital provision.

In 1962, the *Hospital Plan* was launched without firm guidelines, but gradually opinion shifted in favour of building large *District General Hospitals* (DGH). However, in the early 1970s, large centralised hospitals went out of favour and a balance between the DGHs and smaller *community hospitals* was advocated. This gave reprieve for many small hospitals destined for closure under the original plan. However, even in the 1980s, it proved impossible to arrive at agreed policy concerning the correct balance of acute, maternity and chronic hospital facilities, and on the more general distribution between institutional, primary care, and community care facilities.

The radical proposals published by the *King's Fund* in June 1992 and by the Tomlinson Report in November 1992, suggesting wholesale closure of hospital facilities in central London, and their substitution by improved primary care facilities indicated the extent to which policies since 1948 have directed investment into vastly expensive and sometimes inappropriate health-service facilities (much as has been the case, as described in the previous chapter, in Third World countries). This example also demonstrates the difficulties experienced in attempting to break away from the *inherited* pattern of health services, involving the dominance of the *teaching* hospitals and *acute* hospital sector.

The search for economy has entailed action on controversial issues such as health charges, 'privatisation', and private health insurance.

Direct health charges

Since their first introduction, **direct health charges** (i.e. cash payments by patients for certain services, such as prescribed drugs, dental treatment, etc.) have been contentious. Under the 1974–9 Labour government, health charges were held down and in 1978–9 constituted only 2 per cent of total NHS expenditure, the lowest percentage yield from charges since 1952. The Conservative government reversed this trend. For instance, the prescription charge was regularly increased from 20p in

1979 to reach £4.25 in 1993. Dental charges have also been substantially increased and, in 1989, a charge for dental *examinations* was introduced. In 1984, the supply of spectacles under the NHS ended and a voucher scheme was introduced to help the needy. In 1989, a charge for *sight tests* was introduced.

The rises in direct charges were offset by exemptions and voucher schemes, but the system inevitably acted as a disincentive to the poor and the elderly. By steadily increasing charges and reducing the subsidy from taxation, the dental and ophthalmic services of the NHS have been eroded beyond recognition. The threat in 1992 of dentists to withdraw from their NHS contracts constituted evidence of the low state of morale surrounding this once-important NHS service.

Privatisation

On grounds of efficiency the government was committed to **privatisation** (i.e. the contracting-out to private business) of activities like NHS ancillary services, especially cleaning and catering. This policy was inevitably contentious, especially with the NHS personnel affected. In the event, privatisation took root extremely slowly, and it has not been pursued enthusiastically even by the service providers. The real savings to the NHS of the small amount of contracting-out of services has turned out to be much less than advocates of privatisation originally anticipated.

The Thatcher administration was pledged to promote *private health care*, but changes in this field have been smaller than expected. The previous government's plan to phase out private beds in NHS hospitals was reversed, but private-bed usage continued to decline. On the other hand, private *out-patient* attendances increased substantially. The real expansion in private-bed provision took place in private hospitals. The number of beds provided increased at an average of about 10 per cent per annum throughout the 1980s.

This growth was paralleled by the increase in *private health insurance*. This market was stimulated by a significant tax concession for employer-paid medical insurance premiums in 1980. The 1989 White Paper led to a similar tax concession for elderly people. In the 1980s the coverage of private health insurance almost doubled to a level of 10 per cent of the population. However, the economic downturn of the 1990s has adversely affected the insurance market. Also, since 1990 the government has noticeably played down its interest in private health care, presumably to avoid undermining public confidence in its NHS changes.

---

[8]Screening is discussed in *Dilemmas in Health Care*, Chapter 9; for the treatment of coronary heart disease, see Chapter 10 of the same book.

The 1974 reorganisation

Between 1948 and the mid-1970s, health services were expanded by increasing expenditure according to agreed priorities. Since that date, expenditure levels remained more static and a growing tide of administrative reforms have been expected to bear the burden of improvement. The first reorganisation, which took place in 1974, was rapidly accounted a failure, with the result that a further reorganisation was required in 1982. Immediately, the Conservative government embarked on a series of management changes, which culminated with a further substantial reorganisation in 1991.

The ambitious 1974 reorganisation was designed to correct the numerous anomalies resulting from the unsatisfactory compromises of 1948. The original ideal of reorganisation was to simplify administration by *uniting all health services* at a local level under *Area Health Authorities* which would coincide with the reorganised local government areas. It was even contemplated that area health administration might become fully assimilated into local government, along the lines of the pre-1948 municipal health services. Figure 7.1 and Box 7.1 indicate the outcome of the 1974 reorganisation.

In 1974 Executive Councils were renamed *Family Practitioner Committees* (FPCs), with formal but only notional links with AHAs. Local government nominally lost its health responsibilities, but in reality the local authorities introduced in the 1974 local government reorganisation remained involved in health-service affairs because of their importance in housing, community care and environmental health.

☐ With respect to Figure 7.1 and Box 7.1, how did the 1974 reorganisation fall short of simplification and unification of the tripartite structure established in 1948? (See Chapter 6, particularly Figure 6.3.)

■ In England, the regional tier was interposed between the area level and the central government department (the DHSS). The areas were subdivided into districts. The intended single-tier system therefore evolved into a three-tier system. Also, separate administration of family practitioner services was retained. At the local level the NHS therefore retained much of its original tripartite character, especially when the continuing health responsibilities of local government are taken into account.

The paradoxical consequence of the 1974 reorganisation exercise was a service more bureaucratically complex and only marginally more unified than the organisation hastily contrived by the Labour government in 1945.

Box 7.1 The NHS in Scotland, Wales and Northern Ireland

Although the health services in these areas broadly resemble the pattern in England (see Figure 7.1), they retain independence and a significant degree of difference. Each is the responsibility of a separate senior Minister. This note summarises the most important differences in local administration.

Between 1948 and 1974 in Wales, the Welsh Regional Hospital Board and in Northern Ireland, the Northern Ireland Hospitals Authority, operated like a single English hospital region, but with generally smaller local hospital management committees. Scotland was divided into five regions, and 85 local bodies known as Boards of Management. Scottish teaching hospitals were part of the regional system from the outset.

In the 1974 reorganisation, the regional tier was retained only in England. Scotland formed 15 Health Boards, Wales eight Area Health Authorities (AHAs), and Northern Ireland four Health and Social Service Boards. Each of these area authorities was divided into districts, as in England administered by multi-professional management teams. Basically the same structure was maintained in 1982 and 1991, but in 1982 the area authorities in Wales were restyled District Health Authorities (DHAs) and the number increased to nine.

Only with care is it possible to detect elements of rationalisation in the 1974 arrangements.

☐ Again compare Figure 7.1 with Figure 6.3. With respect to England and Wales, what major examples of rationalisation can you detect?

■ Teaching hospitals and most of the local authority health services were integrated under AHA administration.

Two further innovations in the 1974 system are deserving of comment. First, at the district level a new form of management was adopted, which gave greater equality to the main professional groups (doctors, nurses, and administrators) represented on the *District Management*

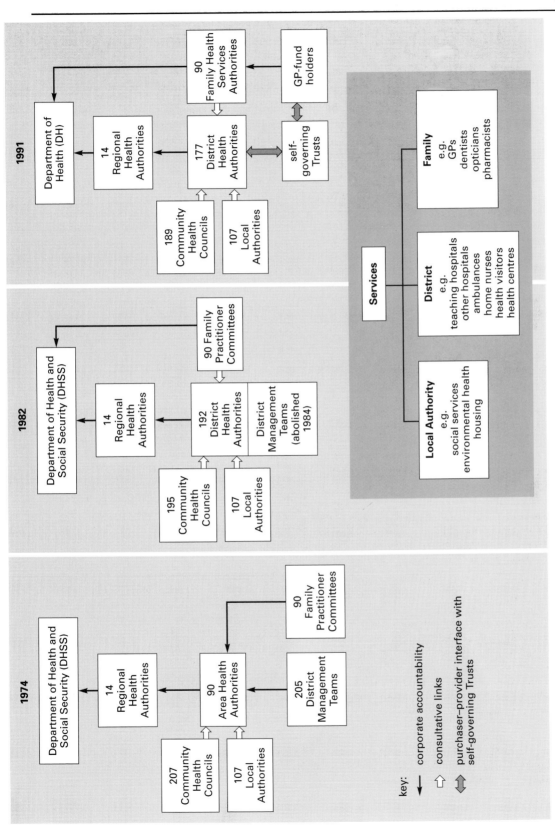

Figure 7.1 *Simplified diagram of the organisation of the NHS in England, 1974–91. The 107 local authorities indicated comprise the local government bodies, which were in 1974 approximately coterminous with Area Health Authorities (32 London Boroughs; 36 Metropolitan Districts outside London; and 39 Non-metropolitan Counties). Outside London and the other metropolitan areas, there are in addition 296 District Councils. London Boroughs and Metropolitan Districts are concerned with social services, housing and environmental health. The Non-metropolitan Counties are concerned with social services, while in these areas the 296 District Councils are responsible for housing and environmental health.*

Teams. Second, to compensate for the greater professional and managerial emphasis of local health services, *Community Health Councils* were introduced to give voice to community groups and to represent individual queries and complaints.[9]

Cash limits

A further important change occurring in the health service in the 1970s was the introduction in 1976–7 of *cash limits* for health-authority budgets. Authorities were no longer automatically compensated for inflation. Henceforth budgets tended to be set with low estimates of inflation with the result that the cost of such items as wage settlements above the rate of inflation were met by economies, including periodic cuts in service and closure of wards.

The effects of cash limits were exacerbated in some areas, especially in London, by the simultaneous application of the *RAWP* formula (so-called because it was evolved by the *Resource Allocation Working Party*) designed over the long term to adjust funding for health services in favour of regions (especially in the North) which had in the past received less than their fair share of resources. RAWP represented a minor response to the problem of regional inequality, but unintentionally it added to the difficulties of sustaining health services in inner-city areas such as central London, which lost out in the redistribution.

Abandonment of plans for expansion and modernisation, cash limits, RAWP,[10] pay disputes, and a wrangle over the government's plan for phasing out of private beds in NHS hospitals, all contributed in the late 1970s to an atmosphere of crisis in the NHS. The incoming Conservative government in 1979 was therefore faced with intractable problems in the field of health care.

The 1980s

There was widespread expectation that the Thatcher administration would take the axe to the NHS, along with the rest of the welfare state. The shorter-term reality proved to be less drastic. The government's immediate room for manoeuvre was limited by the *Royal Commission on the National Health Service*, which reported in 1979. The Commission gave a strong impetus to main-

taining the NHS in its inherited form, subject to simplification of its administrative structure, and a continuing search for improvement, efficiency and economy.

The first interventions of the Conservative government were minor and relatively uncontroversial. As indicated by Figure 7.1, the area tier of administration was abolished in 1982, and FPCs were given a greater degree of independence. The latter represented a concession to the BMA.

You have seen from Chapter 5 that GPs jealously guarded their status as independent contractors. They therefore insisted on separate administration for their sector (and succeeded in sustaining it through several changes of title: National Insurance Committees before 1948, Executive Councils 1948–74, Family Practitioner Committees 1974–91, and Family Health Services Authorities (FHSAs) from 1991). GPs traditionally resented being drawn into centralised health administration. More important, they feared that closer links would facilitate extension of cash limits to general practice budgets.

The main, if unintentional, long-term effect of cash limits was to shift the balance between spending on *hospital services* and *primary health care.* Hospital expenditure was rigidly contained, but spending on primary health care remained *demand-led,* i.e. spending on medicines, vaccines, etc. was determined by the level of patient demand. Continuation of *demand-led* budgets proved greatly to the benefit of GPs. Of course, this demand increased on account of economies in the hospitals. The result is demonstrated in Table 7.1.

> ☐ What does Table 7.1 tell you about the balance between spending on hospital services and on primary health care in this period? How does the balance change if you look instead at their relative purchasing power?

> ■ Spending on hospital services was around three times greater than on primary care, but purchasing power within primary care advanced substantially in the 1980s, whereas hospital purchasing power remained relatively unchanged in most years.

Thus, the funding system helped the primary care services to make up some of the ground lost to the hospitals in the early years of the NHS. Later in this chapter, we return to the discussion of developments in general practice when we consider GPs alongside other health-care occupations.

After the 1982 changes, the emphasis of the government switched towards implanting industrial-style management into the NHS and industrialists were employed to supervise this transition. The changes have become

---

[9]The relative influence in the 1990s of doctors, managers and representatives of the local citizens (such as Community Health Councils) are discussed in *Dilemmas in Health Care,* Chapter 2.

[10]For further detail on the rationing of NHS expenditure, see *Dilemmas in Health Care,* Chapter 3.

Table 7.1 Growth in public expenditure on the NHS in England, selected years, 1980–91 (current spending only, excluding capital expenditure, in millions of pounds sterling)

	1980–1	1982–3	1984–5	1986–7	1988–9	1989–90	1990–1[1]
hospital services							
total spending (£m)	£6 999	£8 251	£9 208	£10 421	£12 758	£13 765	£15 099
cash increase (%)	–	7.3	5.7	7.4	10.9	7.9	9.7
inflation rate (%)	–	6.5	5.8	6.9	10.5	8.0	7.4
purchasing power (%)	–	+0.8	–0.1	+0.5	+0.3	–0.1	+2.1
primary health care							
total spending (£m)	£2 173	£2 894	£3 421	£3 877	£4 871	£5 240	£5 957
cash increase (%)	–	15.6	10.0	7.6	13.3	7.6	13.7
inflation rate (%)	–	11.6	6.9	5.0	9.6	6.5	5.9
purchasing power (%)	–	+3.6	+2.9	+2.5	+3.4	+1.0	+7.3
NHS current total							
total spending (£m)	£9 402	£11 478	£13 050	£14 808	£18 181	£19 657	£21 570
cash increase (%)	–	9.4	7.2	7.5	11.2	8.1	10.7
inflation rate (%)	–	7.4	6.0	6.3	10.0	7.3	6.9
purchasing power (%)	–	+1.9	+1.2	+1.2	+1.1	+0.3	+3.6

[1]Data for 1990–1 are projected. (Data from National Association of Health Authorities and Trusts, *Health Care Economic Review, 1990*, (Birmingham: NAHAT, 1990, p. 22), adapted from Day, P. and Klein, R., 1991, 'Britain's health care experiment', *Health Affairs*, Fall, p. 42, Exhibit 1)

particularly associated with the name of Sir Roy Griffiths, the deputy chairman and managing director of Sainsbury's, the food retailer. Following the publication of the *NHS Management Inquiry* (known as the *Griffiths Report*) in 1983, a strengthened management structure was introduced in the DHSS, and so-called **general managers** were appointed at regional, district and hospital unit level, in place of the *consensus* management teams which had obtained since 1974. Relatively few of these general managers were formerly health-care practitioners. Development of the management function in the wake of the Griffiths Report prepared the way for the more radical management changes introduced in April 1991.[11]

Public frustration combined with medical indignation in a growing resentment of alleged underfunding of the NHS under the Thatcher administration. The strict cash limits regime involved enforcement of regular rounds of cuts and some much-resented hospital closures, which in some cases prompted occupations, one of which is shown in Figure 7.2.

[11]See *Dilemmas in Health Care*, Chapter 2, for discussion of health-service management in the 1990s.

In response to adverse media publicity and demands from the Presidents of the Royal Colleges of Physicians and Surgeons for urgent action over resources, in January 1988 the Prime Minister instigated a high-level, confidential review. The expectation was aroused that this

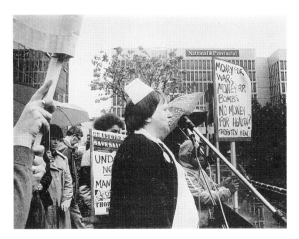

Figure 7.2 *The campaign to halt closure of the Thornton View hospital in Bradford in August 1983. (Source: Bradford Telegraph & Argus)*

would result in a substantial injection of additional funds, either from Exchequer sources, or by some substantial alteration in the method of funding health care. In the course of the review, the DHSS was split into its component parts, leaving the *Department of Health* (DH) in charge of the NHS.

You should now read the first section ('Pressure for Change') of the Reader article by social policy analysts Patricia Day and Rudolf Klein.

□ According to Day and Klein, the stimulus for another shake-up of the NHS stemmed from three interacting factors. What were they?

■ They were:

1   Budgetary constraints on the NHS, which experienced a lower rate of growth in expenditure in the 1980s than in the 1970s.

2   Rising public expectations and increased demand for health care, especially those forms of care which enhance the quality (rather than the quantity) of life and which were subject to long NHS waiting-lists; and

3   Government pressure on the NHS to increase productivity, largely through target-setting and general managers appointed to achieve those targets by exerting pressure in turn on the medical profession.

The point made by the authors under 2 above is not as straightforward as they argue. They emphasise rising expectations, rather than the desire to hold on to existing services against pressure to erode them. They also stress services that enhance quality of life, but many would argue that the pressure for screening for cervical cancer, renal dialysis or cardiovascular surgery (all subject to long waiting lists in the 1980s) are not simply 'quality' issues.

The 1991 reorganisation

The White Paper *Working for Patients* (published in January 1989, but implemented in April 1991) surprisingly by-passed the question of health-service funding. The NHS would continue to be available to all, regardless of income, and to be financed mainly out of general taxation.

Like previous Conservative governments, the Thatcher administration rejected the idea of reverting to American-style private health insurance. The government had evidently accepted that private medicine would occupy no more than a marginal role, and few incentives were given to its further expansion. Instead,

both the Thatcher and the Major administrations placed their expectations on the continuing search for efficiency gains, by further exploiting the potentialities of the newly installed NHS management structures and opening up new opportunities for competition between provider units in a so-called **internal market in health care**[12] (discussed below). They also envisaged a wider provider market, giving greater opportunities for the private sector.

Most of the 1991 package of reorganisation represented pursuit of long-standing objectives. A whole range of measures were designed to relate the *income* of consultants and GPs more closely to services performed for the NHS. This effort represented merely a fresh permutation of alternatives which had been under consideration since the beginning of the NHS.

Removal of local authority and Trades Union members of health authorities and FHSAs (formerly FPCs—see Figure 7.1) also completed a long process of transition in which health authorities were converted from agencies of *local democratic accountability* into arms of the *management* structure. Some compensation for community involvement was allowed by the decision in both 1982 and 1991 to spare the lives of the *Community Health Councils* (CHCs), which both individually and collectively through the Association of Community Health Councils, were apt to produce outspoken criticisms of government policies.

The contentiousness and radicalism of the 1991 reforms rested on the intention to break with the tradition whereby health authorities were planners, owners, employers and providers of all health services within their catchment areas, and were funded on the basis of the integration of these comprehensive functions.

In 1946, Aneurin Bevan concluded that 'universalising the best' required *full integration*: 'This cannot be done effectively if each hospital is a separate, autonomous body' (quoted in Webster, 1991, p. 66). The 1989 White Paper came to the opposite conclusion: 'To bring all parts of the NHS up to the very high standard of the best' required *separation* of purchasing of health services from provision of health services (the so-called **purchaser–provider split**) in order to stimulate competition and provide 'markets'. This internal market in health care was expected to allow the most productive units to prosper and the least effective to wither away. Adoption of a formal contractual relationship between purchaser and provider was expected to yield more precise benefits from the provider.

[12]The internal market in health care is also discussed in several chapters of *Dilemmas in Health Care*.

This principle seemed to offer the key to achievement of more effective yield from scarce resources. In the words of the American health economist, Alain Enthoven, who was an influence on government thinking:

> In medical care, quality and economy usually go hand in hand.... When resources are limited, such as in the NHS, greater efficiency...can be translated directly into more and better services. More spending is not necessarily the only route to more and better care. (Enthoven, 1991, p. 64)

☐ Can you see the attractiveness of Enthoven's proposition to the Thatcher administration?

■ The purchaser–provider split offered the means to square the circle. The NHS could in theory be greatly improved without prejudicing the government's aim to reduce taxes and public expenditure.

You should now carefully study the rest of the article by Patricia Day and Rudolf Klein in the Reader, which contains a brief assessment of the 1991 changes.

☐ Day and Klein identify the key principle of the purchaser–provider split as 'money follows patients'. Explain the importance of this principle by answering the following questions:

(a) In 1991, what were the major 'purchasers'?
(b) How was their budget calculated?
(c) From whom could they purchase health care?
(d) How was this arrangement supposed to be better for patients?

■ The purchaser–provider plan involved the following:

(a) The DHAs were converted into *purchasing authorities*.

(b) They were given a budget by the Department of Health according to the size and demographic composition of their populations.

(c) DHAs could buy services from *any* provider, both in the public and in the private health-care sector, within their own district or elsewhere, so 'money follows patients'.

(d) By utilising their expert knowledge of local conditions to exercise choice on behalf of local communities, DHAs could in theory obtain the most appropriate and economical packages of services from providers.

DHAs were not the only purchasers. DHAs still operated on behalf of GPs who remained contracted to the FHSAs—these were mainly the smaller practices—but from 1991, GPs belonging to larger practices were given the discretion to manage their own budgets for the first time since 1948. These **GP fund-holders**' budgets were not only intended to cover the cost of providing primary care to the patients on their lists, but also the purchase of non-emergency treatment, out-patient services (for example, physiotherapy) and diagnostic tests from hospitals and other providers and from 1993, community care or mental handicap services (as they are still officially known).

In another innovation under the 1991 reorganisation, hospital and other health authority agencies, such as mental health or community care services, were invited to divide up into a multiplicity of **self-governing NHS Trusts** (often referred to as SGTs), which would remain within the NHS and be subject to regulation. Nevertheless the Trusts have been given greater discretion than hospital units under the previous regime. They would for instance decide on their range of functions, determine pay and conditions of staff, and manage their own finances. These changes can be expected to enhance the importance of the *general managers* of NHS hospitals still further—a subject to which we return later in this chapter.

The new system is designed to reward hospitals according to the volume of work performed, so correcting the notorious defect of the past funding system which tended to penalise the most productive hospitals and reward those making least use of their facilities. Trusts successful in competing for contracts are likely to become dominant centres of specialisation, attracting patients from far afield and employing a well-remunerated workforce, whereas their less successful competitors are likely to face contraction and unemployment of their staff, and they might well be threatened with closure. Consequently the hospital system is entering into a critical phase of rehabilitation which is likely to constitute the largest reorganisation of services since the beginning of the NHS. The proposals made in 1992 by the King's Fund and the Tomlinson Report for widespread hospital closures and reorganisation of health services in London provide some indication of the magnitude of the changes begun in 1991.

When the purchaser–provider proposals were first launched, there was ambiguity concerning the scale of the exercise. It was unclear whether the opting-out of DHA control by hospital and other NHS Trusts, and the uptake of GP fund-holding, were intended as a provisional, small-scale experiment, or a precedent designed for universal application. Subsequent events have indicated an escalation towards general implementation. Although the first two waves of Trusts and GP fundholders in April 1991 and April 1992 represent a minority, it is likely that these independent providers and purchasers will predominate during the last decade of the twentieth century.

At the time of writing, in 1992, it is still too early to assess the results of the purchaser–provider system. Sceptics point to the high cost of implementing a market system. Significant spending is being incurred in hospitals and group general practices on elaborate *information systems* required to support *competitive tendering*. New contracts have involved concessions to GPs designed to attract their compliance.

☐ What are the financial advantages of the new contract with GPs, according to Day and Klein in the Reader article?

■ The following sources of new income were noted:

1   Bonus payments were introduced for GPs who met targets for preventive health care, such as vaccination and screening, which Day and Klein assert that most GPs were already carrying out.

2   GPs who practised in inner cities qualified for 'special deprivation' payments and received extra compensation for difficulties in meeting the above targets among their mobile population.

3   Subsidies to GPs for employing practice staff were greatly enhanced under the new contract.

4   GPs could add to their income by engaging in fee-for-service activities, such as minor surgery and health-promotion clinics.

GPs also fought off an attempt to enforce 'indicative prescribing budgets' (a ceiling on the cost of prescribed drugs), which would have represented a move towards cash limits. Such control was devised to curb expenditure on pharmaceutical products, which has for long been the most rapidly expanding area of primary health care expenditure.

In the financial year 1991–2, additional resources were injected into the hospital service on a larger scale than at any time since 1979. It is therefore arguable that improvements in performance were connected to additional income rather than to the purchaser–provider system. It is likely that after the initial brief phase of leniency, the NHS will revert to the more characteristic regime of economy. Although RAWP was abolished in 1991, district budgets were still determined on a population basis, which provided strict limitations for the operation of the competitive system.

A further unfortunate consequence of the 1991 reforms has been to force attention on the *acute* hospital sector, while much less concern was devoted to primary care, community care, public health and preventive medicine. Although these areas are intended for priority development in the 1990s and are being subjected to changes, as will be indicated in the following sections of this chapter, there is no sign that in reality they will be able to bear the burden which is being placed on them. This difficulty will be exacerbated if the Hospital Trusts absorb an increased share of NHS resources.

Finally, it is doubtful whether practicality and political constraints will allow the market system in health care to develop unimpeded. In practice it is likely that service users will notice few changes,[13] and little real competition will take place, the only significant difference being the contractual relationship underlying treatment. Thus, as in the case of previous reorganisations, the promised revolution may turn out to represent an unexpected degree of historical continuity.

Care by the community

At this point, we turn back in time to the beginning of the period covered by this chapter, to consider what effect the reorganisation of formal health services was having on the volume and type of lay care. In the 1950s and 1960s, *community care* was intended as an alternative both to institutional and to informal lay care. But its focus changed sharply in the 1970s and again in the 1980s. Lay care became much more central. During the 1970s, another dimension was added to community care. Instead of just care *in* the community, it was redefined as care *by* the community.

For example, sociologist Michael Bayley, in a study of mentally handicapped people and their care in Sheffield, published in 1973, pointed out that many dependent people needed 24-hour care which could not be met by statutory or voluntary services alone, but depended also on the informal network of support provided by friends, family and neighbours. Evidence such as this fuelled a resurgence of policy-making interest in the use of *volunteers*. The *Wolfenden Report on the Voluntary Sector* in 1978, for example, drew attention to a 'mixed economy' of welfare. It stressed that there was a plurality of caring agencies involving statutory agencies,

[13]See *Dilemmas in Health Care*, Chapter 5, for further consideration of the 'consumers', as health-service users have come to be known.

the commercial or private sector, the voluntary sector and the informal sector—i.e. family, friends and neighbours.

The policy intention at this stage was to ensure a balance between these component parts. But in 1979 the coming to power of a Conservative government committed to a strong pro-family ideology, saw a major shift of emphasis.

> It all really starts in the family, because not only is the family the most important means through which we show our care for others. It's the place where each generation learns its responsibilities towards the rest of society.... I believe that the volunteer movement is at the heart of all our social welfare provision. That the statutory services are the supportive services underpinning where necessary, filling the gaps, and helping the helpers. (Margaret Thatcher, speaking as Prime Minister in 1981, quoted in Digby, 1989, p. 90)

□ What did the Prime Minister see as the cornerstone of community care?

■ She saw two components of the 'mixed economy'—the voluntary sector and the informal sector—as the primary sources of community care. (Although Mrs Thatcher does not mention the private sector in this speech, the 'mixed economy' was intended to include it.)

This particular emphasis on unpaid and voluntary caring was modified in subsequent policy documents. Concern also began to rise about the chaotic and defective machinery of community care; the sight of people begging in British cities, including those who appeared to be mentally ill, proved increasingly embarrassing to the government. In the main, these people have been victims of the 'revolving-door syndrome', in which facilities for in-patient care for predominantly young people with acute mental problems have been reduced and they are rapidly returned to the streets. This concern provoked an intervention by the *Audit Commission* in 1986, the *Griffiths Report on Community Care* of 1988, followed by the *NHS and Community Care Act* of 1990 which handed primary responsibility for community care to local authorities.

The local authorities were given a key role as 'commissioners' of community care services, with public and private organisations actually providing the care. Under the legislation, 'care plans' must be drawn up for people discharged from institutions and a variety of professionals from different agencies are expected to join forces with

voluntary bodies and informal carers to make sure these needs are met. There was much criticism of the delay in implementing this legislation and of the lack of resources. Critics maintained that, without a much higher level of resources than anticipated, community care would retain the negative connotations it has assumed in the decades since its inception.[14] After a series of false starts, the new system was eventually introduced in April 1993.

□ Look at Figure 7.3. What changes strike you in the balance of funding between hospitals and community care since 1979?

■ Hospital expenditure has risen, but that on community care has risen faster. Social security payments contribute a large proportion of the increase. Hospital expenditure still remains very high. (The balance, in terms of the number of people looked after, still remains in favour of hospitals.)

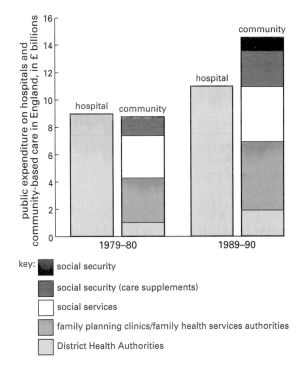

key:
- ■ social security
- ▨ social security (care supplements)
- □ social services
- ▨ family planning clinics/family health services authorities
- ▨ District Health Authorities

Figure 7.3 *Public expenditure (in £billions) on hospitals and community-based care in England, 1979–80 compared with 1989–90. (Data from Audit Commission, 1989–90 prices)*

[14]The future prospects for community care are discussed in *Dilemmas in Health Care*, Chapter 8.

Who cares?

The continued reliance on informal care, which remained a feature of government policy in the late 1980s, was based on assumptions that a plentiful supply of female labour existed in the family, and also that women were somehow 'natural carers'. In 1979, the sociologist Hilary Graham wrote an article which she titled 'Prevention and health: every mother's business'. According to Graham, the burden of community care was placed primarily, if not exclusively, on women's shoulders. However, a study of informal carers by Hazel Green (1988) showed that among adults in Great Britain 3.5 million women and 2.5 million men were acting as informal carers for someone who was physically or mentally disabled. Prevention policy (discussed later in this chapter), with its emphasis on individual responsibility for health, also saw a pivotal role for women in relation to family health. But this was a role which women were increasingly unable to fulfil.

The prospects of turning to 'the community' and in particular its female members, were more limited than ever before. The proportion of working married women rose sharply from the 1970s. Increasing mobility combined with decreasing family size meant that elderly people often lived at a distance from relatives. In inner London, the proportion of elderly people who had a child living within five minutes' walk halved between the late 1950s and the late 1970s. Ties with neighbours were less close, more short-lived and also now compounded by racial divisions in some areas.

But families nevertheless did try to maintain their caring role. In one study of pensioners over the age of 75, carried out in the late 1970s, over three-quarters of those with surviving children saw them at least once a week. Elderly people are the largest group in the community who need care as a result of physical or mental disability (see Figures 7.4 and 7.5), but young people need care too.

However, the burdens on carers, often themselves elderly, are considerable. The sociologists Ann Bowling and Ann Cartwright have made several studies of carers of elderly people. Their article 'Caring for the spouse who died',[15] focuses on the experience and attitudes of about 360 elderly widowed men and women (you should read it now).

[15]The article 'Caring for the spouse who died' by Bowling, A. and Cartwright, A. (taken from a study published in 1982), appears in *Health and Disease: A Reader* (second edition 1995).

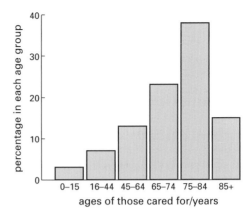

Figure 7.4 *The ages of mentally or physically disabled people who rely on informal care in the community from relatives or friends. (Data from Green, H., 1988, OPCS Social Survey Division, Series GH5, No. 15, Supplement A, HMSO, London, Table 3.5, p. 18)*

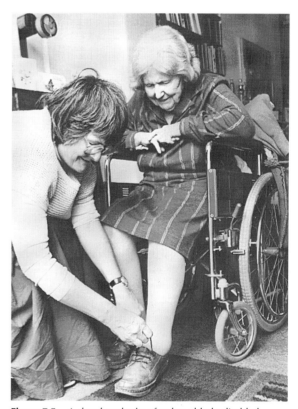

Figure 7.5 *A daughter looks after her elderly disabled mother at home. (Photo: Vicki White, Photo Co-op)*

▢ What does the Bowling and Cartwright research demonstrate?

■ It shows that the bulk of caring is carried out *by* elderly people *for* elderly people. The proportion of wives caring for husbands is considerable. A smaller proportion of husbands care for wives.

Another study by Ann Bowling, published in 1984, shows the emotional demands of caring:

> I had to practically reorganize my own life. As soon as I left home I had to go straight down and make breakfast and do the housework, see to her…and things like that. I got the lunch and the shopping and then came back to anything that had to be done here. I went back again in the evening. It was almost like not living. We all gave up communicating with each other. I had trouble with the children. I had trouble with my mother…because I hit her. I got really angry one day because she just laughed when she made a mess of the bed. I just lashed out at her and hit her across the bottom. It was all trouble, trouble all the time. (Quoted in Bowling, 1984, p. 442)

An *Equal Opportunities Commission* (EOC) study, 'Who cares for the carers', published in 1982, commented:

> The expectation that a woman will provide the necessary care within the family whatever the cost to herself, still underpins the reality of community care. Cuts in health and social services and cash benefits intensify the demands placed on carers, they mean there are less physical resources to aid them, less alternatives to relieve them, and less money to support them. Savings in public expenditure increase the cost to the carer in terms of her social life, her employment prospects and ultimately her physical and mental well being. These costs are borne individually and do not figure in any public expenditure account. The price paid is the restriction placed on women's opportunities. (Quoted in Allsop, 1984, p. 120)

It was not until 1986 that financial help was available for married women carers. In that year the European Court ruled that they were entitled to the *invalid care allowance*. Previously this allowance, payable to a relative staying at home to care for a disabled individual (it was assumed that single women would be willing to forego career and pension opportunities to do this), was not payable to a married woman, who was assumed to be at home in any event. As the EOC had concluded, this effectively excluded 99.5 per cent of those actually giving care. This victory was subsequently negated by changes in the regulations which made it more difficult for *anyone* to obtain the allowance.

Feminist perspectives on lay care

Questions of the organisation of health-care delivery brought the issue of women as carers to the fore. That informal female care was recognised as a form of health and welfare service owed much to feminist analysis. In the 1970s, feminism had mounted a searching challenge to the role of biomedicine in general, arguing that biomedicine was actively involved in sustaining a male-dominated gender order. This was part of a more general critique of medicine, discussed later in this chapter. Feminist studies of caring, in particular those by the sociologists Janet Finch and Dulcie Groves, and by Hilary Land and Clare Ungerson, pointed out that the assumption underlying state health and welfare policy was that women do the caring.

This assumption was related to the problem of defining informal care and establishing what the relationship between it and collectively provided services should be—issues which were discussed with new force in the 1980s. Local schemes, for example that in Kent where volunteers were paid, increasingly blurred the boundaries between informal and formal care.

The feminist critique also focused on the role of lay people in *childbirth*. The *medicalisation* of childbirth had proceeded apace after World War II, as you have seen in Chapter 6. Feminists criticised modern obstetrics for an over-emphasis on the physiology of pregnancy and birth and the medicalisation of a normal biological event, excluding the family and turning the woman into a passive and dependent patient.[16] There was a tendency in these accounts to romanticise patterns of lay involvement in childbirth in the past, but also a necessary assertion of female autonomy. The suspension of Wendy Savage, consultant obstetrician in Tower Hamlets in April 1985, appeared to stem in part from disapproval by male colleagues of her support for women making decisions about how they would give birth (e.g. in the use of drugs, or choice of birth-position).

Childbirth was only part of a wide-ranging feminist analysis of gender issues around health care, epitomised in the self-help text *Our Bodies, Ourselves: A Health Book by and for Women*, by the Boston Women's Health Book Collective, originally published in the USA in 1971 and subsequently republished in Britain and other countries.

---

[16] *Birth to Old Age: Health in Transition*, Chapter 3.

Informal networks of care and advice

The feminist arguments around community care and the role of women in health care marked a more general tendency in the 1970s and 1980s—the emergence of lay care and self-help as a radical issue (from both Left and Right perspectives), appealing to the middle class. The rise in popularity of 'alternative medicine' (discussed later) was part of this trend. Perhaps its clearest manifestation in the 1980s came through the gay response to AIDS (Acquired Immune Deficiency Syndrome).

Informal 'buddies' provided lay care and support for people infected with HIV (the Human Immunodeficiency Virus), or with AIDS, where—at least initially—formal statutory provision was non-existent. The widespread use of 'alternative' drugs without official approval by people with AIDS caused difficulties during clinical trials of 'official' pharmaceuticals. The use of these drugs has been backed by networks of lay information and advice. Such developments have often been in self-conscious opposition to official medicine, much as occurred with popular medicine in the nineteenth century.

AIDS also drew attention to long-established patterns of lay belief about disease, which persisted into the 1980s. The popular views of AIDS as contagious and of moral responsibility for disease, which permeated more general public reactions, was not new, for those attitudes towards infectious disease had a long history.[17]

Other studies also showed how important lay beliefs about health remained in the 1970s and 1980s. For example, the social anthropologist and general practitioner Cecil Helman demonstrated how what he called the 'folk model' of disease both differed from and resembled orthodox medicine.[18]

Lay networks of information and advice also continued to operate. In the early 1970s, Christopher Elliott-Bins studied patients attending a general practice in Northampton. He found that 96 per cent of the patients had received some advice or treatment before consulting their GP. One, a village shopkeeper with a persistent cough, had received advice from her husband, an ex-hospital matron, a doctor's receptionist, and five customers, three of whom recommended a remedy: Golden

Syrup, a boiled onion gruel, and the application of a hot brick to the chest. Elliott-Bins repeated this study fifteen years later in the same general practice; the pattern of self-care and lay health advice had remained largely unchanged.

There have nevertheless been developments in lay care. A wide range of *self-help groups* has flourished since World War II. *Alcoholics Anonymous* was one of the first, arriving in the United Kingdom from the USA in the late 1940s. 'AA' has remained a 'non-political' organisation, avoiding input into alcohol policy. Its model, of encouraging heavy drinkers (or alcoholics) to develop the will-power to cease drinking through mutual self-help, was widely copied by other self-help groups.

☐ Can you suggest other self-help, health-related groups which operate along similar lines to the AA model?

■ You might think of Narcotics Anonymous (for drug users); Weight Watchers (for overweight people); Tranx (for tranquilliser users). The range of self-help groups is enormous, e.g. Cancerlink, and Body Positive (for HIV-positive people).

Overall, self-help and lay care and advice remain the major source of health care in the United Kingdom in the 1990s, with no sign of diminishing participation in this informal sector of the health-care system.

The health-work hierarchy: questioning medical dominance

In the decades since 1974, health-care occupations have continued the shifts of boundary and of status that we described in the previous chapter. The 'end of medical hegemony', predicted as the result of changes in the 1960s, was announced in both the 1970s and the 1980s. In particular, the advent of *general management* in the NHS has been seen as heralding medical decline. But in some areas, the power of the profession increased in the 1970s. General practice, for example, continued to enhance its status and increased role in medical politics.

GPs and the primary health care team

In the 1970s, GPs allied themselves with the concept of **primary health care**. This doctrine, enshrined in the 1978 *Alma Ata Declaration* of the WHO, was elaborated initially as a reaction against the application of inappropriate high-technology medicine in Third World countries (this is discussed in detail in Chapter 8). What was needed, it was argued, were simple dispensaries, basic health advice and basic personnel. The same arguments

[17]HIV infection and AIDS are discussed extensively in *Experiencing and Explaining Disease* (revised edition 1996), Chapter 4.

[18]The article by Cecil Helman, 'Feed a cold, starve a fever', appears in *Health and Disease: A Reader* and is set reading for Open University students during study of *Medical Knowledge: Doubt and Certainty*, Chapter 2.

were then applied to industrialised countries: GPs in the United Kingdom were seen as the allies of their patients, their protectors against science, technology and bureaucratic growth.

Momentum for improved standards and adoption of the primary health care philosophy built up in the 1980s. However, despite tortuous discussions, the government and the profession failed to reach agreement on translating this philosophy into a system of incentives built into the GPs' NHS contracts. The government insisted on a more rigid system of incentives and audit than the profession was willing to concede. Failure to agree resulted in the unilateral imposition of a new contract in 1989, followed by the introduction of the fund-holder arrangement in 1991. The GP has thus been coerced into change to a greater degree than was the case in 1911 or even 1948. This has naturally produced an adverse reaction on the part of the profession, as mentioned in the previous section, but the Reader article by Day and Klein suggests that the balance of advantage in the new arrangements lies on the side of the GP.

This primary care development was at one with the previous emphasis on a holistic philosophy within general practice. It went along with an elaboration of the division of labour in general practice and changes in GPs' working arrangements. In this period, there was an acceleration of the move away from single-handed practice into group practices. Table 7.2 gives information about the numbers of general practices of various sizes in Britain in 1990.

☐ What do these figures tell you about the pattern of general practice?

Table 7.2 Estimated numbers of general practices in Great Britain (excluding Northern Ireland) in 1990, showing the number of GPs per practice, and the number and percentage of GPs and practices in each category

No. of GPs in the practice	No. of GPs	%	No. of practices	%
1	3 382	11.0	3 382	31.4
2	4 543	14.8	2 242	20.8
3	5 511	18.0	1 813	16.8
4	5 607	18.3	1 384	12.9
5	4 962	16.2	980	9.1
6 and over	6 636	21.7	969	9.0
total	30 641	100	10 770	100

Data from British Medical Association, based on Department of Health (1992) Statistics for General Medical Practitioners in England and Wales, 1980–1990, *Statistical Bulletin*, **4**(2).

■ The proportion of doctors working single-handedly in Britain as a whole is low (11.0 per cent). Small-group practice appears to be the norm, but note that over one-third of all GPs (37.9 per cent) work in practices containing 5 or more GPs.

The concept of the **primary health care team** replaced that of the single-handed GP (compare Figure 6.4 in the previous chapter with Figure 7.6). The days when a GP's wife acted as receptionist, chaperon, nurse, and accountant (in addition to the domestic role) were ended. Between 1964 and 1977, the proportion of practices with an attached nurse increased from 12 to 84 per cent. Only 1 per cent of GPs did not have a receptionist in 1977, compared with 25 per cent in 1964.

The male (predominantly) GP was joined by members of middle-stratum occupational groups: nurses, health visitors, receptionists—occupations which had a predominantly female image. The idea was that the GP should remain in charge: as one GP, Dr J. S. Norell, put it:

> …he would rather be recognised as the most versatile of medical social workers than the least of medical men. (Quoted in Honigsbaum, 1979, p. 305)

To the role of 'medical social worker' was added the possibility of specialism in other areas: GP paediatrician was suggested by one report in the 1970s, also GP obstetrician.

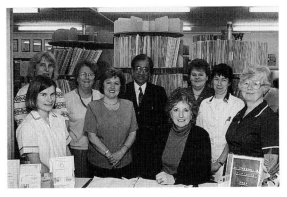

Figure 7.6 *Part of the primary health care team in a large group general practice in England in the 1990s. From left to right (front row): dietician, medical secretary, clerical receptionist (seated), senior practice nurse; (back row) medical secretary, practice manager, GP, fund-holding manager, liaison nurse for the elderly. Not shown: four more GPs, two more practice nurses, two stress counsellors and a physiotherapist. (Photo: Mike Levers)*

By the 1980s, then, the strategy to revive general practice had been largely successful at one level. By 1980, general practice was the first choice of 37 per cent of doctors as they left medical school. The *College of General Practitioners* had become a powerful medico-political body, obtaining its Royal Charter in 1972. The power of the GP had been successfully advanced. Whether the strategy was so successful as far as the patient was concerned was more doubtful. In the 1980s, GPs became involved in a 'ragbag' of health care and maintenance activities, some of which, (preventive screening, for example) had never been properly evaluated.[19]

Nurses

Nurses were not as successful as GPs in achieving increased power and status, and the structural problems that beset the profession continued. The 1974 reorganisation of the NHS (building on the Salmon Report of 1966) gave *nurse managers* equal status in planning with doctors and administrators. The *male* sector of the nursing profession predominated among the ranks of nurse managers, out of proportion to the number of male nurses. Nurse managers had a guaranteed place as an integral part of the *consensus management teams* throughout the NHS regional administration.

In practice, this opportunity to advance the status of nursing was lost. The assertion of managerial authority by nurses was often ineffective because many nurse managers found it difficult to adopt new techniques and roles, and few nurses had sufficient retraining to be able to grasp critical issues of service policy and planning. Within nursing, the nurse managers were criticised by 'professionally' minded nurses for pursuing managerial objectives to the detriment of the development of the professional status of registered nurses.

The uncontroversial reorganisation of the NHS in 1982 did not alter the management structure, and the Pay Review Board improved the status of nurses by increasing their earnings. However, following the Griffiths-inspired introduction of general management from 1983 onwards, nurses lost their hard-won managerial authority and their representation on key management boards. Nurses lacked the embedded foothold in health service administration at all levels which doctors had secured for themselves. Griffiths, in his 1983 report, made no mention at all of nurses, although they were numerically the single largest component of the health-care labour

force. A few nurses have subsequently been appointed as district and unit general managers.[20]

Militancy among health workers

Reorganisation in the 1970s brought other tendencies in the division of health labour to the fore. A trend which was to emerge strongly over that decade was deepening divisions within the medical profession itself.

In 1966, the *Junior Hospital Doctors' Association* was formed, successfully initiating a campaign to raise salaries. In October 1975, junior hospital doctors in Leicestershire took industrial action over pay and this subsequently spread to the rest of the country (Figure 7.7).

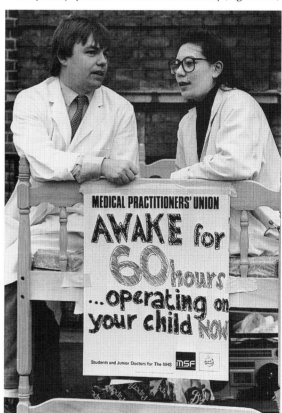

Figure 7.7 *The dispute in the 1970s over long working hours among junior doctors and consequent danger to patients surfaced again in the 1990s when the BMA publicised the fact that a working week of over 80 hours was still the norm. (Source: Times Newspapers Ltd)*

[19]Prevention and screening are discussed in *Dilemmas in Health Care*, Chapter 9.

[20]The role of managers in the NHS is discussed further in *Dilemmas in Health Care*, Chapter 2; Chapter 6 addresses the ways in which other occupational groups (particularly nurses and midwives) have attempted to enhance their professional status.

The tactics of the junior doctors largely represented a grassroots revolt against the leadership of the BMA. Many belonged to the smaller *Medical Practitioners' Union* which had merged with the white-collar trades union ASTMS (Association of Scientific, Technical and Managerial Staffs) in 1970. The outcome of the dispute was an industrial type of contract for the junior doctors, with (tiny) overtime payments for hours worked over the basic 40-hour week. This was at odds with the notion of the doctor as 'professional'; and, in turn, the system of overtime payments led to the erosion of differentials between senior registrars and consultants.

The consultants were aggrieved at this threat to their financial and other status. But they, too, were embroiled with the government in disputes about their contracts and about private pay-beds within the NHS. Increasingly, the *Hospital Consultants' and Specialists' Association*, founded in 1948 but largely dormant until the end of the 1960s, began to challenge the right of the BMA to act as the voice of the consultants. In 1974, it unsuccessfully applied to the Industrial Relations Court for negotiating rights. The role of the BMA as the doctors' trades union was under threat. In 1972 it was anxious enough to invite a former chairman of ICI, Sir Paul Chambers, to investigate its constitution and organisation.

The political scientist Rudolf Klein has expertly summed up the problems which faced a divided profession:

> On paper, the structure was highly corporate, with the medical profession being organised in clearly defined associations and with a highly centralised negotiating structure…under the veneer of disciplined corporatism, however, the reality was an anarchic syndicalism. The leaders of the medical profession—the bureaucrats of the BMA and others—faced precisely the same nagging difficulty as the paternalistic rationalisers at the Ministry of Health—how to influence, let alone control, the individualistic practitioners at the periphery. (Klein, 1983, pp. 89–90)

Klein is here contrasting the apparently *corporate* structure of the profession with the reality. By 'corporate' he means a close relationship between official central structures and related interest groups which work together to make policy. The reality, according to Klein, is medical *syndicalism*; a term usually used to describe movements of industrial militancy based on direct action, and here signifying the ability of individual practitioners to take power into their own hands, as in strike action.

Militancy was not confined to the medical profession. The 1970s brought a rise in trades union activity among ancillary workers as well. When they went on strike in 1973, many felt that the character of social relations within the division of labour in the hospital service had been radically altered. Ancillary workers had ceased to be the docile servants of doctors and no longer accepted that the privilege of working in hospitals justified low pay.

Table 7.3 shows the average weekly earnings of a range of health workers in the mid-1980s.

Table 7.3 NHS health workers in full-time employment: average gross weekly earnings, 1985–6

	Men	Women
medical practitioners	£406	n.s.
nursing administrators and executives	£199	£170
registered and enrolled nurses and midwives	£148	£128
nursing auxiliaries and assistants	n.s.	£102
average for class III non-manual workers	£221	£155
ambulance men	£166	n.s.
hospital porters	£124	n.s.
hospital ward orderlies	n.s.	£104
average for manual workers	£130	£94

n.s. = not sampled. (Data from Department of Employment, 1986, pt D, Tables 86 and 87, reproduced from Stacey, M., 1988, *The Sociology of Health and Healing*, Unwin Hyman, London, Figure 13.2, p. 188)

☐ What do you notice about pay differentials between health-care workers shown in Table 7.3?

■ There are large differentials between different sectors. Medical practitioners earn on average more than twice as much as nursing administrators and executives. This group in turn earn a quarter as much again as registered and enrolled nurses and midwives. Nursing auxiliaries' earnings are on a par with those of ward orderlies. Gender differences are also apparent with women consistently earning less than men even in 'traditional' female occupations. (The figures for the medical profession also conceal big differences between the top and bottom of the profession.)

Militancy was compounded by the fact that trades unions such as COHSE (Confederation of Health Service

Employees) and NUPE (National Union of Public Employees) were competing against each other for members. They were also competing against professional organisations. In particular, they increasingly challenged the *Royal College of Nursing's* role of acting both as a professional organisation and as a trades union.

Once again the cry of the 'end of medical hegemony' went up. There were theoretical as well as organisational reasons for this. From different perspectives the work of writers such as Ivan Illich and Ian Kennedy, the feminist critique of medicine, and the arguments of Thomas McKeown, were mounting a powerful attack in the 1970s on medicine's claim to ideological hegemony and effectiveness.

Alternative medicine: a growing challenge?

Alternative or **complementary medicine** (which uses therapeutic techniques that fall outside orthodox medicine) benefited from this trend in thinking. From the mid-1970s, there was a widespread revival of interest in older healing modes. In February 1986, *Which?* magazine asked nearly 28 000 of its subscribers whether they had used any form of alternative or complementary medicine in the previous 12 months. One in seven said they had (osteopaths predominated). The *British Holistic Medicine Association* was formed in 1983. Prompted by an intervention of the Prince of Wales, in 1986 the BMA produced a report on *Alternative Medicine*, which was predictably antagonistic; but in 1993 the BMA revised its ideas and issued a further report entitled *Complementary Medicine: New Approaches to Good Practice*, which, as the title suggests, was more conciliatory.

Nevertheless, the practitioner status of alternative therapists was rising. There were moves towards formal registration (already well advanced in continental Europe). *The Research Council for Complementary Medicine* actively fostered these developments and some GPs were already receiving training in alternative therapies such as acupuncture and homeopathy.

Table 7.4 shows the number of practitioners of alternative or complementary medicine in the United Kingdom in 1980.

□ What strikes you about the data in Table 7.4 and the balance of practitioners?

■ A considerable number of practitioners in some therapies are qualified in orthodox medicine.

Many medically qualified doctors became more interested in alternative methods in the 1980s. There were also claims that the numbers of alternative practitioners were increasing by 11 per cent each year.

Table 7.4 Number of complementary or alternative practitioners in the United Kingdom in 1980

Therapy	Medically qualified	Lay members in professional association	Lay practitioners not in professional association
acupuncture	160	508	250
chiropractic	1	140	400
herbalism	10	103	200
homeopathy	272	130	230
hypnotherapy	1 000	460	170
massage	350	1 150	11 500
naturopathy	5	115	106
osteopathy	202	650	150

Data from Fulder, S. and Monro, R. (1981) *The Status of Complementary Medicine in the United Kingdom*, Threshold Foundation, London, p. 35.

Nevertheless, the alternative sector of health care remains a fraction of the size of the orthodox sector.[21]

General management: the real threat?

Far more threatening to the structure of health-care occupations, at least in theory, was general management, introduced into the health service in 1984 following the Griffiths Report. A managerial tendency had been apparent in health service reorganisation since the 1960s; in 1984, it reached its peak. The administrative sector of the hospital structure moved centre stage and became *management*: hybrid posts were created which combined two or even three functions. One aim of general management was to reduce the power of the medical profession. But how far this happened in practice is debatable.

One study of the impact of general management by the political scientist Christopher Pollitt concluded that the 1984 reorganisation had failed to face up to medical power; it was almost impossible for managers to remove hospital doctors. Other analysts have found that little changed. The health-service analyst, David Hunter, for example, has found that:

[21]The status of alternative or complementary medicine is discussed further in the second edition of *Medical Knowledge: Doubt and Certainty* (Open University Press, 1994), Chapter 2.

...most doctors and managers continue to inhabit a shared culture of medical autonomy. Managers will on occasion challenge the doctors but it remains the exception rather than the rule. (Hunter, 1991, p. 448)[22]

Promoting the public health

Community medicine: a failed experiment

The position of public health, as you saw in Chapter 6, was at a cross-roads at the end of the 1960s. The old MOH was gone; the new *community physician* was rising out of the ashes. Many in the public-health profession were not averse to this change. Bringing public health into the NHS mainstream seemed to offer tangible advantages, in particular that of specialist status. The establishment of the *Faculty of Community Medicine* in 1972 and the broadening of the public-health training curriculum both suggested that their status would be improved.

Community physicians approached the 1974 reorganisation of the NHS with high hopes; posts for them were created at region, area and district level. But by 1976, many community physicians were asking publicly whether there was any future for their specialty. When the next reorganisation of the NHS took place in 1982, fully 20 per cent of the profession took early retirement and many posts remained unfilled.

What caused this rapid disillusionment and the crisis in community medicine? Both the concept and its practitioners were pulled in a number of different directions. First, community physicians remained low in *status* in relation to other sections of the medical profession. Their influence on the new consensus management teams was limited.

Second, community medicine's greater *integration* in the NHS was a source of weakness as much as strength. Its practitioners were beset by the financial problems of the health service in the 1970s and 1980s and found it difficult to develop an independent role. The loss of the local government base had also seen the demise of the old role of community advocate or watchdog; in addition, there was no longer any direct contact with the local community.

Third, there were unresolved tensions over the *definition* of community medicine. It was difficult to reconcile the management and specialist/adviser roles which were both meant to be part of the remit. Much time

was spent managing health services rather than in analysing health problems. The community physician, like the MOH in the 1930s, was more preoccupied with administration than with promoting a broader mandate for community medicine.

Health education and prevention of ill-health

One consequence of their largely administrative role was that the *prevention of ill-health* was largely left out of the community physician's work. There were also important differences of view about the meaning of **prevention** and hence the targets at which preventive services should be aimed. Community physicians thought in terms of the *personal* and *environmental health services* which had been delivered by the old MOH. But the major definition, which was established in the 1970s, saw prevention in terms of remedying perceived defects in *individual lifestyle*.

A key document setting out this individualistic, 'lifestyle' approach was the *Lalonde Report* (called after the Canadian Minister of Health), *A New Perspective on the Health of Canadians*, published in 1974. Lalonde was influenced by the work of Thomas McKeown who argued that the overall health of the population bore less relationship to medical advances than to overall standards of living and of nutrition.[23] Many countries followed in publishing similar prevention-oriented documents and there was a rapid growth of interest in preventive medicine and health promotion. In Britain, the DHSS's policy document, published in 1976, was entitled *Prevention and Health: Everybody's Business*.

□ What do you think is the significance of this title?

■ It appears to imply that prevention of illness is a personal matter, not primarily the business of governments, nor of industry, nor does it bear much relation to structural and economic factors.

The Royal Commission on the NHS, reporting in 1979, concluded that a significant improvement in the health of all people of the United Kingdom could come through prevention policies.

Health education was part of this resurgence of disease prevention. Like the public-health doctors, it moved from local authority to health-service control in the 1970s. The *Central Council for Health Education*, founded in 1927 by the Society of Medical Officers of

---

[22]The impact of the 1991 NHS reforms on this relationship is discussed in *Dilemmas in Health Care*, Chapter 2.

[23]McKeown's ideas were mentioned earlier, in Chapter 4 of this book, and are extensively discussed in *World Health and Disease*, Chapter 6.

Health, had been developing its role in conjunction with the local authorities in the post-war period, in particular through the appointment of specialist health education officers to local authorities (there were 24 of them by 1960). In 1968, a new *Health Education Council* (HEC) was established, funded directly by the newly established Department of Health and Social Security (DHSS). The Council's role was a difficult one. The removal of local-authority funding made it remote from local participation and it was funded by governments that were ambivalent, or inconsistent, in their attitudes to health-education issues.

The emphasis of health education (like other forms of prevention) was on the *individual's* responsibility for his or her own health, rather than on *structural* causes of ill-health. The focus was therefore on *single-issue campaigns*, in particular those concerning smoking, alcohol and healthy eating in relation to heart disease, but presented in terms of changing individual behaviour.

The pioneering epidemiological research of Richard Doll and Austin Bradford Hill, published in the 1950s, had established the link between smoking and lung cancer. The Royal College of Physicians' first report, *Smoking and Health*, appeared in 1962. The economic benefit which governments continue to receive from tobacco (in the late 1980s, tobacco was the Chancellor's third largest source of consumer revenue) ensured that government policies focused on the role of individual consumers rather than that of the tobacco companies. Campaigning was left to 'outsider' bodies, such as the Royal College of Physicians, and ASH (Action on Smoking and Health). In 1981, Sir George Young, then a junior health minister and a keen anti-smoker, was moved to the Department of the Environment. It was said that the tobacco industry had brought pressure to bear when it looked as though his enthusiasm for anti-tobacco policies might be effective.

Similar pressures affected other areas of concern to health educators. A report on alcohol, produced by the government's own 'Think Tank' in the 1970s, which recommended a broad approach to the reduction of alcohol consumption, was never officially published. Instead, the government produced a much milder document, *Drinking Sensibly*, in 1981, which took a less comprehensive stance and did not challenge the alcohol industry.

The food industry was also influential in structuring the discussion of problems affecting nutrition and the food supply. Nutritionists such as John Yudkin attacked the power of the sugar industry. The resignation of the Conservative Health Minister, Edwina Currie, in 1988 over the 'salmonella in eggs' furore was one demonstration of the power of the farming lobby in nutrition questions.

□ What do you consider to be the main limitations of single-issue, health-education campaigns aimed at changing individual behaviour?

■ They suffer from an inability to present health problems as at least partly the result of broader structural factors in society, and hence to develop policies aimed at social change. They were also likely to be obstructed by interests exercising powerful political influence. (The extent to which health education has been successful at changing personal behaviour is another contentious issue.)[24]

Attempts to broaden the health debate also ran into government opposition in the 1980s. The attempt by the incoming Conservative government in 1980 to restrict circulation of the *Black Report* (named after its Chairman, Sir Douglas Black), *Inequalities in Health*, provoked a successful paperback edition, with the result that the report's conclusions about widening inequalities became better known than they otherwise might have been.[25] Critics of government policy saw a connection between a follow-up report (*The Health Divide* by Margaret Whitehead), produced in 1987 under the auspices of the HEC, and the demise of the HEC. It was replaced by a new *Health Education Authority* (HEA), which was designated a Special Health Authority[26] directly linked to the health department, and given responsibility for a mass-media AIDS education campaign.

The 'new' public health

The desire to integrate the twin perspectives of personal prevention and the growing concern to protect the environment, led to the development in the 1980s of what has been termed the **'new' public health**. The term has been associated with the WHO's strategy of *Health for All by the Year 2000*, adopted by the World Health Assembly in 1981. In Europe, the strategy of *Health for All* was taken further, and a set of WHO targets for *Health for*

[24]This is discussed in *Dilemmas in Health Care*, Chapter 9.

[25]Inequalities in health in the United Kingdom, and competing explanations for these patterns, are discussed in *World Health and Disease* and also in a television programme for Open University students entitled 'A tale of four cities'.

[26]Certain functions which do not fit into the regional and district framework are designated as Special Health Authorities and come directly under central government.

All were produced. The WHO's *Healthy Cities* project had an impact on several countries, and a number of local authorities in England (Oxford, Liverpool, Nottingham and Sheffield among them) established local strategies for promoting health, which went beyond educating individuals and addressed such issues as industrial pollution, traffic congestion and facilities for leisure.

The meaning of 'new public health' is best conveyed in a *Health Promotion Glossary* commissioned by WHO Europe. It is:

> Professional and public concern with the effect of the total environment in health.
>
> *Note* The terms build on the old (especially 19th century) public health which struggled to tackle health hazards in the physical environment (for example, by building sewers). It now includes the socio-economic environment (for example, high unemployment). 'Public health' has sometimes been used to include publicly provided personal health services such as maternal and child care. The term new public health tends to be restricted to environmental concerns and to exclude personal health services, even preventive ones such as immunisation or birth control. (Quoted in Draper, 1991, p. 10)

☐ What strikes you about this definition?

■ It professes a very wide definition of public health, including the economic environment as well as the physical one. It places less emphasis on formal health-service provision.

Largely in response to international pressures, public health in the United Kingdom therefore seemed to be undergoing something of a revival in a new guise in the 1980s. After a period when chronic and degenerative disease had dominated policy discussions around mortality and morbidity, *communicable disease* came back on the political agenda. Outbreaks of salmonella food poisoning at Stanley Royd Hospital in Wakefield in 1984, and 'legionnaires' disease' at Stafford in the following year, highlighted the shortage of specialists in this field. The advent of AIDS as a potentially epidemic disease began to dominate the health agenda in the mid-1980s. Listeria and bovine spongiform encephalopathy (BSE) were added to the list.

Community medicine was in no state to deal with these new challenges to the public health. The move away from consensus management into general management in the 1980s undermined the specialty's already uncertain role. There was also continuing confusion about conflicting responsibilities for environmental health. For these reasons, an inquiry was held into the future of the public health function, chaired by the Chief Medical Officer, Sir Donald Acheson, which reported in 1988.

The *Acheson Report*, strongly influenced by the history of public health in England, made a determined effort to upgrade the status of public health. It proposed the appointment of *Regional Directors of Public Health*, the revival of annual public-health reports (abandoned in 1974 with the demise of the old MOHs) and the development of more collaboration between sectors such as health, education and social services, rather than an exclusive focus on health services. The Acheson Report placed primary emphasis on the maintenance of parity with other medical specialisms. The specialty became known as 'public-health *medicine*' and the independent 'watchdog' role was avoided.

The role of public-health doctors, already reduced, has been still further contested in the response to the Acheson Report. Environmental health officers, health education officers, and GPs have all maintained that they too, have a role in formulating healthy public policies. There was also little evidence that public-health doctors wanted a broader mandate, which would entail a willingness to intervene on politically sensitive issues. The future of public health was therefore not resolved by the Acheson Report.

The publication of a government White Paper on *The Health of the Nation* in 1992, while setting targets for key areas such as sexual health and coronary heart disease, also continued the avoidance of contentious health issues: for example, it did not advocate a ban on tobacco advertising.

In the next chapter, we return to the Third World, where the role of doctors in public health was being eroded by a revolution in health care. You will notice some similarities with developments in the United Kingdom in the same period: the importance of volunteers, the focus on primary care at the expense of high-technology medicine, and an emphasis on the individual rather than on structural change.

OBJECTIVES FOR CHAPTER 7

When you have studied this chapter, you should be able to:

7.1 Describe the general pattern of reorganisation of the NHS from 1974 to the early 1990s, and comment on the extent to which there was continuity with, or a decisive break from, earlier forms of health-service organisation.

7.2 Give examples of ways in which changes in the health service have been influenced by political, professional and economic pressures.

7.3 Analyse the changes in the concept of community care after 1974, and its relationship to lay, and especially female, care.

7.4 Assess the changes in the health-care division of labour since 1974, especially the changes wrought by the professionalisation and unionisation of occupations and the introduction of managerialism.

7.5 Assess the changes that took place in the concept and practice of public health after 1974, especially the rising interest in prevention and health education.

QUESTIONS FOR CHAPTER 7

Question 1 (*Objective 7.1*)

A group of health experts commenting on the drift of NHS reorganisation have concluded that:

> While modelling health authorities on boards of directors or water authorities may be in keeping with the Government's business model approach to the NHS, the result could well be a reduction in local accountability (limited as it is) and public participation in health service policy making...this is precisely the aspect of consumerism which *Working for Patients* does not address. (Harrison, *et al.*, 1989, p. 19)

To what extent have changes in the administration of the NHS from 1974 onwards undermined the accountability of the NHS to local communities and individual patients?

Question 2 (*Objective 7.2*)

The economist Julian le Grand and colleagues conclude that:

> ...the most striking feature of policy towards the NHS, at least until 1988, was its continuity. There were ideological skirmishes on the periphery (over paybeds, tax concessions to private medicine, and contracting out), but the main concerns of all the governments involved were broadly the same: managerial reorganization, regional and other inequalities, and the Cinderella services. However, all this was apparently to change in 1988. (le Grand, *et al.*, 1990, p. 93)

Do you agree with this hypothesis of fundamental continuity, or 'consensus' as it is often called? Were the changes introduced after 1988 a decisive, politically-motivated break with tradition, altering the NHS beyond recognition?

Question 3 (*Objective 7.3*)

> Their responsibilities within the domestic health services unavoidably bring them into contact with professional welfare workers: the doctor and health visitor, the social worker and the district nurse. Their caring role places them at the interface between the family and the state, as the go-between linking the informal health care system with the formal apparatus of the welfare state. (Graham, 1985, quoted in Stacey, 1988, p. 210)

The sociologist Hilary Graham has drawn attention to the important role women play as unpaid carers at the interface between paid and unpaid care. How did the continuing role of women as carers intersect with policies of community care in the period after 1974?

Question 4 (*Objectives 7.4 and 7.5*)

> Dr Joe Smith beamed an inward smile as he left the General Manager's comfortable office. His contract as Director of Medical Services for Southern Cross NHS Hospital had been extended for a further term but, more to the point, he had just negotiated a substantial salary increase, on the strength of his department's performance in exceeding its cost and quality targets for the second year running. He now had approval to reinvest his budget in a new Endoscopy Suite, with the latest Japanese equipment. (Liddell, 1989)

What does this hypothetical scenario tell you about some of the tendencies in the organisation of health-care occupations in the late 1980s? Is it an accurate representation of these tendencies?

Question 5 (*Objective 7.5*)

Read the following extract by Christopher Pollitt, a health and social policy analyst:

> What is remarkable…is that amid all this controversy is to be found one small island of consensus upon which weary policy makers can be observed taking refuge in large numbers. This refuge is health education…. There are not many problems of public policy that can attract such a degree of consensus of approach from so wide a range of interests. (Quoted in Baggott, 1990, pp. 77–8)

The speaker was referring to health education about alcohol. Why do you think there was the consensus he describes? What does it tell you about the general focus of public-health campaigns in the 1970s and 1980s?

8 Health care in the Third World, 1974 to the 1990s

> **This chapter builds upon your knowledge and understanding of health and disease in Third World countries, based on the study of World Health and Disease. In particular, we suggest that you refresh your memory of the diversity of health experience between and within Third World countries by referring back to Chapters 2 and 8 of that book, and revising the complex connections between economic development, population growth and social inequality.**
>
> **During your study of the present chapter, you will be asked to read an article in the Reader by David Werner, 'The village health worker: lackey or liberator?'. A television programme about health care in Zimbabwe relates directly to this chapter, but an earlier television programme and audiotape—both entitled 'Health and Disease in Zimbabwe'—are also relevant.**

Introduction

This chapter continues the discussion of contemporary diversity in health care by providing a broad overview of health and health-care systems in the Third World and the way in which health policies have changed. It covers the period from the 1970s to the 1990s and focuses on a revolutionary change in health policy—*the primary health care movement*. The main questions addressed are:

- Why was there such a significant change in Third World health policy? What led to the introduction of the primary health care approach?

- How was primary health care interpreted when ministries of health in Third World countries tried to put policy into practice?

- What have been the main problems in the implemention of primary health care in the Third World?

Although the primary health care movement was by no means limited to the Third World (its counterpart in the industrialised world, as you have seen in Chapter 7, was in health-centre expansion, primary health care teams, health promotion, and the new public health), this chapter focuses on developing countries.

The many faces of the Third World

Although it is useful to use the term 'Third World' as shorthand, it is important to remind you that it represents a heterogeneous grouping of nations, not a bloc in terms of income and wealth.

☐ Summarise some of the main dimensions of diversity within and between Third World countries.[1]

■ You might have thought of some of the following categories (to which we have added examples in brackets):

1 *GNP per capita* (ranges from 120 US$ in Ethiopia to 2 970 US$ in Gabon).

2 *Under-five mortality rates* (226 per 1 000 population in that age-group in Ethiopia, 167 per 1 000 in Gabon).

3 *Population size* (Nigeria has a population of over 100 million; Botswana, which is almost the same geographical area, has just over 1 million people).

[1]As discussed in *World Health and Disease*, Chapters 2, 3 and 8.

4   *Rural–urban differentials* (infant mortality rates in Mozambique's capital, Maputo, are about 90 per 1 000 live births but in some rural areas are 173 per 1 000 live births).

5   *Intra-urban differentials* (in Manila the infant mortality rate in the urban slums is three times higher than in other parts of the city).

Infant and under-five mortality rates declined in the first decades after World War II, and continued decreasing into the 1970s. Since the mid-1980s, however, the position is not clear in the poorest countries. Economic stagnation and recession have led to deteriorating health conditions, and in some countries it is feared that there will be a significant increase in child mortality in the 1990s.

Consequently, when we look at indicators of health in the Third World we look at a world of huge contrasts. And those differences are reflected in many other ways. A worker in Benin described two faces of Africa, but he could just as well have been writing about Asia or Latin America:

> There is the educated, literate, charming and welcoming Africa where the tourists go, where the business people trade and where project coordinators hatch their schemes. There the five star hotels, exotic cuisine, swimming pools and safari clubs with telexes, telephones and faxes. There the ministries of health or development, there the besuited people with power and influence. But there is the second Africa, usually beyond the city boundaries, beyond the tarmac and neon lights, perhaps 50 km away along dusty or muddy tracks where there are no banks or telephones and children are taught in crumbling mud brick shelters that pass for schools. There where English or French is hardly spoken, where the locals babble away in tongues unknown to Western ears, where clothing is faded and torn, where grins are so often toothless. There where chickens and goats scratch for food around the family cooking pot and naked babies play in the dirt. (Potter, 1991, p. 1 558)

Differences between rural and urban populations persist. But it is *urbanisation* that has increased over the past decades, and which demands attention because of the huge inequalities between groups within cities. For many urban dwellers in slum areas, environmental conditions are damaging to health—housing overcrowded, roads and thoroughways squalid, sanitation and water supply inadequate. Access to the existing health services, medicines, doctors and nurses may be limited. Not only do poor urban dwellers have to cope with violence and injury in cities (both major causes of death), but they also suffer from infectious diseases and malnutrition as well as the chronic cardiovascular diseases and cancers typical of modern Western societies.

Data from many countries suggest a single explanation: access to the conditions that improve people's health are highly inequitable. Both rural and poor urban populations lack sufficient and clean water supplies and sanitation. Education, although widespread, is seldom available beyond primary school, and its quality is variable; employment opportunities are few, especially in rural areas. Shortage of food adds to people's vulnerability. In urban areas violence and overcrowding are threats to health. And health care is patchy: in both city and countryside, people continue to turn to practitioners of traditional or folk medicine for help when ill, sometimes because formal 'Western' care is not easily available, sometimes because they prefer, or have more confidence in, the traditional sector.

The evolution of Third World health policy, 1970–8

Although there had been many reports about developing comprehensive health services based on health centres during and after World War II, what was actually implemented during the following decades were *centres of excellence* in many Third World countries: the university hospitals emulating the teaching hospitals of the industrialised world. As you will recall from Chapter 6, these were all in urban areas, usually in the capital, and absorbed a high percentage of the health budget. By the late 1960s, however, a real shift in thinking about medicine was occurring, although it was only in the 1970s that widespread dissemination of new ideas occurred.

Four areas of influence and changing ideas that laid the basis for primary health care, particularly in the Third World, are discernible in this period, although any such division is to some extent arbitrary and overlapping. Policy change occurs as the result of a complex series of events and ideas not easily distinguishable over time. However, it is possible to focus on four areas:

• experiments in particular countries to find alternative means for improving health;

• changing ideas about poverty, health and development;

• concern about population growth;

- activities and policies of the international organisations such as the WHO and United Nations Children's Fund (UNICEF).

We will look at each in turn.

Experiments with basic health services in Third World countries

By the late 1960s and early 1970s, there was considerable disillusion in both the industrialised world and the Third World with the role of medicine and the way in which health services were organised.

The commonly held assumption that disease could be fully accounted for by a model based on molecular and cellular biology as its basic scientific discipline was increasingly challenged. Anthropologists, sociologists, and psychologists interested in the medical area, showed the importance of socio-economic, cultural and life-history factors in explaining ill-health. They also demonstrated the utility of non-Western systems of health care. As in the West, people predominantly treated themselves or sought care from friends and relatives or indigenous practitioners. In the Third World, lay care networks were even more extensive than in the industrialised world, partly because of well-established indigenous systems of care, partly because of the limited concentration of Western medical systems.

Although sulphonamides and antibiotics had greatly increased medical effectiveness in the treatment of infectious disease, some medicines had damaging effects, some were costly but useless, and some multi-national drug companies used dubious means to promote their products, especially in the Third World (we return to this subject in Chapter 9). There were also immense problems caused by side-effects and unintended consequences of prescribed and over-the-counter drugs (e.g. thalidomide could be bought freely).

Much of the debate centred around the diffusion of medical technology: how and why independent developing countries retained colonial health infrastructures and aspired to ideas that were inappropriate to the health situations in their own countries. For example, an Indian doctor, Debabar Banerji, suggested that the colonial inheritance had had damaging effects on health services. The inappropriateness of selection and training, he suggested, had alienated health workers from the people they served. The costly emigration of newly graduated doctors to the Western developed world was indicative of a professional identification reinforced by irrelevant training (the scale of emigration is assessed in Chapter 9).

The inappropriateness of aspects of Western-type medical training and service delivery was increasingly recognised. Maurice King's *Medical Care in Developing Countries* (1966, reprinted seven times between 1967 and 1973) became the bible for English-speaking health workers in developing countries. The book was the result of a symposium held in East Africa, at which a number of doctors argued that health services were not reaching those in need, for several reasons.

☐ Do you recall David Morley's 'three-quarter's rule' (Chapter 6)?

■ Three-quarters of the health budget was spent on hospitals which served less than one-quarter of the population.

In *Medical Care in Developing Countries* another concern was that health services were attempting to treat illnesses which were preventable. There were no 'medical' solutions for malnutrition, a major complicating condition in many children's illnesses. The underlying cause of much disease was poverty, and other solutions—social, educational, economic and political—had to be sought. King's book therefore emphasised the need for more *preventive health measures* (such as immunisation or ante-natal care), and to move health services nearer to the population by building health centres and clinics in rural areas. In order to increase access to health services, the use of *medical auxiliaries* was strongly advocated. This laid the first step towards accepting lay care, by acknowledging that biomedical training for doctors was not necessarily the only, or even the best, way to provide health services.

In Tanzania, such ideas were actually implemented in the late 1960s. The *Arusha Declaration* of 1967, which set the framework for social and economic policy for the whole country, emphasised the need to give priority to rural areas. Tanzania introduced a comprehensive system of rural health posts, dispensaries, health centres and hospitals, emphasised the need for preventive services, and began to train a variety of health workers for different levels of services: for example, the village health workers and medical assistants. Although there were shortfalls in Tanzania's innovative approach, it was for many a shining example of what a developing country could do to try to meet its people's basic needs. In 1972 the government health expenditure ratio between urban and rural areas was 80 : 20—by 1980 it was 60 : 40. This shift reflected a real improvement in the rural health infrastructure, as shown in Table 8.1.

Table 8.1 Growth in rural health-care infrastructure in Tanzania, 1972 and 1980

	1972	1980
health centres	99	239
dispensaries	1 501	2 600
medical assistants	335	1 400
rural medical aides	578	2 310
maternal and child health aides/midwives	700	2 070
health assistants	290	681

Data cited in Heggenhougen, K., *et al.* (1987) *Community Health Workers: the Tanzanian Experience*, Oxford University Press, Oxford, p. 28.

☐ What else does Table 8.1 tell you?

■ While the number of *facilities* roughly doubled, the number of health *workers* increased between three and five times.

China too, inspired many to look for alternatives to existing health services. The Cultural Revolution of 1966–9 placed emphasis on developing the rural areas, and information about the mass mobilisation of the Chinese people against endemic diseases was beginning to be disseminated by the early 1970s. Doctors such as Joshua Horn, who worked in China for many years after Mao TseTung's revolution, described the system of **barefoot doctors**—health workers in their time off from the fields. The symbiotic relationship between the community and its barefoot doctors caught the imagination of many concerned about how to increase the rural populations' access to health care. Although China was a low-income country (GNP per capita in 1980 was US$290), life expectancy had improved from 47 years in 1960 to 67 years in 1980, infant mortality rates were similar to those in the industrialised countries, and preventive programmes had greatly decreased the prevalence of diseases such as schistosomiasis (bilharzia).

For many the Soviet Union was another source of inspiration. The *feldshers*, who had been introduced in the nineteenth century in Russia, were school leavers who were trained to provide care to rural populations. Popular images included them riding off on horseback into the bleak and thinly populated steppes. Borrowing from this example, Venezuela introduced a system of auxiliary health workers to extend health care to remote areas of the country, where it was difficult to attract doctors. In Guatemala, in the hub of the Indian highlands, an American doctor—Carroll Behrhorst—helped to train ordinary villagers to provide basic health care to their own communities.

Although admired by many, such schemes were not without their critics, and the conservative medical establishment took a decade to be convinced that health care could be provided by any other than a doctor trained over six or seven years. Behrhorst describes one such medical specialist taken to see the health promoters in Chimaltenango, Guatemala.

> He was sceptical that men with so little formal education could dispense adequate medical care, but as the day wore on and he found the promoters dealing knowledgeably with one ailment after another, his scepticism wilted. Finally, he thought he had caught one of the promoters giving incorrect treatment. 'You have the right disease but the wrong remedy,' he said to the promoter. 'The specific indicated here is penicillin.' The Indian promoter shook his head 'Ah,' he replied, 'but this patient is allergic to penicillin'. (Quoted in Newell, 1975, p. 36)

A handful of countries made radical shifts in health policy and, by the 1970s, were receiving international attention for the resulting improvements in health status. Cuba, which lost one-third of its doctors after the revolution, reconstructed its basic health services, building up a network of polyclinics or health centres, and brought down its infant mortality rate to the lowest in Latin America. Costa Rica was another exception in Central America, with health status levels comparable to those in the developed world. Sri Lanka had much lower infant mortality rates than neighbouring India. In all these countries there was some involvement of the community in health, whether through local organisations or education campaigns. It seemed that even relatively poor countries could improve the health of their people, through a redistribution of resources that emphasised access to education and health services and food security.

However, a *caveat* is in order here. The reasons why health improves (or mortality declines) are extremely complex. The countries mentioned above also had some, or all, of the following features: a substantial degree of autonomy for the female population; a dedication to education; an open political system; a largely civilian society, without rigid class structures; a history of some egalitarianism. Other countries which did not apparently introduce radical political or social changes in the 1960s and 1970s also experienced improvements in health, probably because they displayed some of the features mentioned above. In contrast, countries in which mortality remained high during the 1970s lacked the above characteristics.

Table 8.2 Infant mortality rates per 1 000 live births relative to income and female education in selected Third World countries, 1988

Country	GNP per capita/US$	IMR/1 000 live births	% female age group in primary school
low mortality			
Sri Lanka	420	32	102[1]
China	330	31	124[1]
Jamaica	1 070	11	106[1]
Thailand	1 000	30	(94)[2]
high mortality			
Saudi Arabia	6 200	70	65
Algeria	2 680	73	35
Ivory Coast	740	95	58
Morocco	610	80	56

[1]Figures are expressed as the ratio of female pupils to the population of female school-age children. Countries differ in what they consider primary school age. For some countries, school enrolment ratios exceed 100 per cent because some pupils are younger or older than the country's standard primary school age (usually 6–11 years, but not always). [2]In lieu of numbers of females enrolled in primary school (not given for Thailand) the figure in brackets refers to the percentage of adult females who are literate. (Adapted from Caldwell, J. C., 1986, 'Routes to low mortality in poor countries', *Population and Development Review*, **12** (2), p. 174, using data from World Bank (1990) *World Development Report* and UNICEF (1990) *The State of the World's Children*, Oxford University Press, Oxford)

Table 8.2 is a reminder of the relationship between infant mortality rate (IMR) and female education.[2] The high IMR countries are largely Muslim, or have large Muslim minorities, and are characterised by the separate and distinctive position of women.

Changing ideas about poverty, health and development

Soon after World War II, development theories had stressed the over-riding importance of investment in the physical elements of national growth—industry, roads and dams—and saw health and other social services such as education as non-productive consumption sectors. Thus government money expended on such services was perceived as a dissipation of national savings.

By the late 1960s these theories were increasingly challenged. There was growing scepticism about who was benefiting from development. In many countries with high rates of economic growth, the rapid rise in income per capita was firmly concentrated in the hands of fairly small numbers, and many groups were worse off than they had been in the previous decade.

A decade later, experiences of low-income countries like China and Sri Lanka, as well as middle-income countries like Cuba and Costa Rica, suggested that it was possible to have reasonable rates of growth *and* to redistribute some of the benefits to the poor. It was not necessary to wait for the benefits of growth to 'trickle down' from richer to lower income groups.

In 1976, a conference held at the *International Labour Office* (ILO)—one of the specialised agencies of the United Nations—most clearly rejected past strategies for development and identified a new priority based on the eradication of poverty, the provision of basic needs and productive employment for the whole population. The ILO conference turned from a narrow focus on industrialisation to setting minimum targets for *basic needs*: food consumption, clothing, housing and the provision of essential services in the areas of water, sanitation, education, health and public transport. People's health would improve if their basic needs were met: one of these needs was health care, and it was apparent that there were gross inequalities in access to health services (the scale of which is assessed in Chapter 9).

Concern about population growth

During the 1960s, one of the common explanations for poor countries' slow rates of development was that economic growth was being dissipated because it had to be divided among ever more people. The growth in population was seen by many as a fundamental brake on

[2]For a full discussion, refer to *World Health and Disease*.

development.[3] Concern was expressed that the world's resources were finite, and that pollution, misuse of existing resources, and consumption demands were all increasing. Robert McNamara, then President of the *World Bank*, also noted in 1979 that uncontrolled population growth could lead to high levels of poverty, stress and overcrowding which would threaten social and military stability.

The developing world's view of the population 'explosion' did not always coincide with the developed world's view, but by 1970 many billions of dollars were being spent on population control activities by international, national and private bodies. Three-quarters of the funds went into family planning activities, often employing lay women for information and promotion of family planning methods among their neighbours. By the end of the 1970s, family planning (or family spacing) was seen as an essential element of primary health care services.

Activities and policies of the international organisations

The ideas and experiences described above were brought together by two international agencies which played a particular role in promoting what has come to be known as the primary health care approach. Both were specialised agencies of the United Nations: the WHO and UNICEF, the latter initially playing the supportive role to the health professionals in WHO. These multilateral organisations played an important part in developing and disseminating health policy, in offering technical assistance to Third World countries to implement health programmes and in funding such programmes. How did these two organisations take a critical part in the shift of health policy?

In the early 1970s, WHO experts were trying to explain apparent failures in the malaria eradication programme. Technical reasons for the difficulties in malaria eradication were acknowledged, but the dominating cause of failure was the lack of a complete and continuing health-service infrastructure which could reach every household *and* remain in place. Malaria eradication had been introduced as a **vertical programme**—that is, a programme with its own funds, workers, vehicles and supplies, which worked separately from all other health services. When the campaign had finished in one area, it moved on to another and, because it was not integrated into the basic health service, there was no continuing

---

[3]For a full discussion of population growth and the measures by which countries have attempted to control it, see *World Health and Disease*, Chapter 8.

activity so the mosquitoes returned. One of the WHO instigators of the primary health care movement, Ken Newell, writing in 1988, argues that primary health care owes its genesis to this failure.

A special working group set up within WHO to look at problems in basic health services reported that not only was access to health services very uneven, especially between urban and rural areas, but also:

> …there appears to be widespread dissatisfaction of populations with their health services…. Such dissatisfaction occurs in the developed as well as in the third world. (WHO, 1973, p. 106)

The report went on to enumerate the reasons for such dissatisfactions, which included failure of health services to meet people's expectations, inadequate coverage, great differentials in health status within and between countries, rising costs and:

> …a feeling of helplessness on the part of the consumer who feels (rightly or wrongly) that the health services and the personnel within them are progressing along an uncontrollable path of their own which may be satisfying to the health professions, but which is not what is most wanted by the consumer. (WHO, 1973, p. 106)

The report had two important effects: first, it defined the **primary health care approach**. Although it concentrated almost totally on health services and the health sector, it emphasised the need to involve the consumer, to tap local resources, to 'make medicine "belong" to those it should serve' and called for a 'national will' as well as 'international will' for positive health. Second, it legitimised WHO's leadership role in changing health policy. The report drew attention to WHO's role as 'world health conscience':

> It is possible to use WHO not only as a forum to express ideas or dissatisfactions, but also as a mechanism which can point to directions in which member states should go. (WHO, 1973, p. 108)

As part of the search for new solutions in health services, a joint WHO–UNICEF committee commissioned a study of successful programmes using alternative strategies for providing health care. As you have seen, a number of countries (Tanzania, the Soviet Union, Guatemala, Cuba) and many non-governmental organisations had experimented with innovations in health services, through expanded use of auxiliaries, health centres and community involvement. Some of these radical approaches were disseminated in two books widely publicised by WHO—both published in 1975: *Alternative approaches to meeting basic health needs* (Djukanovic and Mach, 1975) and *Health by the people* (Newell, 1975).

In the meantime, WHO began to take a much more active role in persuasion and promotion of a particular health message, firmly orchestrated by Halfdan Mahler, who became Director-General in 1973. In 1975 he launched the idea of 'Health for All by the Year 2000' as WHO's contribution to the UN's 'New International Economic Order', proposing urgent action now to achieve 'in the twenty-five years of a generation what has not hitherto been achieved at all' (Mahler, 1975). Health had to be considered in the broader context of its contribution to, and as a lever for, social development.

This climate of ideas provided the context for the *International Conference on Primary Health Care*, held at Alma Ata in 1978, and sponsored by the WHO and UNICEF, with a substantial financial contribution from the host country, the Soviet Union. A report on *primary health care* was prepared for the meeting, which was attended by representatives of 134 governments and 67 international organisations. The **Declaration of Alma Ata** outlined the role of primary health care in 'Health For All by the Year 2000':

> A main social target of governments, international organisations and the world community in the coming decades should be the attainment by all the peoples of the world by the year 2000 of a level of health that will permit them to lead a socially and economically productive life. Primary health care is the key to attaining this target as part of development in the spirit of social justice. (WHO–UNICEF, 1978, p. 3)

Primary health care itself was defined as

> ...essential health care based on practical, scientifically sound and socially acceptable methods and technology made universally accessible to individuals and families in the community through their full participation and at a cost that the community and country can afford to maintain at every stage of their development in the spirit of self-reliance and self-determination. It forms an integral part both of the country's health system, of which it is the central function and main focus, and of the overall social and economic development of the community. It is the first level of contact of individuals, the family and the community with the national health system, bringing health care as close as possible to where people live and work and constitutes the first element of a

continuing health care process. (WHO–UNICEF, 1978, p. 3)

Primary health care was understood to include (at least) the following components:

- promotion of food supply and proper nutrition;
- an adequate supply of safe water and basic sanitation;
- education concerning prevailing health problems and ways to prevent and control them;
- maternal and child health, including family planning;
- immunisation against the major infectious diseases;
- prevention and control of locally endemic diseases;
- appropriate treatment of common diseases and injuries;
- provision of essential drugs.

Behind the rhetoric was a serious shift in ideology—at the centre of which was a concern with *equity, community participation*, and a changing emphasis on *prevention* and *health* rather than treatment and disease. It was by no means only applicable to the Third World—industrialised countries were also signatories to the Alma Ata Declaration. But it is difficult to translate an ideology into practical reality, especially in the Third World context, where conceptual confusions about primary health care led to some major problems in implementation.

Implementing primary health care in Third World countries, 1978 to the mid-1980s

Primary health care endorsed at Alma Ata gave the concept of public health an international boost. Reaching 'Health for All by the Year 2000' could only be achieved if new approaches were taken to deal with health problems which stemmed from socio-economic and environmental, as well as biological causes. The broad, equity- and community-based primary health care strategy emphasised the need for *multi-sectoral action*, that is, collaboration between different government sectors such as health care, education and agriculture. But it was difficult to translate this into practical activities. In the industrialised world the call came for a *new public health movement*—reorienting attention *away* from health services, and *towards* the environment, promotion of good health and community participation. (The gap between the rhetoric and the reality in Britain was discussed in Chapter 7). In the Third World, the concept of primary health care focused attention more on *health services* and people's *participation* in them—an approach which soon became known by its acronym—**PHC**—in the agencies promoting it.

In the search for practical programmes of activity in the Third World, the broad concept of PHC was gradually narrowed down and focused on two *assumptions*, outlined in Box 8.1.

Box 8.1   Assumptions underlying the concept of primary health care in Third World countries

1   Conventional medical resources were not available in rural areas—doctors and nurses were unwilling to work outside urban health facilities and their numbers were insufficient. Therefore it was essential to train members of rural communities to deliver basic health care to their own people. The Chinese barefoot doctor and similar village health worker schemes could be universally applied all over the Third World.

2   Most of the health problems in the Third World were preventable and susceptible to elementary methods of care and simple drugs, which could be provided by community health workers. Improving environmental conditions and hygiene, raising awareness about health behaviour, and providing preventive care, such as immunisations against childhood infections, were the most effective means for improving health, but real gains could only be achieved with significant participation of communities. Selecting which of all these activities to undertake was initially assumed to be simple.

Let us look at the practical consequences of these assumptions in turn.

Building on lay care: community health-worker programmes

Many Third World countries confronted their shortages of professionally trained health staff by shifting the boundaries between lay and formal care. Acknowledging that people within communities were already giving care, they argued that, with relatively short training, villagers could both prevent and treat common complaints that had been the remit of health professionals. They would become the link between the formal health services and the community, and stimulate action to involve people in their own health care.

Some countries introduced a *new* cadre of community health worker while others extended programmes initiated long before Alma Ata. Community health workers were given different names: 'village health workers' in Tanzania, 'community health aides' in Jamaica, 'village health guides' in India. The 'catch-all' term **community health worker** (or **CHW**) only came into general use in the 1980s. The important difference between the early programmes that employed community health workers, and those that were introduced after Alma Ata, was that the first were *indigenous* efforts to meet local needs, whereas later initiatives were often motivated more by a government's desire to show a commitment to PHC and were *imposed* on health workers and communities.

On what models did countries base their CHW programmes? Two had by then received significant publicity: *national government programmes* such as the Chinese barefoot doctor scheme, and small, *non-government projects*. These models differed in style and ideology. In his article in the Reader, 'The village health worker: lackey or liberator?', David Werner describes a number of these programmes in Latin America: you should read it now.

Werner contrasts the appropriateness of professional auxiliaries and village health workers.

☐ What does he consider are the benefits of the latter?

■ They are selected from the community in which they live; they are trained for short periods, therefore their training is not expensive; they are supported by the community; and they are often already accepted by the community because of their standing as traditional healers or midwives.

Note that Werner saw such workers as having an important political role, as agents of change. However, it is one thing to nurture a small-scale community health-worker programme with committed, dynamic and charismatic leadership such as that of Werner (and there are many other examples all over the Third World), but it is quite another to provide the same level of support and enthusiasm in a large, national, community health-worker programme that depends on the existing health infrastructure and professions.

By the mid-1980s many countries had national community health-worker programmes (see Figure 8.1, *overleaf*). Many were composed of *unpaid volunteers* with a fairly narrow range of largely educative tasks. For example, Thailand had trained both village health

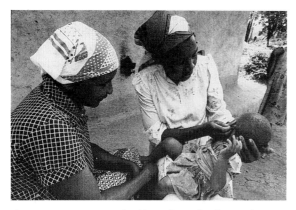

Figure 8.1 *Community health workers often have a few simple medicines such as aspirin and anti-malarial drugs to offer against common illnesses. Here a Kenyan community health worker examines a child who has been brought by her mother. (Source: Panos Pictures)*

volunteers as well as village health communicators for every village inthe country, and other countries had very large numbers of CHWs: 100 000 in Sri Lanka, 40 000 in Zambia, I million in Indonesia. Other countries trained fewer community health workers, but paid them a salary or honorarium: by the mid-1980s Botswana had over 600 in place, Colombia 5 000, Jamaica over 1 200.

Implementing community health-worker programmes

It soon became apparent that CHWs working in national programmes were faced with particular difficulties not always anticipated from previous experience.

First, it was clear that very few CHWs were actually chosen in an open way by their *communities*. In many countries, it was the community *leaders* or *health workers* who chose the CHW. Debbie Taylor, a Third World writer, provides a vivid profile of a village volunteer, Samchai, in Thailand, which is mirrored the world over:

> He had hoped that being trained as a health volunteer would give him more opportunities to help the other villagers. He had been disappointed not to have been selected when the *puyaiban* first chose people for training three years ago. It was only to be expected, he supposed, that the *puyaiban* would choose his relatives and friends first. But it made him feel so frustrated to see them all pocketing their *per diems* and stowing away their piles of training manuals unread—knowing that they had neither the time nor the inclination to use their training properly. What was even worse, the son of the *puyaiban*'s best friend—who had gone for the longer 15 day training to be a health

volunteer—did not live in the village any more. He had gone off to work in Bangkok.... (Taylor, 1986, p. 38)

Gradually it was acknowledged that communities were not homogeneous, and that local politics could affect which community health workers were chosen to 'serve the community'. This raised questions of suitability, commitment and loyalty, with huge variations within and between community health-worker programmes.

Second, it was soon realised that community health-worker programmes were *not cheap*. Although training was short, and community health workers received only basic supplies, large numbers had to be trained. While savings could be made by using unpaid volunteers, drop-out rates were high. This was hardly surprising in those places where all community health workers were women, who are in general heavily burdened with daily tasks.

In some countries *volunteer programmes* seemed to work better than others: religion, among other factors seemed to play a part. For example, in Buddhism, voluntarism is a positive value and countries with large Buddhist populations such as Thailand, Burma and Sri Lanka had large volunteer programmes. However, religion was seldom the whole story. In Sri Lanka, health volunteers were largely young, well-educated women, who had few job opportunities. When asked, the majority said they volunteered in order to give service, but also because they hoped that voluntary work would lead to future employment.

In those national programmes where community health workers were paid a salary by the ministry of health (Botswana and Colombia, for example), the cost of running the programme was much higher, and fewer were trained. Paid community health workers tended to be committed to their job, especially given the paucity of employment opportunities in rural areas. However, research showed that many felt allegiance to the ministry of health and preferred to work in health centres or dispensaries, rather than visiting people in their homes.

> ☐ Can you think why working in the health centre rather than visiting homes may be a problem?

> ■ For all sorts of complex reasons, not everyone attends the health facility, even when they are ill; the community health worker was not necessarily reaching the whole community.

By the end of the 1980s, questions were being asked about the *effectiveness* of community health workers. Many argued that community health workers were captured by the health service professionals and used as 'extra pairs of hands':

The journey from the nearest town took five hours, half of it on a sandy road past nothing but salt pans, baobab trees and the odd fleeting glimpse of a springbok. We arrived at the health clinic in Maun—a large village of about 70 000 people—just before noon. The morning's work was almost over. A nurse was taking a woman's blood pressure, a few mothers and babies were waiting patiently to see another nurse. Outside a small group was sitting under a tree, receiving nutrition education.

The chief nurse was welcoming, and when we explained why we had come her enthusiasm was uninhibited. 'Family welfare educators?' she exclaimed, indicating the woman who was sweeping the clinic floor. 'We couldn't do without them! It's wonderful to have extra pairs of hands in a busy clinic like this!' (Walt, *et al.*, 1990, p. vii)

Others argued that community health workers could not support communities who wanted *drugs* and *emergency services* when they were ill. One writer described the frustration of a community health worker in Tanzania:

On one of our walks we stopped by a crumbling hut of an elderly couple. The wife was sick, ashen looking, lying on her cot with pain in her right leg, terribly thin and anaemic. No latrine, disorder all around. The man was busy building a small spirit house where food would be placed to placate the spirits so that his wife would get better. The CHW suggested to the husband that he take his wife to the health centre—but how, when she could not walk? Under the circumstances, the CHW could offer no other advice.... (Heggenhougen, *et al.*, 1987, p. 76)

The problem was that, by the mid-1980s, many countries were having to cut back on services because of diminishing resources, and the first level of care to be affected was the one furthest away from the capital. Drugs and other supplies became increasingly erratic; in some countries salaries for health workers were not paid for months; fuel and spare parts for transport were increasingly unavailable; visits to peripheral health posts or communities became rare. Staff became demoralised. People soon learned that their health facilities often ran out of drugs and vaccines and the general quality of care was low, so they stopped attending. There was minimal support or supervision for community health workers.

Traditional midwife training

The other group who were given training through the 1970s and 1980s were the **traditional midwives**, who are the main source of help in childbirth in many Third World countries (see Figure 8.2).

A sociologist, Jacqueline Vincent-Priya, who lived and worked in Malaysia for four years, made a special study of traditional midwives:

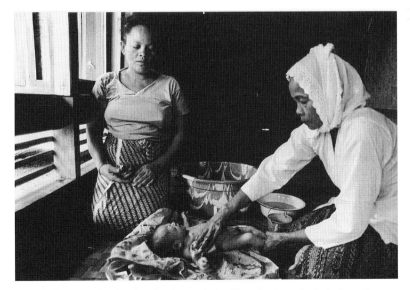

Figure 8.2 *A mother has her first lesson in looking after her new baby from the traditional midwife in her village in Java, Indonesia. (Source: Panos Pictures)*

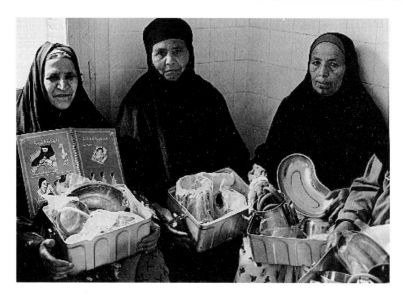

Figure 8.3 *Egyptian traditional midwives who have received a short training display their modern kits. (Source: Panos Pictures)*

Without exception they all had a tremendous range of experience; most had borne children of their own and served a long apprenticeship before they began practising. One of their big advantages is that they share the same ideas and the spiritual and practical life of the mothers for whom they give their services so freely, and they usually know these mothers well. Whatever help the traditional midwife gives is always given according to what the mother feels she needs, and her autonomy is rarely questioned or compromised. Traditional midwives usually have some spiritual calling for their work, which gives them and their clients confidence in their ability to deal with both normal and abnormal births. They use techniques which are appropriate to their situation: bamboo is a good thing to use for cutting the umbilical cord in communities which neither understand nor have the facilities for sterilizing instruments. In every group I visited there were simple, cheap and easily available remedies for most of the common problems associated with pregnancy and birth. (Vincent-Priya, 1991, p. 199)

The rationale for training traditional midwives in elements of *Western obstetric practice* is obvious—and some were known to use unsterile, inferior, and occasionally, harmful practices. But there were, in some countries, underlying tensions between traditional and government practitioners. For example, Vincent-Priya

points out that, according to the local Malaysian newspapers, traditional midwives are 'a bad thing'. Malaysia has trained many government midwives, who are seen to have a superior training (general nursing followed by midwifery) and therefore to provide safer conditions for mother and child.

☐ Can you suggest why large numbers of *traditional* midwives were also trained?

■ In many countries it was simply not possible to train sufficient government midwives or to persuade women in rural areas to go to maternity clinics to give birth. Even in urban areas women sometimes preferred delivery by a traditional midwife rather than go to the clinical surroundings of a city hospital or health centre; traditional midwives were less expensive and would go to the women's homes, so mothers were not parted from their other children.[4]

Many countries, with assistance from WHO and UNICEF, introduced short training courses for traditional midwives, typically lasting one to three weeks. Women learned about family planning methods, antiseptic techniques and detection of high-risk pregnancies. They were often rewarded at the end with a simple maternity kit (for example, a pair of scissors or razor blade, rubber gloves, soap), as shown in Figure 8.3. By the mid-1980s

---

[4]Note the striking parallels with the UK debate about the benefits and limitations of home vs. hospital births—discussed in *Birth to Old Age: Health in Transition*, Chapter 3.

considerable experience with training programmes had been recorded, but increasing scepticism about their value was being expressed.

The sociologist Patricia Jeffery and co-workers, writing about northern India in 1988, observed that *dai* training programmes (*dai* is the Hindu name for traditional midwife) have failed to take into account the complex cultural constraints on Indian women. They are valued essentially for their childbearing capacity, but they do not control any of the decisions that affect pregnancy, such as the use of antenatal services, acceptance of tetanus toxoid, or the need for rest and adequate nutrition. Local understanding about childbearing—which includes strong notions of shame and pollution—are not considered in the training. Even if *dais* have been trained by health professionals, and retain and use their new knowledge (which is difficult to ascertain) they may be limited in where they can help:

> The Harijan dai is welcome only while the new mother is herself unclean: the Caste Hindu *dai* is tainted by her work. Only for a Muslim among Muslims or a Harijan among Harijans, and then not always, are the barriers between a *dai* and her client at a minimum. Government health staff, as urban superiors, are socially distant in one direction, while the *dai*, as a polluted menial, is socially distant in the other. (Jeffery, *et al.*, 1989, p. 219)

Drawing on experience from years of fieldwork with Maya midwives in Yucatan, Mexico, and on participation in government-sponsored training courses for indigenous midwives, the anthropologist Brigid Jordan was scathing in her criticism of the training programmes. In her analysis of instructional methods she draws attention to inappropriate modes of teaching that put emphasis on definitions and irrelevant messages:

> In Yucatan, as in many parts of the world, women believe that the most fertile time is immediately before and after menstruation, because at that time 'the uterus is open'. Women who want to avoid pregnancy will have intercourse at midcycle when they believe the uterus to be closed—exactly at the most fertile time. The medical staff, however, were not aware of this belief, and anyway, there was no space for discussing it in the lesson plan. So the family planning course failed to impart the single piece of information which could be expected to have significant impact on contraceptive behaviour. (Jordan, 1989, p. 297)

Jordan does not gloss over the difficulties of imparting knowledge that challenges traditional views but argues that, at the end of the course, midwives will graduate successfully because they have learned to give their trainers the 'right' answers, although these will bear little resemblance to how they will later practise.

However, there are huge differences between training programmes, and some may be more successful than others. One report from Zimbabwe described a programme as highly successful because of the positive relationship between the formally trained maternity assistants at health clinics and the traditional midwives, or *vanambuya*, who were trained once a fortnight over a five- or six-month period.

> The great advantage of the programme is that it is locally administered. The maternity assistants get to know the traditional midwives well, and in many of the clinics collaboration between them has been enthusiastic. Maternity assistants noted that many traditional midwives have been encouraging women to go to antenatal clinics, and to take children for immunizations. (B. Booker quoted in WHO, 1984, p. 21)

Primary health care: comprehensive or selective?

From the beginning there was a divergence of opinion on how far PHC could be implemented.

☐ Can you think of one major hurdle to overcome if PHC was to be implemented equally across a whole population?

■ The cost of meeting the basic health needs of the whole population would be immense.

In 1979, just one year after the Alma Ata meeting, two specialists in tropical medicine, Julia Walsh and Kenneth Warren, argued that PHC was idealistic and that it would cost too much to guarantee basic primary health care to all. They suggested that what countries should do was to identify their most common diseases, ascertain what low-cost or cost-effective technologies existed to deal with them, and then concentrate resources on these. They gave an example by comparing lassa fever, *Ascaris* (round worm) and malaria. Lassa fever, they argued, would be a low priority because it was fairly rare, and although often fatal, there was little that could be done about it. On the other hand, although *Ascaris* was extremely common, people suffered little direct morbidity, and it would need such continuous treatment and improvements in basic hygiene, that it too, was of low priority. However malaria was very common, did cause significant morbidity and sometimes mortality, and was preventable or treatable through a number of different methods. Therefore, countries should give priority to activities in malaria control programmes. Walsh and Warren called this **selective primary health care**.

However, many argued that selective PHC diverted attention from the original concept of primary health care. One of its early protagonists, Ken Newell, said that PHC represented a revolutionary change, which highlighted the environmental and social aspects of health, removed it from the dominance of the medical profession, and encouraged people's participation. In this sense of PHC—later called **comprehensive primary health care**—health and development were closely aligned.

☐ How did selective PHC contrast with comprehensive PHC?

■ The principles of equity, prevention, multisectoral collaboration and community involvement underpinned comprehensive PHC and yet were hardly mentioned by those in favour of selective PHC. The selective approach to PHC was much more focused. It concentrated upon specific diseases or interventions and special groups (children under five, mothers, the poor). It was health-care oriented.

Selective PHC also had the advantage of being relatively easy to implement. Within a few years of the Alma Ata meeting, many international donors were re-defining PHC as a *package of low-cost interventions*, which were based on assumptions about the most effective methods of improving the health of young children. The four most widely adopted assumptions are shown in Box 8.2.

The activities that flow from these four assumptions—called the **GOBI interventions** (growth monitoring, oral rehydration, breast-feeding, immunisation)—were imaginatively and energetically promoted by UNICEF in particular, but also by many other aid donors who supported health programmes in Third World countries. Later, other factors that had a link with health were added to the list: family spacing, female education and food supplementation.

Many donors of financial and technical assistance favoured *selective* PHC programmes.

☐ Can you think why?

■ They appeared relatively easy to monitor and evaluate: numbers of immunisations or oral rehydration sachets given could be counted, growth charts examined. It was more satisfying for aid donors (who had to persuade their constituents at home that their money was being sensibly spent) to focus on a

---

Box 8.2 Assumptions about low-cost interventions to improve children's health

1 If children were *weighed* regularly during their vulnerable first years, those who were not growing as they should (because of illness or poor nutrition), could be identified at an early stage, and preventive action could be taken. Weighing a child, and marking its progress on a growth chart was not difficult (see Figure 8.4).

2 As many as one-half of the deaths from diarrhoea among infants and children could be averted if *dehydration* was prevented or treated. This could be achieved by giving them **oral rehydration solution (ORS)**, a relatively simple mixture of water, salt and sugar. ORS could be mixed at home or distributed in sachets by community health workers or volunteers; mothers could be taught how to make it, and when to administer it.

3 There was a clear link between *breast-feeding* and health. Those children who were exclusively breastfed for at least 4–6 months were protected from contracting diarrhoeal diseases and some other illnesses. In some countries, especially in Latin America, mothers were only breast-feeding for very short periods (a few weeks) and they had to be encouraged to lengthen this.

4 *Vaccines* were increasingly efficient, especially against the infectious diseases of childhood (measles, diphtheria, tuberculosis, tetanus, polio and whooping cough), and these killing or maiming diseases could be prevented if significant numbers of children could be immunised against them.

---

specific disease and intervention than try to take account of all the common problems presented at health clinics.

Selective PHC in practice: a fading dream?

For many countries, such selective interventions were equated with PHC, and were implemented widely through training community members to undertake them. However, enthusiasm for selective PHC was faltering in the late 1980s, largely as a result of negative experiences. For example, the four 'pillars' of the GOBI interventions were starting to collapse.

Growth monitoring was increasingly criticised as being seen as an end in itself, rather than as a means of identifying vulnerable children and acting to improve their nutrition. Screening requires accuracy in several sequential steps: reading the weight, plotting it on the child's growth chart, and interpreting the child's growth pattern. Establishing the *reasons* for growth faltering is usually done by talking to the mother. A number of studies suggested that none of these things was being done very well, and indeed, some health workers expressed a helplessness in knowing how to intervene, even if they did recognise that a child was malnourished. A health education talk, as given in Figure 8.4, was not always particularly helpful when families simply lacked food.

A similar anxiety was growing about *oral rehydration*. Initial euphoria at the ease with which women learned to make oral rehydration solutions at home safely and effectively, was later challenged because knowledge did not necessarily lead to use. Even if mothers used oral

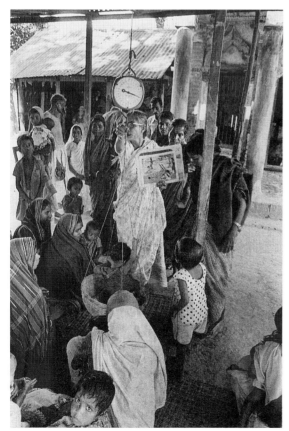

Figure 8.4 *A Bangladeshi community health worker takes the opportunity, while weighing babies, to give a short health education talk. (Photo: Tom Learmonth/Christian Aid)*

rehydration solutions, it was often used only for specific *sorts* of diarrhoea. Chowdhury and Vaughan (1988) showed that the terms health workers used for diarrhoea meant: 'very severe diarrhoea' to mothers. Women believed that *less* severe diarrhoea could best be cured with traditional remedies. So ORS was only given in a small percentage of cases.

A study in Bangladesh after ten years of a well-supervised oral rehydration programme, showed that most mothers thought oral rehydration solution would *stop* diarrhoea, whereas ORS prevents dehydration, but may make diarrhoea *worse* initially. This may have discouraged mothers from giving it to their children (it is also extremely time-consuming to feed a sick infant with oral rehydration solution, which does not taste particularly good). Commercial companies also saw an opportunity to market fruit-flavoured sachets of ready-mixed ORS powder, which was often unsuitable and expensive (see Figures 8.5a and 8.5b, *overleaf*).

Concerns about the decline in the number of women *breast-feeding* in the Third World—and the resulting increase in infant morbidity and mortality—led some countries to introduce health education campaigns to encourage women to continue breast-feeding for longer periods (see Figure 8.6, *overleaf*). But, however attractive, television, radio and poster campaigns were pitted against the powerful influences of the multinational food industries. Thirty per cent of the revenue of Bangladesh television comes from baby food adverts. One such advertisement is described as follows:

> The chubby baby on the television screen is heading for the plate of food on the table by his mother's chair. Glancing up from her newspaper, she smiles indulgently. 'No, this isn't for you. For you, Cerelac'. Cut to the same baby, grinning happily, with the remains of his meal smeared around his mouth. Cut to tins of Nestlé's Cerelac. (Burgess, 1990, p. 45)

Other, more subtle promotion methods are also used by the infant food industries, by, for example, providing maternity services with free samples for all recent mothers:

> Mothers coerced into bottle feeding in this way leave hospital with a tin of formula and a dwindling supply of breast milk. If they persist in bottle feeding, their babies are 25 times more likely to die of a gastrointestinal, respiratory, or other infection. The cost of purchasing further formula poses an enormous financial strain and puts the nutritional status of whole families at risk. Typically, artificial milk consumes around 50% of the household income. (*The Lancet*, 1990, p. 1151)

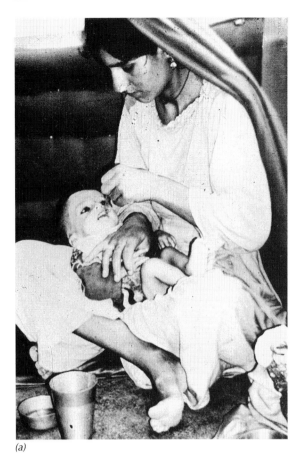

(a)

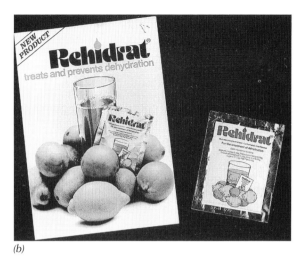

(b)

Figure 8.5 *(a) This woman in Afghanistan is spoon-feeding her severely dehydrated baby with oral rehydration solution (ORS) which she mixed herself from sugar, salt and water. (Photograph courtesy of Teaching Aids at Low Cost (TALC), P. O. Box 49, St Albans; details of TALC materials sent free on request). (b) This commercial ORS packet was sold in Sierra Leone and advertised in an attractive promotional leaflet. It has twice as much glucose and half as much salt as the solution recommended by the World Health Organisation—and it is sixteen times as costly. (Source: OXFAM)*

Although the WHO passed an *International Code on Breastmilk Substitutes* in 1981, it has been difficult for countries to implement in its entirety, and international organisations such as WHO or UNICEF cannot police the promotional activities of multinational companies.

Immunisation—a successful selective programme?

The fourth 'pillar' of GOBI—immunisation—raises even more complex issues. The huge effort and resources put into immunisation campaigns in many of the developing countries may well deserve to be seen as the *public health revolution* of the less developed world. Indeed, some countries have coverage figures that are better than those in the United Kingdom. In the mid-1970s nearly 5 million children were dying every year of six infectious diseases: measles, tetanus, whooping cough, diphtheria, tuberculosis, and polio. Millions more were permanently disabled. In 1980, only about 5 per cent of children in the Third World were immunised against these six diseases.

By the end of the 1980s, well over half were fully immunised by the time they were one year old (see Figure 8.7). Clearly aggregate figures like these tell a partial story. Some countries still have very low coverage, but others could, for example, boast in 1989 that between 80 and 90 per cent of all children under one year had received the three doses of polio vaccine they need to protect them: Botswana, Brazil, China, Cuba, Egypt, Nicaragua, Republic of Korea, Saudi Arabia and Tunisia are among those named by UNICEF.

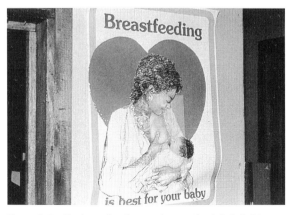

Figure 8.6 *Posters exhorting mothers to feed their babies with infant formula milks are being replaced in many Third World countries by posters encouraging mothers to breastfeed. This one is from Belize. (Source: Panos Pictures)*

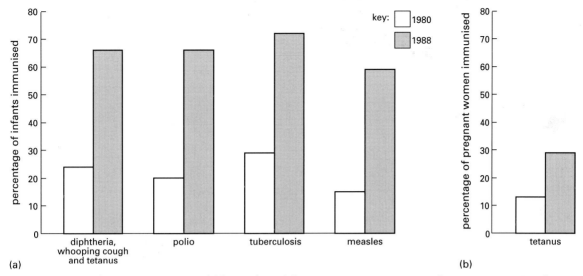

Figure 8.7 *During the 1980s aggregate world figures showed dramatic increases in coverage of immunisation against the main diseases of childhood for which vaccines exist. (Source: WHO/UNICEF: UCI Reports, cited in UNICEF, 1990,* The State of the World's Children, *Oxford University Press, Oxford, Figure 3, p. 15)*

However, in order to eradicate polio—it is almost eradicated in the industrialised world—it is essential to maintain high immunisation coverage levels (90 per cent) among children under the age of one year, for some years even after no further polio cases have been reported.

□ Can you suggest why this is necessary?

■ If even a single source of infection remains, it can spread quite rapidly if there are sufficient non-immune children in the population in which the polio virus can multiply. But if almost everyone is immune, isolated cases will not be able to spread.

Achieving high immunisation rates can be difficult and expensive in countries with large rural populations. Many aid donors believed that the best way of reaching the majority of the population was through *vertical* immunisation programmes.

□ Can you recall how a vertical programme is organised?

■ It is separate from the basic health service, and has its own funds, health workers, vehicles and supplies, all of which are used solely for that particular programme.

The great drive throughout the Third World to immunise children was spearheaded by WHO and UNICEF. A typical campaign would show the President of the country on the front page of the national newspaper, 'giving the first shot' in a national two- or three-day campaign, which involved teachers, policemen and priests, as well as health workers. Posters promoting immunisation would be widely distributed (see Figure 8.8, *overleaf*). As we said earlier, in some countries the results were spectacular.

□ But such campaigns also have their drawbacks—can you suggest the main pitfalls?

■ Children missed by a three-day annual campaign, or born just after it, have to receive their immunisations elsewhere. If immunisations are not part of the basic health services, then campaigns may have only transient effects.

A number of other concerns about immunisation programmes have been expressed:

1 That the momentum will not be able to be sustained in the face of major economic recession.

2 That not withstanding the benefits to many children, the *poorest* countries have actually achieved very little in terms of population coverage.

3 That the energetic drive to immunise may have diverted resources—both human and financial—from other services which were also needed.

4 That already weak health-care systems have been further fragmented by vertical programmes.

5 That other, perhaps equally important infections for which no vaccine exists—acute respiratory infections for example—have been neglected.

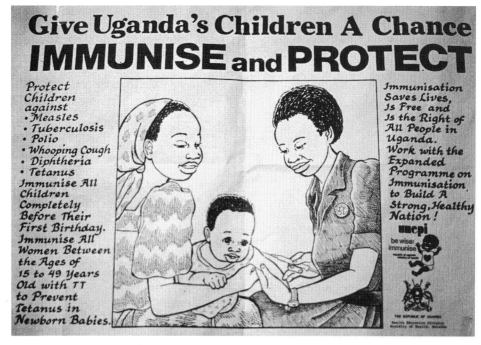

Figure 8.8 *Immunisation campaigns pass on, but the posters reminding mothers to have their children immunised remain on the walls of clinics and other public places. (Source: Panos Pictures)*

Helping or hindering: aid agencies in competition?

One of the arguments against the selective approach to PHC was that it diverted attention and resources away from the *basic health system*, emphasising specific diseases or particular interventions such as oral rehydration. Often international donors exacerbated this, by providing funding only for approved programmes. Sometimes these were organised and delivered completely separately from national health services. Sometimes they were incorporated into ministries of health, but were still run like vertical programmes, with their own staff, vehicles, logos, incentives and accounting systems.

This tendency created some tension between UNICEF and WHO in the early 1980s, and led to what many saw as unnecessary competition at the country level. WHO's Director-General, Halfdan Mahler, did not hide his irritation at what he saw as UNICEF's selective approach to PHC. In an address to the World Health Assembly in 1983 and without naming names, he said:

> Honourable delegates, while we have been striking ahead with singleness of purpose in WHO based on your collective decisions, others appear to have little patience for such systematic efforts. I am referring to such initiatives as the selection by people outside the developing countries of a few isolated elements of primary health care. (Mahler, 1983, p. 4)

The public quarrel between the two organisations was short-lived. By the end of the 1980s, much of this tension had been smoothed out, and there was greater consensus on the need to integrate health activities. But the fear was that the essential infrastructures for delivering *comprehensive* PHC had been significantly undermined by the diversion of funds to *selective* programmes.

Summary

We have focused on PHC in this chapter because it was promoted as a radical change in health policy, even if it was not always understood or was implemented as if it meant simply introducing a community health worker programme, training a few traditional midwives, or selecting a few health activities. But does this suggest that the concept was flawed? Is PHC is 'our sacred cow, their white elephant'? (Reidy and Kitching, 1986).

Many would concur that PHC was adopted with much enthusiasm and haste, but with insufficient attention to planning and management; that the complexity of delivering even simple services and interventions was underestimated; that it was often imposed in a 'top-down' manner where what was needed was extensive dialogue with health workers and communities in order to change attitudes; that the real costs of implementation were not sufficiently considered.

But for most, the basic concept of PHC retained its moral imperative. However, PHC was introduced into a fast-changing world, which threatened many of its premises. In the final part of this chapter, we look at the contemporary dilemmas facing the PHC initiative.

The promise and the threat: PHC in the 1990s

When PHC was launched in 1978 the prevailing climate was hopeful and optimistic. Its architects could hardly have imagined the negative trends in economic growth, the extent of borrowing and the changing ideology which would reinforce political thinking in the capitalist world, and bring about the demise of the communist bloc. Many ministries of health (especially in the newly independent Third World countries) had enjoyed increases in resources during the 1970s and thought (erroneously) that PHC would be inexpensive.[5] At the international level, donor agencies accorded health more attention than ever before, and the two UN agencies that promoted PHC had committed directors who pushed for change decisively and forcefully. Other key professionals in international agencies, non-governmental organisations, and ministries of health soon accepted the persuasive arguments in favour of PHC in the Third World.

PHC in crisis

Within a few years of the endorsement of PHC, however, the global economic, political and social environment had changed dramatically. By the mid-1980s *economic growth* had slowed or even reversed. Of course the effect was not uniform: growth continued in most of East and South-east Asia, but recession has hit many poor countries in Africa and Latin America particularly hard.

Heavy debts and falling incomes led countries to try to reschedule their repayments and this in turn meant that the financial institutions such as the *World Bank* and *International Monetary Fund* (IMF) insisted on **structural adjustment policies** as a condition for rescheduling repayments and getting new loans. Structural adjustment took the form of dampening down demand, devaluation of currency, withdrawal of subsidies on fuel and staple

foodstuffs, and deep cuts in government expenditure. In many countries, charges for education and health were introduced for services previously provided free by the government.

As governments had less to spend, so budgets for different sectors requiring public funding were cut. In some countries cutbacks of over 50 per cent were made in the health sector alone, and, increasingly, health ministries found themselves highly dependent on external aid for even basic equipment and essential drugs. At the level of households, such economic effects were devastating. In the 1980s, average incomes in Africa fell by between 10 and 35 per cent. The slow progress that had been occurring, for example, by increasing access to clean water, education and medical care in the previous decades came to a halt. For many households, living standards slipped back to what they were in the 1970s.

Economic recession was accompanied by *political changes* of huge import. On the one hand, instability, low intensity warfare, refugees and the migration of displaced persons affected numerous countries all over the world. During the 1980s, major armed conflict took place in eleven countries in Africa, six in Latin America, thirteen in Asia and six in the Middle East (Zwi and Ugalde, 1991). In Mozambique, Sudan, Uganda and Ethiopia alone, there were a million deaths and five million people displaced. There were also violent protests at the results of structural adjustment policies—removals of subsidies, increasing costs, rising inflation. In many Third World countries people took to the streets to protest against the rising cost of living.

At the same time, structural adjustment fitted well with the ideological shift to policies that emphasised *individual* over *collective* choice, and *private* sector, *market* provision over *public* sector, *state* provision. This was heightened with the break up of the Soviet Union in 1991, and the widespread disillusion expressed with communist regimes and centrally planned economic policies.

At the time of writing in 1992, the impact of the structural adjustment programmes introduced from the mid-1980s is still difficult to see in available, internationally comparable, statistics. However, evidence from a number of countries suggests that malnutrition is increasing, especially among the poorest groups. School enrolment is falling and drop-outs are rising. Fewer people are utilising health services because they cannot afford to pay higher charges.[6]

---

[5]There are echoes here in the policy of community care in the United Kingdom—see *Dilemmas in Health Care*, Chapter 8.

[6]This is illustrated in a television programme for OU students on health care in Zimbabwe.

The impact of AIDS

Added to the bleak economic outlook from the mid-1980s, was the spectre of AIDS (*Acquired Immune Deficiency Syndrome*).[7] By 1985 it was apparent that the disease affected all countries in the world, but that the epidemic was most advanced in some parts of Sub-Saharan Africa. Studies reported that 30 per cent of women in some ante-natal clinics were HIV-positive (i.e. had antibodies in their blood which revealed the presence of the *Human Immunodeficiency Virus*); that 25–40 per cent of babies born to these mothers would also be infected, and would die before they were five years old.

Projections by WHO in 1992 of total numbers infected with HIV (estimated to be 10 million), relative to the number diagnosed with AIDS (350 000 formally notified but estimated to be over 1 million), predicted that 40 million people would be infected with HIV by the year 2000, and over 5 million would have AIDS. Although AIDS in the developing countries was seen initially to be largely an *African* problem, WHO estimated that by the year 2000 one-quarter of people with AIDS would be in Asia, especially India.

Recognition that AIDS was a *global* problem only slowly took force, but by 1987 the WHO, with financial assistance from many donors, established the *Global Programme on AIDS*, and began to fund AIDS programmes in the Third World. Uganda was one of the first countries to launch a national programme, and by 1990 well over 125 countries had established national AIDS programmes, usually administered by ministries of health. Because AIDS was a disease that transgressed the boundaries of the ministry of health, others also became involved, from religious and non-government organisations, to other government sectors such as education or the military. In Uganda, Noerine Kaleeba, whose husband had died of AIDS, courageously joined with others to form the first indigenous AIDS support group:

> When we first began we were just a group of lunatic people, some of whom had AIDS. We met to talk, to cry, to pray, to share, to let off steam. Soon we realised we needed to do more than that, especially in relation to medicine and clinical care, professional support and welfare support. (Kaleeba *et al.*, 1991, p. 44)

[7]The epidemiology of AIDS and HIV infection is discussed in *World Health and Disease*; the biological aspects appear in *Human Biology and Health: An Evolutionary Approach* (Open University Press, 1994); and the sociopolitical and personal dimensions are analysed in *Experiencing and Explaining Disease*, Chapter 4.

The Ugandan AIDS Support Organisation (TASO) began in 1987 with 16 people, 12 of whom had AIDS. Within one year those 12 founders had died, but in the same year 850 other people used TASO's services. By the 1990s, TASO was providing counselling, information, medical and nursing care, and material assistance to over 6 000 families or people with HIV or AIDS. By then many African countries had also introduced such services, including health education programmes for the whole population, sometimes targeting special groups (see Figure 8.9).

For many Third World countries, the burden of care in the 1990s will be overwhelming. With falling GNP and smaller health budgets, the harsh reality is that the expensive antibiotic therapies for 'opportunistic' infections (which flourish only when immunity is deficient) or the therapeutic discoveries of the future such as drugs and vaccines which delay the onset of AIDS or its progress, will not be within the means of either health ministries in

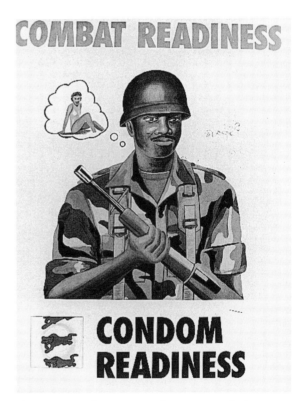

Figure 8.9 *AIDS posters sometimes target particular groups to warn them against risky behaviour. Here Ghanaian soldiers are reminded of their military duty to their country, themselves and their partners. (Source: 37 Military Hospital, Accra, Health Division of Ghana Armed Forces)*

the Third World or most households. But clearly it is not a problem that can be tackled by ministries of health alone—it is a *public health* issue which crosses the normal boundaries of the health sector. And it is not the only environmental problem facing developing countries.

Ecological deterioration: polluting the land

In the 1970s, community health workers were taught the importance of environmental cleanliness at the domestic level. They tried to raise consciousness about clean water, the need to build latrines, to pen animals so that they did not wander inside the house. But the greater environmental problems were ones of deforestation, falling or insufficient water levels, creeping desertification, overgrazed land—all taxing the survival tactics of many rural populations—and threats for which community health workers had no tools or even answers. What else could women do than go further and further afield to find wood to burn, so they could cook?

Since the protection of the environment was raised as a world issue, more than 500 million acres of tropical rain forest have been felled and nearly 500 billion tonnes of topsoil lost (equivalent to the entire cropland of the USA). By the time of the *Earth Summit* in Rio de Janeiro in 1992, two billion more people were living on the Earth than had been twenty years before, the gap between the rich and poor nations had grown, and the recession had cooled industrial nations' interest in taking responsibility for controlling environmental problems.

But it is in the *cities* that environments are particularly at risk (see Figures 8.10a and 8.10b, *overleaf*). By the year 2000 over 80 per cent of the world's people will be urbanised, and many of them will be living in conditions that will gravely affect their health for the worse. Between 30 and 60 per cent of urban dwellers in the Third World live in squatter or tenement areas in cities. The rapid urban growth witnessed over the past three decades has not been accompanied by an investment in services in urban areas. Even though many slum and squatter communities have shown considerable ingenuity and capacity for organisation and planning, they cannot address the problems of providing paved roads, drains, sewers, piped water, garbage collection or services. Governments have been unable to keep up with the need for such infrastructures; nor have they installed sufficient safety mechanisms to avoid the tragedies of industrial disasters:

> Industrial development may bring many bonuses, but it also opens up new possibilities of accidents involving transport accidents, chemical spills, fires and explosions, toxic wastes (including gases) and mass poisonings.

A few dramatic events of recent years, including the accidental release of chemicals at Bhopal (1984) and Seveso (1976), the gas explosions in Mexico City (1984) and the explosion of the nuclear power station at Chernobyl (1986) as well as many other close calls, have served to draw public, governmental and expert attention to the growing problem.... It is in the Third World regions with rapid urban population-growth that urban planners face the greatest problems in managing urban expansion and in so doing, limiting the risks arising from the close proximity of people, industrial production and pollution, risks accentuated by poverty. (Hardoy, *et al.*, 1990, p. 220)

Although there is considerable agreement about the problems facing the Earth's environment, conflicts abound. Writing about the preparations for the Earth Summit held in 1992, *The Observer's* environment correspondent pointed to some of the divergent interests:

> The United States has objected to all references to Western over-consumption. The Vatican and some other countries are causing trouble over population control. Arab Oil producers, who 20 years ago justified price rises as a way of conserving precious oil, want to delete any reference to energy saving.... All Western nations, except the US, are now ready to stabilise emissions of carbon dioxide, the main cause of global warming. (Lean, 1992, p. 20)

Is PHC enough?

Such debates make it clear that primary health care is not sufficient in itself to reduce inequalities in health. More importantly, the danger is that the focus of the debate shifts from *poverty* to population growth and environmental issues. In the 1960s poverty was 're-discovered' as the basis of much ill-health, and the World Bank's *poverty alleviation programme* was aimed to tackle this directly. By the 1980s there was a decline in the attention attached to poverty, since the predominant World Bank ideology was that *economic* reform, in the Third World and elsewhere, was essential. It was accepted that the 'medicine' of structural adjustment programmes would make the poor feel much worse before they felt better.

The World Bank may be a more important organisation for many Third World countries than other donor agencies—its financial assistance (through loans) is often seen as pivotal for certain programmes. The Bank's position has been strengthened because many aid agencies began to tie their aid to policy agreements negotiated by

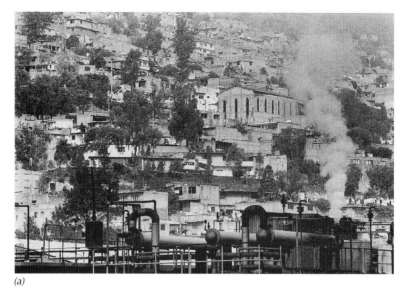

(a)

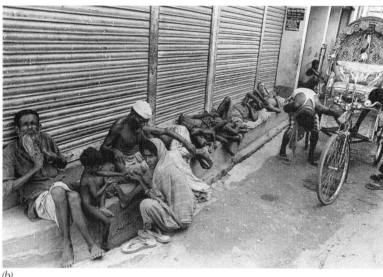

(b)

Figure 8.10 *(a) Urban slum and squatter areas are often unhealthy environments, crowded precariously on steep inclines, unserved by water and sewerage services or electricity, and prone to collapse or flooding during the rainy season. As in this one in Mexico, industrial pollution is a common hazard. (Source: Panos Pictures). (b) In many cities in India and Bangladesh, urban slum dwellers have no choice but to eke out an existence on the narrow pavements—washing, sleeping and eating in the public thoroughfares of the city. (Photo: Tom Learmonth)*

the World Bank and IMF. By the 1990s, significant shifts in health policy were being encouraged. For example, as noted above, some countries which had provided health services free of charge at the time of use, introduced charges to consumers. In many of these countries the provision of health services by the *public* sector is shrinking, with a corresponding increase in *private* sector provision.

Crises often legitimate change. As you have seen, the primary health care movement was diverted during the 1980s into a technology-driven, *selective* approach of low-cost interventions in health care. In poor countries with weak infrastructures, this approach failed miserably, and some of the interventions have been much more difficult to implement than anticipated, and therefore much less effective. The rationale for *comprehensive* primary health care is once more gaining ground. The problem will be to persuade foreign donors to support *integrated* rather than vertical programmes.

Whether PHC will continue to be largely confined to the *health* sector and therefore focus mostly on health services, or will retain its original equity-derived, multi-sectoral and participative orientation, will depend on government policy. If PHC is to be about *more than* health care, then such policy must favour redistribution of resources between sectors. Education and food security are critical to improving health. However, in the absence

of, or with severe retardation of, economic growth, it is likely that PHC will continue to be seen largely as a health sector concern, and will concentrate on the provision of health services.

This is not necessarily bad. People want and need health services, and much has been learned in the primary health care revolution about what needs to be done: improve quality of care, improve management techniques, look more carefully at costs, find ways to harness and coordinate the private sector. Many of these changes can be made without huge inputs of funds, but some reallocation of resources to health will be necessary. Otherwise the health goals set by the WHO and adopted by the world community will steadily move beyond the reach of the Third World.

OBJECTIVES FOR CHAPTER 8

When you have studied this chapter, you should be able to:

8.1 Use appropriate examples to illustrate a discussion of the four main areas of influence on the shift towards primary health care in the 1960s and 1970s: (a) experiments in different countries; (b) changing ideas about poverty, health and development; (c) population growth; and (d) the role of international organisations.

8.2 Describe training programmes for community health workers and traditional midwives in general, and comment on their strengths and limitations.

8.3 Distinguish between the goals of comprehensive and selective primary health care, using appropriate examples to illustrate problems in implementation.

8.4 Discuss the wider implications of, and constraints on, PHC programmes in the 1990s.

QUESTIONS FOR CHAPTER 8

Question 1 (*Objective 8.1*)

Community participation was a basic principle of primary health care. Where did the idea come from?

Question 2 (*Objective 8.2*)

What is the rationale for shifting the boundaries between lay and formal care by training community health workers or traditional midwives in elements of formal practice?

Question 3 (*Objective 8.3*)

Compare the main weaknesses of selective PHC with the main limitations of comprehensive PHC.

Question 4 (*Objective 8.4*)

What are the main hazards that threaten to undermine the PHC approach in the 1990s?

International patterns of health care, 1960 to 1990

9

This chapter builds on knowledge of patterns of health and disease in industrialised and Third World countries as described in **World Health and Disease**, *in particular Chapters 7 and 8, which discuss the effects of economic development on these patterns. The television programme about health care in Zimbabwe and an earlier television programme and audiotape—both entitled 'Health and Disease in Zimbabwe'—referred to in Chapter 8 are also relevant to this chapter. An article in the Reader[1] by A. Ramesh and B. Hyma is set reading for this chapter.*

Introduction

This chapter, like the previous two, is concerned mainly with the period from the early 1970s to the 1990s, but we also look back briefly to the 1960s. The first objective is to try to uncover some recurring patterns within the diversity of health care in different countries. The second objective is to place the United Kingdom within the context of other industrialised countries. The third is to consider some of the main similarities and differences between the industrialised countries and those in the Third World.

The chapter focuses on a set of questions that tend to dominate contemporary comparative research on health care world-wide, and on which at least some information is available:

1   How much do different countries *spend* on their health services, how has it changed over time, and why is there so much variation?

[1]'Traditional Indian medicine in practice in an Indian metropolitan city', in *Health and Disease: A Reader*.

2   What are the main *ways of funding* health care, and what kinds of different organisations are involved in *providing* health services? and

3   Are such things as migration of health workers and multinational pharmaceutical companies reducing diversity and creating a *world health-care system*?

These questions have been studied most closely in the industrialised countries of the world, and especially among the member states of the *Organisation for Economic Cooperation and Development* (OECD): that is, the industrialised countries of the world apart from the former socialist countries of Eastern Europe and the Soviet Union. In addition, published data normally refer only to *formal* health care. However, we have tried where possible to extend the discussion to the countries of the Third World (and the 'Second World' countries that were formerly part of the Soviet bloc), and to include some references to lay, traditional and public-health provision.

The cost of formal health care

Health expenditure per person

We begin by trying to establish what resources are devoted to formal health care in different countries. One way of attempting to measure this is to try to express the total amount spent on formal health care as a *sum per head of population*, converted into a standard currency so that different countries can be compared. The most obvious way of putting everything onto a comparable basis is to calculate everything in terms of one currency such as British pounds or US dollars, using the prevailing exchange rate (as we did in the previous chapter). However, exchange rates between currencies can fluctuate sharply over short periods, perhaps because of an election, political problems or a whole variety of other reasons that have little to do with the actual price levels in a particular country. For example, between 1980 and 1990 the number of French francs one dollar could buy rose

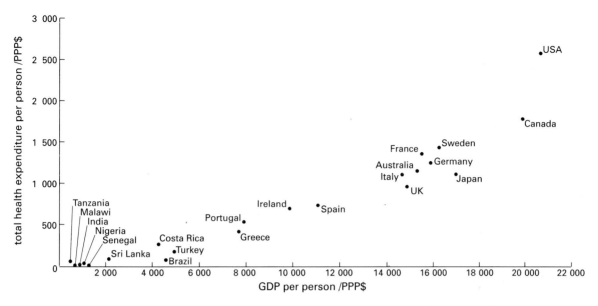

Figure 9.1 *Health expenditure per person, and GDP per person, for 24 OECD countries and eight Third World countries, in US dollars using purchasing power parities, 1988–90. (Data from OECD, 1991,* OECD Health Data, *Version 1.01, CREDOC/OECD, Paris/United Nations Development Programme, 1991,* Human Development Report 1991, *Oxford University Press, Oxford, Tables 4, 8 and 29)*

from 4.2 to 9.0 and then fell again to 5.5. So if French health expenditure had been expressed in terms of US dollars using prevailing exchange rates, the quite misleading impression would be created that it fluctuated sharply.

One way of avoiding such problems with exchange rates is to calculate a *stable conversion rate* between currencies which makes them comparable in terms of the prices for goods and services within different countries, and this rate is called the **purchasing power parity** (**PPP**). Figure 9.1 shows the expenditure per person on health care in a range of countries during the period 1988–90, calculated on the basis of these PPPs. The countries are arranged in ascending order of **Gross Domestic Product** (**GDP**) per person, which, like **Gross National Product** (**GNP**) is a measure of *national wealth.*[2]

Even within the group of mainly industrialised, mostly Western European, and relatively wealthy countries towards the right-hand side of the figure, there are

[2]GDP and GNP are both measures of national income: the money value of all the goods and services available to the nation. The main difference between them is that GDP includes only income from *domestic* economic activity, whereas GNP also includes income from abroad, for example from foreign investments.

wide differences in the amount spent each year on formal health care per person: nearly twice as much in France as in Ireland, for example, or twice as much in the USA as in Germany. The United Kingdom is shown to be at the lower end of this group, spending less on health care than countries such as France and Italy which have very similar levels of GDP per person.

But perhaps the most striking feature of Figure 9.1 is the gulf in health expenditures it reveals between rich and poor countries: whereas the former commonly spent around 1 000 PPP$ per person on health care in 1990, the majority of the Third World countries in the figure had health expenditures of less than one-tenth of this, and in some cases barely one-hundredth, or a mere 12 PPP$ per person per year. And this difference becomes even more striking when the formidable health problems facing most Third World countries are recalled. Not surprisingly in these circumstances, large portions of the population in many Third World countries are effectively not provided with any formal health care.

Using the United Nations Development Programme's definition of *health service access*—the percentage of the population that can reach appropriate local health services on foot or by the local means of transport in no more than one hour—less than two-thirds of the population of the developing countries as a whole had access to health services at the end of the 1980s, falling to less than half in Sub-Saharan Africa. Such very limited resources for formal health care were of course the background for many features of Third World health care discussed in Chapter 8: notably the reliance of many people on lay carers, traditional practitioners and community health workers, and the adoption of the primary health-care strategy in the belief that it would be inexpensive.

An obvious reason for variations between countries in the absolute amount spent on formal health care per person is that countries vary in their level of national income. The broad picture revealed by Figure 9.1 is that as national income per person increases, spending on formal health care rises, just as in richer countries people on average spend more on clothes or cars or food. However, what is interesting is that higher-income countries seem systematically to devote a larger and larger *proportion* of their income to formal health care. Figure 9.2 shows formal health-care expenditure as a proportion of GDP for the same countries listed in Figure 9.1; again, the countries are arranged in ascending order of GDP per person.

If the USA or Canada were each devoting the *same* proportion of their GDP to formal health care as the United Kingdom, health-care spending per person would be much higher in these countries than in the United Kingdom because their GDP per person is in fact higher

than the United Kingdom's. But the *proportion* of GDP these two countries devote to formal health care is also much higher than that of the United Kingdom—12 per cent in the USA and 9 per cent in Canada, compared to 6 per cent in the United Kingdom.

Broadly, therefore, countries with a higher GDP per person also devote a larger share of their national income to health. Figure 9.2 shows that formal health services now consume on average around 8 per cent of the total national income of the richest industrialised countries, and ranging as high as 12 per cent—one-eighth of total national income—in the USA. In the poorer countries, a much lower proportion of national wealth is devoted to formal health services: on average around 4–5 per cent but in some cases as low as 1 per cent.

Findings such as this convey an important message: that there seems to be no ceiling or limit to how much can be spent on formal health care, and the richer a country becomes the more it will tend to spend. Indeed, it has sometimes been suggested that national income is by far the best predictor of formal health-care spending. A number of studies conducted at different times and using different samples of countries (mainly industrialised countries only) have all found that approximately 90 per cent of the variation in formal health-care spending per person could be statistically 'explained' by variations in national income per person.

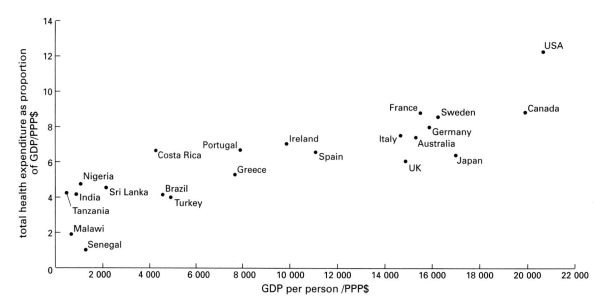

Figure 9.2 *GDP per person, and health expenditures as a percentage of GDP, for fourteen OECD countries and eight Third World countries, in US dollars using purchasing power parities, 1988–90. (Data from OECD, 1991,* OECD Health Data, *Version 1.01, CREDOC/OECD, Paris/United Nations Development Programme, 1991,* Human Development Report 1991, *Oxford University Press, Oxford, Tables 4, 8 and 29)*

Superficially, this would seem to leave very little room for such things as national health policies, or methods of funding, provision and remuneration to exert any influence. However, this would be a quite misleading conclusion. It is clear that very few countries exactly fit the pattern, some spending much more and others much less than might be predicted on the basis of their national income. For example, Figure 9.1 shows Senegal spending less per person on health than Tanzania, although its GDP per person is more than twice as large. Costa Rica spends significantly more per person on health than Brazil, despite having a lower GDP per person. And, as Figure 9.2 shows, the United Kingdom devotes a lower share of GDP to health than do Italy or France, which have similar national incomes per person.

More fundamentally, when examining patterns of health expenditure it is important to remember that many other aspects of a health system may influence the type, amount, quality and distribution of services: there are important differences between the kind of system that developed in Britain in which patients' access to hospitals is controlled by GP referrals, and a system in which the public have direct access to specialists (for example, recall the comparison of methods of referral in Britain and the USA, as described in Rosemary Steven's article which you read with Chapter 4). And, as discussed in Chapter 6, the establishment of the NHS in 1948 did not immediately result in any increase in health spending—if

anything, real spending initially fell—but it nevertheless did fundamentally change many aspects of health provision. So national income is only one factor influencing health expenditure, which in turn is only one factor influencing a health system.

Trends over time

Chapters 6 and 7 traced the way in which a long period of unprecedented economic growth after 1948 was accompanied by a massive expansion of welfare provision, but that this was interrupted by the oil price rise in 1973, after which economic growth deteriorated and welfare policies were placed under increasing economic and political pressure. Figure 9.3 attempts to trace these changes by showing the percentage of GDP devoted to health care averaged across the main OECD countries over the period from 1960 to 1990. The figure also shows the same information for the United Kingdom separately, to assess whether the British experience was in any way untypical.

The figure shows that across the OECD countries as a group there has been a clear trend since 1960 towards formal health care taking a larger and larger slice of national income: in 1960 around 4 per cent of GDP was devoted to health, but by 1990 this had almost doubled. However, the figure indicates that this trend has gradually been becoming less pronounced: on average, the proportion of GDP devoted to health care in these countries

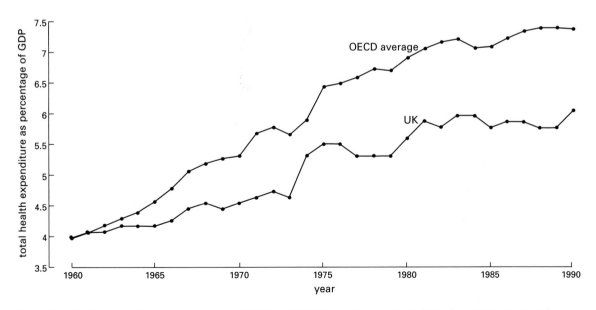

Figure 9.3 *Health expenditure as a percentage of GDP in all OECD countries and United Kingdom, 1960–90. (Data from OECD, 1991,* OECD Health Data, *Version 1.01, CREDOC/OECD, Paris)*

grew less rapidly in the 1980s and late 1970s than during the early 1970s or 1960s.

☐ What does Figure 9.3 reveal about the United Kingdom's health spending compared to that of the OECD as a whole?

■ In 1960, the United Kingdom was devoting an average amount of GDP to health, but since then it has fallen steadily further behind.

Thus the bearing down on health and welfare provision described in Chapter 7, which has formed a constant backdrop to policy towards the NHS in the United Kingdom, is graphically illustrated by Figure 9.3. The 1973 oil crisis was undoubtedly an economic and political turning point, as previous chapters have made clear, but the figure indicates that the impact on health expenditure was delayed by a few years; this delay occurred as governments across the OECD struggled to respond to events and to shake off existing expenditure plans. Indeed, the initial effect of the oil shock was to reduce manufacturing activity, so that existing health expenditures suddenly and temporarily accounted for a *bigger* share of a national 'cake' that had abruptly contracted. A similar phenomenon occurred in Britain during the severe recession in 1980–1, after which the proportion of national income devoted to health care barely changed for 10 years.

Once again, comparable data for Third World countries are very hard to obtain and should be treated with some caution, but Figure 9.4 shows *government* expenditure on health as a percentage of *GNP* for a group of fourteen Third World countries over the period from 1960 to 1990.

It is not possible to draw firm conclusions from Figure 9.4, because the data are fragmentary and refer only to government spending on health, excluding private expenditure. However, it does suggest that health spending was under severe pressure in many Third World countries during the 1980s, for reasons which were discussed in Chapter 8: structural adjustment policies, slow economic growth or even falling incomes, high levels of debt, and a general policy shift away from public provision towards the private sector.

The distribution of health expenditure

So far, we have been comparing *average* levels of formal health-care spending per person in different countries, but the existence of substantial variations in the way this is distributed *within* countries has already been noted at several points in this book: for example, Chapter 5

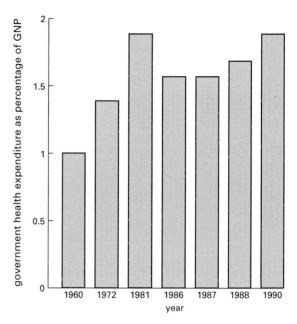

Figure 9.4 *Government expenditure on health as a percentage of GNP, averaged for 14 Third World countries, 1960–90. (Data from World Bank (various years)* World Development Report, *Oxford University Press, Oxford and New York)*

discussed the unequal geographical distribution of voluntary hospitals and local-authority health services in Britain between the two World Wars. Such variations are still commonplace. In 1989, for example, Oxford Region received 18 per cent less than the national average of NHS expenditure per person, whereas North East Thames Region received 13 per cent more than average. Such differences have persisted despite the existence for many years of the RAWP mechanism (named after the Resource Allocation Working Party which developed it) to share out resources more equally, bearing out the conclusion in Chapter 7 that RAWP was a minor response to the problems of regional inequalities, although it had a greater impact in some areas such as London.

Research in other European countries has found even larger variations, for example that within France the best endowed region received almost one-third more than might be expected, while the worst received 57 per cent less (Maynard and Ludbrook, 1981). So France may have spent more per person on health than did the United Kingdom in 1990 (as shown in Figure 9.1), but it is likely that it was distributed more unequally across different regions. Such regional differences in expenditure are only one form of inequality in health care within nations, but they do illustrate the shortcomings of relying on very simple aggregated measures when making international

Table 9.1 Expenditure on health services in parts of the United Kingdom, 1988–9

Country	Expenditure on health services per person/£			
	Total[1]	Hospital services	Community health services	Family health services
England	352	204	34	92
Wales	387	227	35	104
Scotland	468	297	33	97

	Expenditure on personal social services/per cent[2]		
	Administration and fieldwork	Residential care	Day and domiciliary care
England	16	43	34
Wales	16	39	45
Scotland	26	35	27

	Hospital beds per 100 000 population:		
	Elderly	Mentally ill	Mentally handicapped[3]
England	770	160	98
Wales	940	170	86
Scotland	1610	320	139

[1]Includes expenditure on other services not shown here. [2]Allocations to main categories of expenditure only. [3]The term 'people with learning disabilities' is preferred by service-users and their representatives. (Data from DHSS, Welsh Office and Scottish Office statistics.)

comparisons: as the data are disaggregated, so more and more diversity becomes exposed.[3]

The same kinds of differences can be found between the different countries of Britain. For example, as Chapter 6 described, community care was a prominent policy goal of successive British governments in the post-war period, although there was no consistent definition of what it actually meant. But when community care policy and practice are examined in England, Wales and Scotland, it becomes clear that there are large differences from one part of the United Kingdom to another. Table 9.1 shows some of the evidence.

☐ What does Table 9.1 suggest to you about the differing priority given to community care in England, Wales and Scotland respectively?

■ Scotland receives substantially more in total health expenditure than do England or Wales, but seems to give high priority to the hospital-based services when using the additional resources:

community health service spending in Scotland is actually lower than in England or Wales. The table also shows that England and Wales spend proportionately more of their personal social services budget on day and domiciliary care than does Scotland. Finally the table shows that higher hospital spending in Scotland is reflected in the much higher provision of beds for priority groups such as elderly people and those described in official statistics as mentally ill or mentally handicapped.

Faced with such marked differences, one comparative study of community care for mentally handicapped people in Britain concluded that the policies adopted:

...appear as the products of three independent nations rather than as modest differences readily accommodated within a unitary structure of policy objectives. (Hunter and Wistow, 1987, p. 158)[4]

[3]Policies to redress regional inequalities in the provision of health care in the United Kingdom are considered in *Dilemmas in Health Care*, Chapter 3.

[4]Care in the community is examined in more detail in *Dilemmas in Health Care*, Chapter 8.

Such differences in health provision within countries are even more pronounced in the Third World. Table 9.2, for example, displays some data collected from a small number of countries on the distribution of population and of government health spending between the rural and urban areas.

Table 9.2 The distribution of government health expenditure and population in five Third World countries, 1982 or nearest date

Country	Share of government health spending (%)		Share of total population (%)	
	Rural	Urban	Rural	Urban
China	29	71	79	21
Colombia	19	81	38	62
Indonesia	77	23	83	17
Malaysia	57	43	60	40
Senegal	57	43	81	19

Data from Jiminez, E. (1986) 'The public subsidisation of education and health in developing countries: a review of equity and efficiency', *World Bank Research Observer*, **1**, p. 120, Table 9.

☐ What pattern is revealed by the data in Table 9.2?

■ The urban areas generally attract a disproportionately large share of health expenditure. In some instances, the imbalance is fairly small, but in China, for example, four-fifths of the population live in rural areas, but receive less than 30 per cent of government health expenditure. (This may remind you of David Morley's 'three-quarters rule' in Chapter 6.)

Summary

In summary, the main points to note are:

1   Higher-income countries tend to devote a higher *proportion* of their national income to health care than do lower-income countries

2   Among the OECD countries, health care has been taking a growing share of national income for many years, but this trend has become less pronounced since the mid-1970s. In many Third World countries, pressure on health spending was severe during the 1980s.

3   Health expenditures are often distributed very unevenly within countries—for example, between different regions or between rural and urban areas—and this should be recalled when comparing national averages.

Health expenditure: why does it vary, between countries and over time?

So far, we have been concerned mainly to establish *levels* of health expenditure in different countries and how they have *changed*. Amidst the diversity, and the many different policy influences and historical contingencies that have been richly documented in earlier chapters, can any more systematic reasons be discerned for these variations between countries and over time?

Variations between countries

Definitions of health care

One obvious reason for variations between countries in health spending is that they are likely to differ in what they define as formal health care.

☐ In which areas would you particularly expect there to be international differences in what is referred to as formal health care?

■ One of the vaguest boundaries is between formal health care and informal or lay care. In some countries, for example, all nursing work in hospitals is performed by paid staff, whereas in others the relatives of patients may provide a good deal of nursing care, as well as supplying food, laundry and other services. Next, traditional healers, complementary medicine, or health-related activities such as attending health spas may be included in some countries but not others. Community health workers—a sizeable part of the workforce in many countries, as Chapter 8 showed—may or may not be included. Another hazy boundary is between formal health care and the social welfare services. A wide range of social welfare services are included as formal health care in some countries but excluded in others. Similarly, there is often an overlap between formal health care and education services, which often provide some health services for children.

The groups that often straddle such boundaries include physically and mentally handicapped people, elderly people in residential and private nursing homes, and others such as people who are addicted to drugs. However, although these differences do cast light on the way in which the boundaries of formal health care vary, they explain only a small proportion of the variation in spending discussed earlier in this chapter.

Variations in health activities

Another potential explanation for differences in health spending between countries relates to the activities actually undertaken by their health-care systems. In particular, evidence has gradually been amassed that the rates at which many medical and surgical procedures are performed vary widely between (as well as within) countries. Figure 9.5 illustrates this with data on the rate at which people were admitted to hospital for two common surgical operations in a variety of industrialised countries in 1980.

The figure shows very wide variations between countries in the rates at which people were admitted for these two procedures. For example, the rate at which people were admitted for a tonsillectomy was sixteen times higher in the Netherlands than in the United Kingdom.

The reasons for surgical interventions are many and complex, and can be influenced by a range of factors, most obviously the *prevalence* and *incidence* of disease. However, it is not conceivable that this could explain all the variation shown in Figure 9.5. Other factors include clinical judgement, or prevailing customs, traditions and beliefs. It is also plausible to suggest that such variations are connected to different levels of *income*.

In high-income countries such as the USA, operations may be purchased when they offer some measure of reassurance to the patient, who may have no symptoms. The spectre of 'preventive hysterectomy' is alarming, but equally, in a society familiar with the hor-rors of cancer, it would be an economically 'rational' choice for someone terrified of the disease, having a great need for reassurance, and having a high enough income to pay for it. Finally, there is again some evidence that activity rates may be influenced by the way in which health care is funded and provided, the way doctors and hospitals are remunerated, and so on. We will also return to this below.

Variations in costs

Although *purchasing power parities*, or PPPs, as described earlier in this chapter, are a much better basis on which to make international comparisons than are exchange rates, nevertheless they are normally calculated for an economy as a whole, and it remains a possibility that it may be relatively much more expensive in some countries than in others to buy the things needed to run a health system. For example, there are very big differences from one country to another in the prices charged for pharmaceuticals. Similarly, doctors are much better paid in some countries than in others, even after differences in purchasing power are taken into account. In Britain a doctor, on average, earns around two and a half times the national average wage, but in the USA the figure is nearer four times, and in Japan around seven times.

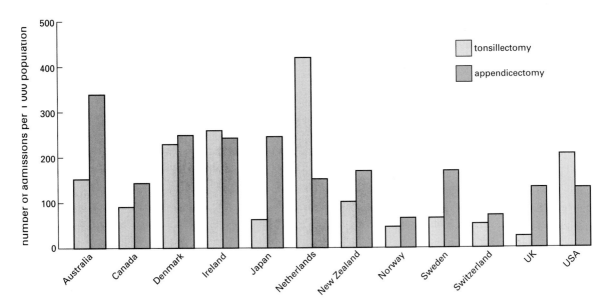

Figure 9.5 *Reported admission rates for two selected procedures in 12 industrialised countries, 1980. (Data from OECD, 1991,* OECD Health Data, *Version 1.01, CREDOC/OECD, Paris)*

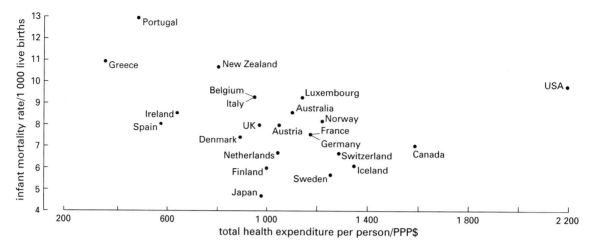

Figure 9.6 *Infant mortality rates per 1 000 live births and health expenditure per person (PPP$) in 23 OECD countries, 1988. (Data from OECD (1991)* OECD Health Data, *Version 1.01, CREDOC/OECD, Paris)*

These differences are the result of many different factors, including the bargaining strength of doctors, the way they are remunerated, and their general social standing and status. Chapter 6 described how the status of GPs tended to decline in post-war Britain, and there is also evidence that the advent of the NHS allowed the British government to put the earnings of doctors under more pressure than they had been in the inter-war period. Whatever the reasons for such variations, the consequence is that in some countries doctors are relatively much more expensive than in others, and this means that more money is devoted to health care. Again, however, this does not explain more than a fraction of the variations in health spending that actually exist.

Variations in ill-health

Another possibility is that variations in health spending are related to the health problems faced by each country. In one sense this seems clearly untrue, in that countries in the Third World with colossal health problems spend on health care a fraction of the amount spent by industrialised countries whose health problems seem minor in comparison. However, many researchers have turned this question round, and asked whether there is any evidence that spending more on health care creates any discernible improvement in health.

The Third World does indeed offer a number of well-documented examples of countries which have attained low mortality rates and high life expectancy by means of a range of policies including relatively well-funded health services: examples such as Costa Rica, Sri Lanka and

Cuba were discussed in Chapter 8.[5] More perplexing has been the poor correlation between the amount spent on health care by Western industrialised countries and commonly used measures of health such as the *infant mortality rate* (IMR). For example, Figure 9.6 is a scattergram showing the IMR per 1 000 live births and health expenditure per person for each OECD country in 1988.

☐ How would you describe the pattern revealed in the scattergram?

■ There is a slight inverse correlation (countries with a low level of health spending have higher infant mortality rates), but the association between the two variables is not very strong. And some countries such as the USA and Japan seem to have much higher or lower IMRs than might be expected on the basis of their health expenditure.

What does this apparently weak correspondence between the level of health-care spending in industrialised countries and mortality mean? There are many difficulties involved in trying to assess the relationship between health care and health. First, the measurement of health-care resources produces many problems, as discussed earlier in this chapter. Second, just because a country spends heavily on health care and does not have comparably low mortality rates, it does not follow that the

[5]These low-mortality countries are also discussed in *World Health and Disease*, Chapter 8.

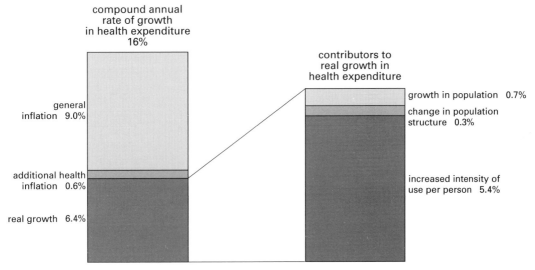

Figure 9.7 *The main components of health-care expenditure, OECD, 1960–84. (Data derived from Culyer, A. J., 1990, 'Cost containment in Europe', in OECD,* Health Care Systems in Transition: the Search for Efficiency, *OECD, Paris, Table 3)*

health care was ineffectual: mortality rates might have been even higher without large amounts of health care. And third, we are only assessing the effect of health care in terms of *mortality*, which might be quite unrealistic. It may be better to focus on specific *causes* of mortality where it is agreed that health care can have some impact, or to examine various measures other than mortality, for example, rates of morbidity or disability.

The problem with measures other than mortality is that it is so much more difficult to measure morbidity, or reductions in anxiety, or the level of comfort and reassurance. Despite such measurement problems, it is evident that it is necessary to consider much more than mortality rates when assessing the effect of formal health care. A significant number of activities are in no way intended to reduce mortality—hip replacement, for example, is an area of formal health-care provision that is intended primarily to improve the *quality* of life.[6]

In addition, there is now virtually no limit to the amount of intensive care that can be provided to a patient in the last stages of life: sometimes with a negligible effect on survival chances. Modern anaesthetics and surgical techniques make it possible to operate on very old people, when gains in life expectancy may be extremely small. Similarly, terminal care for people with cancers may have little impact on life expectancy, but may

nevertheless transform the last stages of life from a painful deterioration into a relatively comfortable decline. Spending on formal health care in industrialised countries, on this account, may well have more influence on *health* that it does on *death*.

Variations over time

Chapters 5 and 6 showed how health and welfare provision expanded fairly rapidly during the long post-war phase of sustained economic growth, but came under increasing pressure after 1973. Some of the reasons for the growth over time in health spending have been examined in the OECD countries, and Figure 9.7 summarises this research.

The figure shows that, over the period from 1960 to 1984, the compound annual rate of growth in health expenditure in the main OECD countries was 16 per cent. Nine per cent of this annual increase was accounted for by general *inflation*, and another 0.6 per cent was accounted for by the fact that inflation in the health sector was slightly greater than in the economy as a whole. The remaining 6.4 per cent was the *real increase* each year, and of this less than 1 per cent was due to population changes—partly a growing proportion of older people who make more use of health care, but mainly a slow increase in the total size of the population. The same broad pattern applies to Britain. So most of the increase in real spending reflected the fact that each individual on average made more use of health services: more consultations, more hospital admissions, more operations, and more prescriptions, which in turn were more

---

[6]The evaluation of quality-of-life interventions is discussed in *Dilemmas in Health Care*, Chapter 3.

expensive because of more advanced equipment, more and better paid staff, higher standards and so on.

The reasons why *rates of use* of health care should be rising so strongly are not clear, but a number of possible explanations have been offered. First, the pattern of disease may be changing, towards more chronic illnesses that are not easily treated. Second, new technologies, procedures and methods of diagnosis have expanded the range of treatments that health care can provide.[7] For example, big improvements in anaesthetics during the 1960s and 1970s made it much safer to operate on people who were old, frail, or very sick. Third, expectations have risen: people not only hear about new treatments and want them, they also expect better food, more privacy, and other facilities for themselves or their relatives when in hospital. And finally, in many countries it has become easier to get *access* to health care, as governments increasingly have accepted responsibility for funding and providing health care, rather than leaving it to individuals to fend for themselves. The next section turns to this issue of funding and provision.

Funding and provision

Chapter 7 discussed the reforms to the NHS after 1989, and in particular the purchaser–provider split. This distinction between *health-care funding* and *health-care provision* is simple but very important. Health services may be funded in one way and provided in another: for example, hospice care may be funded by charitable donations but provided in a building owned by local government and employing staff employed by the government through a health authority. Or, residential care for the elderly may be provided by private homes but paid for by government social security payments. In Britain, awareness of this distinction between funding and provision was for many years obscured by the fact that, before the reforms began in 1989, almost all formal health care was provided by the NHS, a publicly funded *and* publicly provided system of health care.

Sources of funding

There are wide variations between countries in the ways in which health care is funded, and even within a country many different sources of finance may be used in combination. The basic distinction is whether these sources are *public* or *private*. Public sources of funding include general taxation, taxes which are specifically earmarked for health care, and compulsory health insurance schemes,

and it is possible to think of various sub-divisions to these categories: for example, taxation can be raised nationally or locally. However, the essential feature of all these public sources of finance is that they are *compulsory*: people cannot choose whether to contribute the funds or to withhold them, irrespective of the use they may make of health care.

The main private sources of funding include voluntary health insurance, and direct or 'out-of-pocket' payments by individuals, such as over-the-counter purchases of drugs, or charges for particular services or treatments. The common attribute of these private sources of health finance is that they are *voluntary*, or are tied to the *use* an individual makes of a particular service. Unfortunately most countries use different accounting conventions, or publish some pieces of information but not others, so it is extremely hard to obtain comparable data. Table 9.3 shows some information from a study of industrialised countries published in the early 1980s.

Although the data are somewhat old, the basic patterns revealed in Table 9.3 have not changed fundamentally; the table also illustrates well the variations *between* countries, and the use of a variety of funding sources *within* countries.

General taxation invariably plays some role in the finance of health care, but the United Kingdom has been unusually reliant on general taxation: in the past, up to 91 per cent of all health spending has come from this source, but in 1990 the proportion was around 83 per cent.

Compulsory or *social insurance* has become the dominant form of health-care finance in many countries, especially in Europe, where France, Germany, Italy and the Netherlands all draw the majority of their health-care funding from this source. Even in the United Kingdom compulsory insurance—that part of the National Insurance contribution earmarked for the NHS—provided around 5 per cent of all health funds when the table was compiled, a proportion that rose to around 15 per cent by 1990.

The only country not reliant on general taxation or social insurance for the major part of health funding is the USA. There, the single most important source of funds for health care is *voluntary* or *private health insurance*, purchased mainly by people in employment, and often involving contributions from employers. However, reliance on private insurance creates a major problem: not everyone can afford the insurance premiums needed to obtain coverage, and, in particular, people who are old or in poor health (and therefore especially in need of health care) may be the least likely to be able to afford the higher payments they normally face. It is these kinds of problems which have led most European countries down the road towards *compulsory* health insurance.

[7]The impact of new medical technologies on health-care provision is discussed in *Dilemmas in Health Care*, Chapter 7.

Table 9.3 Percentages of total health expenditure funded from different sources in 11 industrialised countries, mid-1970s

	Public		Private		Other
	General taxation	Public/social insurance (compulsory)	Private insurance (voluntary)	Out-of-pocket expenses	Philanthropic, voluntary organisations, etc.
Australia	63	2	14	21	1
Canada	66	9	3	19	3
France	7	69	3	20	1
Germany (West)	15	63	5	13	5
Italy	24	67	(9)		–
Netherlands	15	56	(27)		2
Sweden	79	13	–	8	–
Switzerland	42	25	(33)		–
United Kingdom	87	5	1	6	1
USA	31	12	26	27	5

Figures in brackets relate to joint entries for private insurance and out-of-pocket expenses. (Data derived from Maxwell, R., 1981, *Health and Wealth: an International Study of Health-care Spending*, Lexington Books, Mass., USA, p. 61, Table 4.1)

In the USA, too, the inability of some groups to get adequate insurance coverage against ill-health has resulted in government intervention: the government finances medical programmes for Native Americans, armed forces veterans, poor and elderly people. However, in 1988, around 37 million Americans, or around 15 per cent of the population, were not covered by these programmes and yet had no health insurance or were inadequately insured. Some of these were young people who to some extent were choosing to go uninsured on the assumption that they were a low-risk group, but the majority were low-paid, unemployed or disabled Americans not eligible for government support but unable to afford private insurance.

Out-of-pocket expenses account for a significant proportion of health-care finance in most countries, and again the United Kingdom is unusual in the relatively low share of total expenditure raised from this source, although they are much more important in particular areas such as dentistry or optician services. These out-of-pocket expenses may cover a range of different items: *direct charges* levied on users of health services, for example the prescription charges or charges for glasses provided by the NHS in Britain; *co-payments*, whereby people who are insured have to pay a proportion or a set amount of any claim made on the insurance policy; *fees* paid directly to privately practising doctors or other health workers; and purchase of other health-related products, such as non-prescription or *over-the-counter* drugs. In total, it is not uncommon for such out-of-pocket expenses to provide one-fifth or even one-quarter of all health-care finance.

The final item listed in Table 9.3 is funding from *philanthropic and voluntary organisations,* and funds voluntarily contributed by *employers.* Philanthropic organisations often provide care without formal payment, and hence are often excluded from measures of health-care expenditure, so their contribution is normally underestimated. In fact, they continue to play a significant role in most countries, and in some countries their contribution may be of similar magnitude to funds from private health insurance. In the United Kingdom, one estimate in the early 1980s suggested that voluntary help to hospitals was equivalent to around 300 000 full-time workers, spending around 50 per cent of their time on fund-raising and administration (CIPFA, 1984, p. 33). And this still omits the activities of informal carers in the home, who remain the main source of health care, as Chapter 7 showed.

Back in 1960, public expenditure on health was equivalent to 63 per cent of total health spending in the OECD countries taken as a whole: in some countries such as the USA this share was as low as 25 per cent, with the remainder met privately. But during the 1960s, the public sector share of health expenditure rose rapidly as many governments shouldered additional responsibilities for the health care of their citizens: this was all part of a wider 'mobilisation for total welfare', similar to that discussed for the United Kingdom in Chapter 6. As a consequence, the public sector share of total health spending across the OECD rose steadily, and by the mid-1970s had reached around 75 per cent. Figure 9.8 (*overleaf*) shows these changes, and what happened during the 1980s.

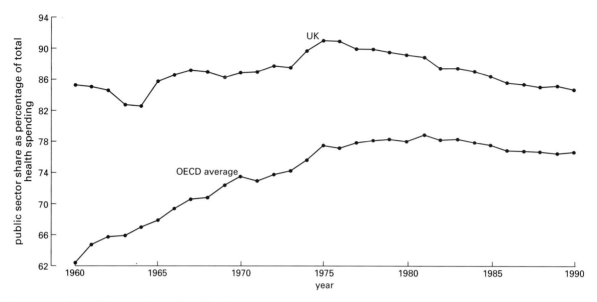

Figure 9.8 *The public sector share of total health expenditure in the OECD countries, 1960–90. (Data from OECD, 1991,* OECD Health Data, *Version 1.01, CREDOC/OECD, Paris)*

□ Recalling Chapter 7, how would you explain the pattern shown in Figure 9.8 from the mid-1970s onwards?

■ After the oil price rise of 1973, many governments became concerned at the ever-expanding importance of public spending in their economies, and attempted to rein back public expenditure in areas such as health while encouraging the private sector. As a consequence, the public share of total expenditure on health levelled off and then began to decline. In Britain the pattern was very similar, although the public share of total health spending remained well above the OECD average.

Third World countries

The same broad categorisation of funding sources can be applied to Third World countries, but if anything there is even more variation between countries. Table 9.4 shows some information from Zimbabwe in the mid-1980s.[8]

□ In order of importance, what were the four main sources of funds for health care in Zimbabwe?

■ Central and local government provides just over half of the total funds (53 per cent). Next in importance are insurance schemes and private individuals (26 per cent), foreign assistance (under 12 per cent), and industry, mines and commercial farms (8 per cent).

If we classify foreign assistance as coming mainly from other governments, then Table 9.4 shows that almost two-thirds of the funds for health care in Zimbabwe come from *public* sources. There is very little information on how health spending is split between public and private sectors in other countries, or on how this may have changed over time, but one estimate for 1980 was that the public sector share of total health spending amounted to 62 per cent in Africa (suggesting that Zimbabwe was fairly typical), 51 per cent in Latin America, but just 30 per cent in Asia (Jiminez, 1986, p. 112). If these estimates are reliable, they indicate that the public sector plays a less important role in health care in the Third World than in the industrialised countries.

You saw earlier in the chapter (Figure 9.4) that the share of national income devoted to public spending on health dipped in the Third World during the 1980s, and the main reasons for this—discussed in Chapter 8—were recounted: problems of low economic growth or decline, and a general ideological shift against the public sector and towards private provision, which has been transmitted to the Third World and reinforced via international agencies such as the *International Monetary Fund* and the *World Bank*.

[8]Zimbabwe is the subject of two television programmes and an audiotape for Open University students. These programmes supplement the discussion presented here.

Table 9.4 Total expenditure on health care in Zimbabwe, 1986–7, by source of funds and by provider (per cent)

Service providers	Source of funds					
	Central and local government	Church missions and voluntary organisations	Industry, mines and commercial farms	Foreign assistance	Insurance schemes & private individuals	Percent of total by provider
Central and local government	51			11	1	**63**
Missions and voluntary organisations	2	<1		<1		**4**
Industry, mines and commercial farms			8			**8**
Private sector					25	**25**
Percent of total by source	**53**	**<1**	**8**	**<12**	**26**	**100**

Data from World Bank (1992) *Zimbabwe: Financing Health Services: A World Bank Country Study*, World Bank, Washington, DC, p. 8, Table II–1.

The World Bank document *Financing Health Services in Developing Countries An Agenda for Reform*, published in 1987, emphasised four main directions for health policy in the Third World in the 1990s (in fact, very much in line with many of the health reforms introduced in the United Kingdom and elsewhere during the 1980s):

- privatisation of health facilities;
- greater reliance on health insurance;
- more use of direct charges to patients or service-users; and
- administrative decentralisation of health care wherever possible.

Direct charges to users are also sometimes described as *cost recovery programmes*. The main arguments used in their favour are that they generate additional income which can be used to expand health care, they provide users and providers with information about the cost of different services, and they deter 'frivolous' use and therefore favour users with the greatest need. They have a long history of use in mission hospitals and clinics, which often provide high quality care to those most in need of it. However, it has also been argued that direct charges can deter the very patients who are at greatest risk and who would benefit most from health care, that they can be costly and difficult to collect, and that often they are not accompanied by any improvement in quality of service.

Ultimately, these arguments will only be resolved by recourse to evidence, which is still accumulating. Studies of a number of African countries in the mid-1980s indicated that on average 5 per cent of the total running costs of the health care could be recouped in this way, with a range of between 2 per cent and 15 per cent (Vogel, 1990). Against this has to be set the cost of collection, which in some instances is considerable. Moreover, in many instances part or all of the income generated from direct charges is not retained for use in the health sector but returned to government finance ministries. Overall, therefore, direct charges are not yet a proven way of making a major contribution to health service finance.

The best documented effects of imposing direct charges are on the *use of services*.[9] One study in Ghana found that a large increase in charges for health care in 1985 did lead to almost 15 per cent of health service operating costs being recouped, but at the cost of sharp drops in usage: two years later, utilisation rates at rural clinics were still half the level they had been before the charges were raised (Waddington and Enyimayew, 1989). In another study in Swaziland, charges at government health clinics and hospitals were raised sharply to the levels charged by mission providers, but there was no matching improvement in quality. Consequently, use of

[9]For example, the television programme 'Health and Disease in Zimbabwe' highlighted the fall in attendances after the introduction of charges to women at antenatal clinics. This may have contributed to the slowing down of improvements in the infant mortality rate which were previously evident.

government facilities fell by a third, and of mission facilities rose by 10 per cent. The most important consequence, however, was that the patients who were most deterred by the charges were people with sexually transmitted diseases, respiratory diseases, and other infectious diseases (Yoder, 1989). This severely handicaps policies to control infectious diseases such as AIDS, the rapid spread of which was noted in Chapter 8. Thus there may well be longer-term health losses to set against any short-term increase in funds, which suggest that more information is needed before direct charges are adopted even more widely.

Methods of provision and remuneration

The diversity in the ways that health systems are funded is matched by a tremendous amount of variation in the ways they are provided and the methods by which providers are paid. And these differences in turn can exert a major influence on the degree of access to health care, the cost of providing it, and the type and quality of services provided.

Categories of provider

Providers of health care fall into three basic categories. The first is *government institutions*, such as hospitals owned and managed by public bodies. In comparison with most other European countries, the United Kingdom has been unusually reliant on this method of provision, whose historical origins—culminating in the nationalisation of almost all hospitals in 1948—has been traced in earlier chapters. In Zimbabwe (Table 9.4), central and local government providers account for just over 60 per cent of the total.

The second main category of providers—*non-government institutions*—can be subdivided into two sub-groups: *not-for-profit* and *profit-making*. Not-for-profit providers, including charitable hospitals and homes, seldom account for a large proportion of health expenditure in industrialised countries, but in the USA *Health Maintenance Organisations* (HMOs)—non-profit associations which provide health care to subscribers—had expanded to cover around 29 million Americans, or 12 per cent of the population, by 1989. In Zimbabwe, the charitable missions and voluntary organisations are responsible for a very small proportion of health expenditure—around 4 per cent. *Profit-making institutions* include private hospital chains and insurance companies. The third category consists of *individual practitioners in private practice*. In the United Kingdom, for example, GPs are independent self-employed individuals, who have contracts to provide certain services to the NHS. This category also includes the *self-employed indigenous and traditional practitioners,* such as the traditional midwives discussed in Chapter 8, who comprise the bulk of people involved in health care in many countries of the world. These traditional practitioners are discussed by A. Ramesh and B. Hyma in an article entitled 'Traditional Indian medicine in practice in an Indian metropolitan city', which is in the Reader.[10] Read this article now and then consider the following questions:

☐ What proportions of health care are estimated to be provided by indigenous practitioners, Western medicine and lay care?

■ About 40 per cent by indigenous practitioners, 20 per cent by Western medicine, and 40 per cent by lay care.

☐ How did patients obtain access to these practitioners?

■ They self-referred, and paid a fee for each visit.

☐ How specialised were the indigenous practitioners?

■ There appeared to be little formal specialisation; most practitioners treated a wide range of disorders.

Paying the doctor

The way in which *doctors* are remunerated has already been discussed at various points in this book: for example Chapter 6 described the way in which GPs held out against the salaried service to which specialists agreed in 1948. In practice, there are three main ways of paying doctors (although they may be used in various combinations):

- a *salary* agreed in advance;

- *capitation*, in which payment is related to the number of people a doctor is responsible for, for example in a general practice; or

- *fee-for-service*, where a doctor receives payment according to the services she or he performs.

The British system of remunerating GPs has involved a mixture of capitation payments, fee-for-service payments for particular items, and a salary element. By the mid-1980s these three elements contributed roughly equal shares to an average GP's total remuneration, although the NHS reforms are likely to increase the importance of capitation payments in the 1990s. Most other OECD countries pay GPS on a fee-for-service basis or—if working from health centres—by means of a salary. And although the NHS system of salaries for hospital-based

[10] *Health and Disease: A Reader* (revised edition 1995).

specialists is found in a number of other OECD countries, including France, Italy and Germany, fee-for-service is also widespread, as it is in British private hospitals, although the details vary considerably.

Paying for hospitals

The other major category of health provider that can be reimbursed in various ways is the *hospital*. In countries such as the United Kingdom, Sweden and the Netherlands, most hospital costs are paid for on the basis of an *annual global budget* which is set *prospectively*. This system makes it easier to control health spending, although it may achieve this by reducing access or quality, or by passing costs on to patients, for example in the form of long waiting times for admission. In a number of other European countries hospitals are not controlled by any global budget, but instead are refunded their running costs *retrospectively*, for example by insurance companies on the basis of a set rate per patient per day: this is known as *per diem* payment (from the Latin word *dies*, day). Retrospective payment systems avoid some of the problems associated with global budgets, but they also remove incentives for hospitals to keep costs down. For example, in West Germany where the per diem system is widespread, average lengths of stay are comparatively long and by the 1990s there were far more hospital beds relative to the population than in most other European countries, which reduced bed capacity during the 1980s. This in turn makes the health system expensive to operate.

Because of these problems, a number of countries, such as France and the Netherlands, dropped the per diem system during the 1980s in favour of setting annual global budgets for hospitals. And in the USA, where the Medicare programme for elderly people involved the government in picking up the bill retrospectively for any treatment that hospitals saw fit to provide, concern over rapidly rising costs led in 1984 to a system in which hospitals are paid *prospectively* the amount deemed reasonable to treat particular problems, classified by *Diagnosis Related Groups* (DRGs). This system, which is intended to give providers more incentive to keep costs down, is likely to play a part in the contracts that will increasingly be agreed between purchasers and providers in the reformed NHS. It is still too early to say with any confidence what effect this form of hospital reimbursement will have on the quality or volume of care, on access, or indeed on costs in the United Kingdom.

Influence of funding and provision on health spending

It seems clear, therefore, that the way in which health care is funded and provided may influence the quantity and quality of care. An example of this is given in Figure 9.9, which shows trends in the percentage of GDP taken by health spending in the USA, Canada and the United Kingdom.

☐ Compare health expenditure trends in the USA and Canada, using data from Figure 9.9.

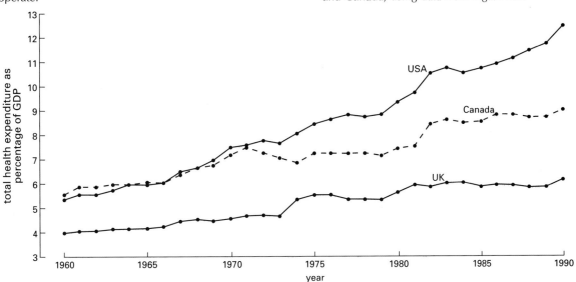

Figure 9.9 *Health expenditure as a percentage of GDP in the USA, United Kingdom and Canada, 1960–90. (Data from OECD (1991) OECD Health Data, Version 1.01, CREDOC/OECD, Paris)*

■ From 1960 until the early 1970s, health expenditure as a percentage of GDP was very similar and grew in an almost identical fashion in the USA and Canada. However, from the early 1970s the proportion of American GDP devoted to health care continued to grow quite rapidly, while in Canada it suddenly slowed and thereafter followed a path similar in shape to that of the United Kingdom (though 2–3 per cent higher).

Figure 9.9 in fact gives a very clear example of the importance of *health policies*, for in the period up to the early 1970s Canada had a health system very similar to that in the USA, with a low level of government involvement, and a dominant role taken by private health insurers and independent, voluntary hospital providers. However, during the early 1970s Canada decided to introduce a system of nationwide compulsory national health insurance, similar to that found in many European countries: in other words, it extended public control over the *funding* of health care, leaving the *provision* of health care largely in private hands, but within annual prospective total budgets. These changes had the effect of slowing the rate of growth of health expenditure quite dramatically. Moreover, there was no clear evidence that these changes were accompanied by reduced quality of health care, poorer access, or poorer health.

The influence of the remuneration system on a doctor's activity, mentioned above, raises a more general issue concerning the doctor's ability to *influence the demand* for his or her own services. In most instances where goods or services are being exchanged, the roles of the person demanding and the person supplying are taken by two people assumed to be equally well informed about the item being exchanged. The patient 'demanding' formal health care, however, is frequently in a bad position to know what to demand.

□ Why might this be so?

■ First, the patient may be unconscious or in need of emergency treatment. Second, the patient will frequently be at a disadvantage over information: about what is wrong, or the range of options for dealing with the problem, their availability and their likely consequences. Even after treatment, the patient may find it difficult to assess the outcome, or the quality of the work performed.

In short, there is an *asymmetry* in the information available to doctor and patient, which places the doctor in the position of having to make the key decisions about what to supply to the patient. This is sometimes referred to as an **agency relationship**, in which the doctor acts as the agent of the patient, making decisions on the patient's behalf. But once this situation exists, the possibility arises that the doctor will supply more health care than the patient would have chosen had the patient been fully informed. The doctor in such circumstances can be said to be inducing a demand for her or his own services, and hence this phenomenon has come to be called **supplier-induced demand**.

□ Under what circumstances might doctors have particular incentives to create supplier-induced demand?

■ If they are paid according to the number of services that they provide, then they will have a financial incentive to induce as much demand for their services as possible.

It is fairly clear that the existence of a fee-for-service payment system, as in West Germany or the USA, has a significant influence over the rates of *surgical intervention*, which are considerably higher than rates in the United Kingdom's National Health Service, where surgeons are paid by a salary that is independent of the volume of work done. This is one factor in the variations in surgical intervention rates discussed earlier. But the crucial question that the discussion of supplier-induced demand raises is not whether the rates of surgical intervention in, for example, the USA, are higher than in the United Kingdom, but whether they are higher than patients in the USA *would be willing to tolerate if they were fully informed*, and so far research on this question has not provided any unambiguous findings.

Summary

In summary, you should note the following points:

1   There are many possible reasons for variations in health spending between countries. Factors such as different definitions of health care or rates of activity explain only a small part of the variation. Level of national income is a very important influence, but by no means the only one.

2   The correlation between levels of health spending and levels of mortality are fairly weak, especially among the industrialised countries. This may be because mortality is not the best or only way of measuring the effect of health care.

3   Health expenditure has grown mainly because of rising utilisation rates: higher admission rates, operation rates, and so on.

4   The basic distinction in methods of funding health care is between public and private sources of funds. The public share of health expenditure in industrialised countries rose rapidly during the 1970s to around three-quarters of the total, but began to decline during the 1980s. The public-sector share of health spending is lower in Third World countries.

5   The way in which health care is provided, in particular the way in which providers such as doctors and hospitals are remunerated, can have a powerful effect on the quality and quantity of health care.

Contemporary health care: an international trade

So far, the main concern of this chapter has been to explore the *diversity* of health systems around the world, particularly in terms of their funding and type of provision, and to assess the extent to which the United Kingdom is typical of or different from systems elsewhere. But you have repeatedly seen how health systems have been subject to influences from other countries: ranging from the colonial interventions described in Chapters 3–6 to the policies of international organisations such as the WHO discussed in Chapter 8.

   □ Drawing on earlier chapters, can you suggest some ways in which such international influences on health care occur?

   ■ There are many, but four of the main ones are:

   1   The migration of health workers, in particular doctors and nurses.

   2   The movement of ideas and knowledge via journals, books and conferences.

   3   The trade in drugs and medical equipment.

   4   The provision of health services by international agencies such as the World Health Organisation (WHO).

This final section of the chapter considers such *international exchanges*, and whether they might have the effect of *reducing* health-care diversity. We will look in more detail at two aspects of these exchanges—the migration of health workers and the pharmaceutical trade.

Migration of health workers

The migration of doctors and nurses from the Third World was discussed in Chapter 6, and the basic conclusion was that it represented a huge donation from poor to rich

countries. These flows from poorer to richer countries are also found within the European Community. Although EC doctors have in theory been free to work in any other EC country since 1977, by 1992 fewer than 1 per cent of the Community's 750 000 doctors had taken the opportunity to do so. Language barriers were one reason, but perhaps more important was that the countries of the EC are quite similar in terms of national income, so that there are fewer incentives to move. Among nurses, there was even less movement within the EC: for example, in 1991 fewer than 600 nurses came to the United Kingdom from other EC countries to join the United Kingdom labour force of almost half a million, and most of these arrivals were from Ireland.

   The reasons for migration can be divided into two broad categories: factors that tend to *push* health workers out of donor countries, and factors tending to *pull* health workers into recipient countries. Among the push-factors, the fundamental one is that some countries train more doctors and nurses than they can afford to employ. This lack of connection between the number of doctors or nurses a country trains and the number it can afford to employ is compounded by the fact, mentioned in Chapter 6, that the type of training is often based on teaching curricula that have been transferred from much richer countries.

   On the other side of this equation, the main pull-factor is that some of the richer countries train an insufficient number of doctors for their needs, and can therefore offer employment opportunities to immigrants. In the 1960s, the lowering of immigration barriers and the granting of employment permits by richer recipient countries brought forth a large increase in the number of doctors and nurses migrating. However, in the late 1970s and early 1980s, immigration barriers were raised again and qualification criteria tightened to reduce the flow. This was because the rich industrialised countries of Western Europe and North America were then producing enough, or even too many, of their own doctors.

   The movement of a health worker between countries is likely to involve various losses or gains to the countries involved, but these may be hard to assess. If we were to assume for a moment that all migrant workers stayed in their country of origin, then broadly the industrialised countries would be slightly worse off and Third World countries better off than they are in reality. But these differences are insignificant in comparison with the gulf in the overall level of provision between the industrialised and Third World countries. With or without migration, the former have between five and ten times as many doctors and nurses per head of population as the latter. In any case, as you saw earlier, a fundamental reason for migration is the lack of employment in donor countries. This would still be the case if every migrant doctor or nurse were to go back to the country they trained in. So the loss to donor countries is not so much the loss of a doctor or nurse; rather, it is the loss of the scarce resources invested in their training, which could have been used for other purposes.

The world pharmaceutical industry

The world pharmaceutical industry merits attention not least because its products have had a significant impact on mortality and morbidity patterns in most parts of the world. The industry performs in a very political and highly regulated environment, where the safety, effectiveness, prices and marketing of its products may all be subject to public scrutiny and legislation. This has contributed to an atmosphere of secrecy around most large drug companies, and so detailed information on the industry is limited. Much of the empirical information given below has been gleaned from a detailed international study, sponsored by the *UN Industrial Development Organisation*, which was published in the early 1990s (Ballance, *et al.*, 1992).

The pharmaceutical industry has a very unusual structure, with the actual production of drugs sandwiched between a powerful scientific research effort and a vigorous and sophisticated marketing system. The marketing end of the industry is genuinely global, in that the largest companies increasingly operate around the world and sell products in almost all national markets. However, research and production remain concentrated in a few countries, and the pattern of consumption is also highly uneven.

The most striking area of concentration is in research. One standard measure of research effort and success is the number of new products or *new molecular entities* which are developed by a company and then marketed on a world-wide basis (that is, on at least six of the world's major national markets). Between 1970 and 1983 there were 170 such products, and no fewer than 127, or 75 per cent of them, came from companies based in just four countries: the USA, Switzerland, Germany and the United Kingdom, with the USA by far the dominant country.

Most of the manufacture of pharmaceuticals also remains concentrated in a core group of countries in which the modern industry emerged, in North America, Western Europe and latterly Japan. Together, these regions account for almost 70 per cent of world production. Other industrialised countries accounted for a further 12 per cent of world production, with the developing countries producing the remaining 18 per cent.

This pattern of production has changed very little despite a rapid expansion in the world pharmaceutical industry throughout the post-war period. Between 1975 and 1990 the value of world production (measured in US$ at constant 1980 prices) more than doubled from $70 billion[11] to $150 billion, a more rapid rate of growth than for manufactured goods generally, but the only country outside the core group that was able to build a substantial pharmaceutical industry of its own was China. No fewer than 46 countries in the Third World lacked a domestic pharmaceutical industry in 1989 and were entirely dependent on imports: these were mainly the smaller and poorer countries, such as Dominica, Botswana, Chad, Mauritania and Bhutan. And even in Third World countries where a substantial part of drug consumption is domestically produced, local producers are often foreign-owned: for example, in Chile, Mexico and Pakistan, foreign-owned firms were responsible for around 50 to 80 per cent of domestic drug production, and for more than 80 per cent in Brazil, Indonesia and Nigeria (Redwood, 1987, p. 262).

The pattern of world consumption of pharmaceuticals closely parallels the pattern of production. In 1990, around 85 per cent of total world sales of pharmaceutical products were to the industrial countries, with the remaining 15 per cent sold in Third World countries (Figure 9.10). Put another way, the United Kingdom, with a population of 56 million in 1990, consumed twice as many pharmaceuticals (measured by value) as all of Africa, with a population of over 640 million.

Although many thousands of small and medium-sized companies are involved in the pharmaceutical industry, the top 25 companies accounted for 44 per cent of total production in 1990. At a global level, this concentration of production is not strikingly different from that of many other large industries, and at the national level the degree of concentration is much less than would be the case in car manufacture or electrical engineering: on average in 1988 the top four pharmaceutical firms in any developed or developing country had around 15 per cent of the market. However, unlike the market for cars or television sets, the market for pharmaceuticals is very fragmented, with almost as many sub-markets as there are diseases and treatments (for example, one sub-market would be antibiotics, another would be anti-depressants, or drugs to combat malaria). And in these sub-markets the degree of concentration is substantially greater: typically there may be 50 competing brands, but the top brand will have up to one-quarter of the market, while the top five will account for more two-thirds (Burstall and Senior, 1985).

[11]thousand million.

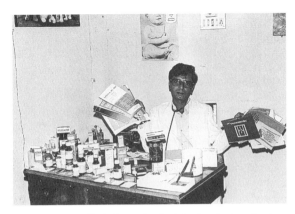

Figure 9.10 *A GP in Secunderabad, India, displays the free samples and promotional materials he has been sent in just two weeks. Manufacturers' promotion of their products can exert a particularly powerful influence on prescribing patterns in Third World countries, which often cannot afford to regulate promotional activities or to provide objective information on new drugs. (Photo: OXFAM)*

☐ Why might a lack of vigorous competition in sub-markets for drugs be of concern to policy makers or to consumers?

■ The main concern is that the prices charged for drugs may be higher than would be the case if markets were more competitive.

Concern over the price of drugs has led a number of industrialised countries to introduce some form of price regulation. However, the dominant issue in the industrialised countries has tended to be the *safety* and *effectiveness* of the drugs coming onto the market, and in general these factors have tended to take precedence over drug prices. The price of drugs is much more of a priority in Third World countries, where far less money is available for drug purchases, and proportionately far more of the health budget is spent on them—up to half of all health-care expenditure, compared to an average of 10 per cent or less in industrialised countries. Measures to keep costs to a minimum include price freezes, encouraging the use of generic drugs, and refusing to recognise patents, but the countries involved are frequently too poor to enforce or monitor these policies, or find that they do not work in the ways intended.

Another policy that has gained ground in many Third World countries is to obtain better value for money by cutting back on the purchase of non-essential drugs and concentrating on a limited number of *essential drugs*. In 1991, for example, the *United Nations Development Programme* estimated that drug consumption per person in developing countries was $5.40 in 1985, but that basic and essential drugs could be provided for around $1.00 per person. Any savings could be used to improve access to essential drugs, and to spend more on other health interventions—such as improved sanitation and water—which may have a bigger impact on health than do medications. This approach has been encouraged by the World Health Organisation, which has produced a list of 275 medicinal chemicals judged to be essential to the therapeutic needs of developing countries. Although much less radical, there have also been moves within a number of industrialised countries including the United Kingdom to create *limited lists* of drugs, concentrating on those with proven effectiveness and, where effectiveness is similar, on those that are cheaper.

Sri Lanka was one of the first countries to adopt this policy in the 1960s, and in Mozambique the same process cut the list of routinely supplied drugs from 13 000 to 355. In Zimbabwe, an Essential Drugs List was launched in 1981, and has helped to contain drug costs while making essential drugs more available to the mass of Zimbabwe's population.

But despite the gradual adoption of such policies in many countries, the United Nations Development Programme estimated in 1991 that between 1.5 and 2.5 billion people world-wide had little or no access to essential drugs (see Figure 9.11).

So the global configuration of the modern pharmaceutical industry mirrors the distribution of world income: drug research, production and consumption are concentrated in the countries with the largest markets. But once such patterns are established, they tend to become self-reinforcing. So, for example, the research effort of pharmaceutical companies tends to be focused

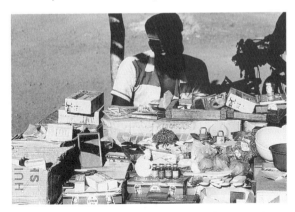

Figure 9.11 *A range of drugs and other products on sale on a market stall in Upper Volta. The small jars in the centre of the picture contain penicillin: it should be refrigerated, so exposure to heat in this fashion will have destroyed its effectiveness. (Photo: OXFAM)*

on the chronic or degenerative diseases that are prevalent in the industrialised world rather than on the infectious and parasitic diseases that prevail in developing countries: in 1989 less than 20 per cent of the 4 300 new medical entities in pre-clinical development around the world were antibiotic or anti-parasitic products. Thus low incomes in developing countries lead to a lower research priority on relevant drug products, and in turn to a mismatch between the drugs coming onto the market in the future and the medical needs of these countries.

A world health-care system

These briefly considered aspects of international health care suggest that, although some common patterns and trends can be detected in the health-care systems of different countries, the degree of diversity remains almost overwhelming. Moreover, as noted at several points, apparent similarities seem to dissolve or slide out of focus on closer inspection. Nevertheless, there does exist something that might be called a *world health-care system*. Western models of health care and medicine tend to dominate in this system, and this is reflected in pharmaceutical production, consumption and research priorities, medical education and technology, the migration of health workers, and the organisation of health care.

This dominance is partly related to the comparative effectiveness of Western medicine in dealing with specific diseases, but it also reflects patterns of economic strength and weakness, custom and culture. Not least, it is an example of how the modern world reflects the past, for many aspects of international health care can be traced to developments discussed earlier in this book, particularly to the gap which opened up between Europe and the rest of the world from around the late fifteenth century. When studying the diversity of health care in the contemporary world, the consequences of this gap form a constant accompaniment.

OBJECTIVES FOR CHAPTER 9

When you have studied this chapter, you should be able to:

9.1 Discuss variations between different countries and over time in the resources committed to formal health care, and the difficulties involved in making comparisons.

9.2 Summarise the main ways in which formal health care may be financed and provided, using examples to illustrate variations between and within countries.

9.3 Describe ways in which methods of funding and providing health care may influence the volume or quality of services.

9.4 Use the examples of migration of health workers and the international pharmaceutical industry to illustrate international influences on health care.

QUESTIONS FOR CHAPTER 9

Question 1 (*Objective 9.1*)

'Spending on formal health care increases in direct line with national income.' Is this statement true?

Question 2 (*Objective 9.2*)

On the evidence of this chapter, to what extent is the British way of funding health services typical of other industrialised countries?

Question 3 (*Objective 9.3*)

Under what circumstances might a 'shortage' of doctors not be overcome by increasing the number of doctors at work?

Question 4 (*Objective 9.4*)

'Pharmaceutical companies will develop products if markets for them exist. Therefore they will not neglect common diseases.' How true is this statement?

10 *Conclusions*

There was a period—the years following the Second World War in particular—which was marked by an extreme optimism concerning prospects for health among other aspects of human existence. That is no longer the mood today. Yet it is important that we do not succumb to the predominant pessimism which the size and complexity of present-day threats seem to warrant. There is a danger that defeatism can act as a self-fulfilling prophecy and paralyse the effort needed to find solutions. (Jefferys and Lashof, 1991, p. 318)

This book has reviewed the effort to contain disease and optimise health in both the developed economies and the Third World. This final chapter summarises some of our main points of emphasis under six headings.

Health care: a universal phenomenon

Preoccupation with health and with health-care systems formed in response to this concern is a universal phenomenon, applying as much in the past as the present and not confined to the developed world. Although we have limited ourselves to events since 1500, it is clear that the expanding empire of Western Europe was drawing on a cultural tradition of long ancestry. Europe as the seat of the Renaissance took over a system of medical ideas which was formed before the time of Aristotle and Plato. European Christianity traditionally placed primacy on obligation to the poor and treatment of the sick, and believed on New Testament authority that the miracle of healing was available to believers. The Reformation and the fragmentation of the church did nothing to obscure the healing and charitable mission of the church.

Magical healing associated with the Christian church provides a link with traditional societies, which also evolved parallel and elaborate frameworks for coping with distress and disease, involving modes of treatment which were integrated into their frameworks of religious belief and magical practice.

In all societies the health-care system reflects the delicate system of values devised for maintaining social equilibrium. Accordingly, health-care systems are not a modern creation dependent on the existence of operating theatres, intensive care units, or doctors with scientific training. Early Christianity and Islam made use of hospitals for the sick, and highly educated corps of doctors were common in remote antiquity. But neither doctors nor hospitals were essential to health care, the greater part of which has always been a function of the family or local community. Consequently this book has attempted to avoid equating health care with formally constituted health services and professions, although it naturally draws attention to the growth of health services and health-care professions as an important element in modern Western society.

The continuing involvement of family, community, and many facets of the social infrastructure in health maintenance, have determined that health services reflect all the diversity of our cultural and political atlas. This variety accounts for the difficulty pointed out in Chapter 9 in evolving simple typologies of health care for the purpose of international comparison.

The characteristics of British health care

Our account of developments in Britain has provided a specific and detailed insight into the manner in which the informal and formal aspects of the health-care system have been moulded by the values, cultural norms and institutions prevailing in a modern nation state.

Sober reflection on Britain (latterly the United Kingdom) as a case history, with special attention to the longer-term record, dispels much of the complacency which has dominated earlier representations, typified by Sir George Newman's *The Building of a Nation's Health* (1939), from which we quoted in Chapter 1. Such reconstructions projected a view of the evolution of health care designed to complement Britain's imperial status. Arguably, some of this complacency carried forward into the period of the National Health Service and contributed to the myth that the United Kingdom was characteristically first in the field and a model for others to follow.

Setting aside untenable notions concerning priority and linear progress associated with the triumphalist view of history, you have discovered some features which have contributed to the characteristic conformation of health care in the United Kingdom. For instance:

(a) *Secularisation* began early in the Reformation and proceeded quickly. Britain's medical charities, voluntary hospitals, university medical schools, nursing organisations and training agencies, were certainly affected by religious inspiration and they retained generalised religious links. But they were predominantly non-denominational in character and administered in a largely secular manner. Britain was unusual in Europe in possessing no religious denomination sufficiently dominant to play the leading role in medical philanthropy.

(b) The absence of church ascendancy contributed to the dominance of *lay organisations* in the administration of poor relief and medical care. The parish became the major provider, and in the later nineteenth century parishes were superseded by newer forms of local government. These developments were supported by local taxation. A mounting body of national statutes were required to ensure uniformity of the local government effort. In the twentieth century, state involvement expanded rapidly, and increasingly entailed direct subsidy from general taxation. Health and welfare services thereby offered opportunities for redistribution of wealth and reduction of inequality. This trend culminated with the establishment of the NHS, which, as pointed out in Chapter 9, was the first major health service in the Western world to be supported almost entirely by general taxation. The United Kingdom therefore provides one of the main examples of strong state involvement in health care (both at central and local government levels), and this generalisation also applies to other social services.

(c) You have discovered from Chapter 9 that the United Kingdom demonstrates the perhaps unexpected combination of high state involvement in health together with low expenditure relative to countries with comparable incomes, measured by a number of separate criteria. This parsimony is deep-rooted historically and it is arguably explained by the traditionally strong links between health care and the poor law. This conclusion was reached in consideration of each of the periods discussed in Chapters 2, 3 and 4. The state assumed responsibility for the care of the sick, but the close ties between sickness, poverty and social deviance entailed invasion of the principle of *less eligibility* into health care. Because the treatment of the poor was financed by taxes levied on the rich, the secular authorities were always vulnerable to political pressures to minimise this imposition, even if this acted to the detriment of the health of the poor. Appeals to altruism with implications of higher taxation to support health care may ultimately have gained general assent, but the temptation of low taxation has prevailed at the ballot box. Britain has thus evolved a system of health services which is notionally generous, guaranteeing a high level of access, but in practice is less kind to the poor than systems founded on less enlightened principles.

The diversity of health care

The British case study underlines the phenomenon of diversity. Even within the United Kingdom, despite the modern cults of efficiency and rationalisation, you may have noticed the separate administration of the health services, as well as independence on policy and resource allocation in England, Wales, Scotland and Northern Ireland, and the persistence of a high degree of autonomy at the local level. When the informal sector is taken into account this diversity is even greater. The pattern is even more diverse within the European Community, and as indicated in Chapter 8, it is bewilderingly complex in the Third World.

Consequently, although this book has attached importance to the process of *modernisation*, and to such associated phenomena of secularisation, rationalisation, bureaucratisation and professionalisation, we are constantly reminded of the *pluralism* of health care, even extending to the persistence of beliefs and practices which are rooted in the pre-modern era. Paradoxically, while Western medicine has been advancing in developing countries, a plethora of alternative medicines of ancient, and largely religious origin from China, India and Japan, have been making notable headway in the West. Although, as indicated in Chapter 9, it is difficult to quantify such changes in the pattern of health care in any country, it is obviously unrealistic to confine attention to developments connected with Western biomedical science, as if all other dimensions of health care are an irrelevant and obsolete legacy from a discredited pre-scientific past.

Even in cases where Western high-technology medicine is supreme, a purely technical approach to health care has proved impracticable. Ethical problems impinge on health care at so many points that the practice of medicine and conduct of health service personnel are regulated on the basis of codes evolved with respect to legal, philosophical and religious criteria.

☐ Select some notable examples in health care where the application of technical innovations has been influenced by the above criteria.

■ Birth control and abortion provide the most obvious examples. Numerous other examples mentioned in this book or others in the series include: enforced confinement and treatment of people who are mentally ill or have learning disabilities; questions of consent raised, for instance, in transplantation; *in vitro* fertilisation and experiments on embryos; or compulsory blood-testing for HIV infection. Immunisation, blood transfusion, and water fluoridation have all met with opposition on ethical grounds.

These examples demonstrate that, even in its most secularised phase, health care and medical practice have become exposed to controls stemming from religious or quasi-religious sources.

Limits to a world health-care system

This book has underlined the *persisting* diversity of health care. This argument needed to be developed to combat the once dominant opinion in Western social science that economic development and modernisation were irrevocably producing a large measure of social and economic uniformity. As a general theory this idea of convergence is misleading, but the case of medicine and health care illustrate its usefulness for limited descriptive purposes. The tried successes of biomedical science have given Western medicine an assured standing throughout the world. Numerous conditions are treated everywhere in the same manner, by medical personnel trained similarly, and all linked by a universal system of professional organisations and a body of advanced knowledge enshrined in academic journals. The examples of migration of all types of medical personnel given in Chapter 9 are made possible by the convergence of medical training. 'Western' medicine has therefore become something of a misnomer: 'Western' relates to remote historical origins. Since the beginning of the twentieth century biomedical science has provided the universal language of medicine, used and understood throughout the world, and applied with dramatic effect. The advancement of medicine is the work of scientists of every nationality. Uniformity of standards and practices has permitted the mobilisation of medical expertise on a massive scale, as witnessed by the campaigns of immunisation and vaccination described in Chapter 8.

☐ What major infectious diseases have been brought under effective control in both developed and Third World regions by immunisation and vaccination?

■ Diphtheria, measles, polio, smallpox and whooping-cough and, until recently, tuberculosis.

The definitive triumph for preventive medicine was announced in 1980 when WHO declared that its global campaign to eliminate smallpox had been successfully concluded.

Vaccination for smallpox was the single most effective medical discovery made before 1900, and perhaps the only one to have had perceptible demographic effect. Most of the advances in immunology, chemotherapy and surgery which have transformed the capacity of medicine to save lives and improve the quality of life were introduced in the twentieth century, although they were based on researches begun in the previous century. For much of this century medical advance has proceeded at an almost exponential rate, until in the 1970s the application of innovations became limited by the financial capacities of the health services, even in the most wealthy economies. This stark economic reality reminds us of the limitations of the thesis predicting convergence towards a global health-care system. Owing to powerful economic, political and social constraints, the world-wide system of medicine achieves only a fraction of its potential, and its effectiveness tends to be least where its resources are most needed. The failure of the malaria eradication campaigns mentioned in Chapters 6 and 8 indicate that relatively simple interventions have failed owing to the absence of stable, elementary welfare infrastructure.[1]

Insufficiency of health care

This book has demonstrated that medicine alone is incapable of controlling disease and disability, a great part of which is attributable to poverty and exploitation. Low family income, unemployment and adverse working conditions have always been passports to malnutrition and diseases associated with bad housing conditions and unhealthy occupations. Of course, entirely different diseases stem from affluence, but the burden is nothing like that carried by the poor. Indeed, the poor in all parts of the world are also afflicted by impediments to health connected with affluent lifestyle and imported or even imposed on them from the richer economies.

☐ What examples of such imports to Third World countries spring to mind?

■ Feeding babies with dried milk, the fashion for canned soft drinks, or Western food habits. Even more pernicious: alcohol, organised prostitution,

[1] A further example is provided by the failure of tuberculosis eradication campaigns, discussed in *Medical Knowledge: Doubt and Certainty* (Open University Press, revised edition 1994), Chapter 4.

changes in nutrition consequent on enforced transition to cash crops including tobacco, or involvement in the production of other addictive drugs.

Of course, alcohol, addictive drugs and prostitution are not creations of the advanced economies, but the scale of their adversity has been exacerbated by Western influence.

For the above reasons, it is clear that any realistic programme of health maintenance must be based on achieving an optimal level of subsistence for the entire population. Consequently our historical review has paid attention to environmental regulation, sanitation and water supply, and also education and the wider economic and political sources of inequality. Chapter 4 reminds us of the benefits stemming from the Victorian sanitarian programme which gave priority to environmental regulation. The subsequent decline of the status of public health in the West shows the subsequent failure to exploit the potentialities of this preventive approach. As indicated in Chapter 2, the traditional 'best practices' of the religious institutions of poor relief embodied the ideas that social support and maintenance of independent subsistence were the main guarantee of sound health.

Appreciation of the unity of factors relevant to health prompted the famous dictum by Rudolph Virchow, the German pioneer of health reform: 'Medicine is social science, and politics is nothing more than medicine on a grand scale.' (quoted in Rather, 1985, p. xiii). In the 1930s the conception 'social medicine' encapsulated this idea. In Britain, the Black Report (1980) and the World Health Organisation primary health-care initiative (1973), discussed in Chapters 8 and 9, have represented recent statements of the inseparability of social justice and health care. This principle is easier to annunciate than to follow. Extreme social adversity ceased to apply on a large scale in Europe only after World War II. Events of the 1990s remind us that destitution and poverty are by no means things of the past, even in Western Europe.

Nevertheless, the problems of the poor in Europe and other Western economies are on nothing like the scale experienced in the Third World. Long ago the influential Swiss medical thinker Henry Sigerist warned that 'to immunise coloured people against disease with the one hand and to exploit them into starvation with the other is a grim joke' (Sigerist, 1943, p. 236). As our book demonstrates, despite all the urgent efforts of relief agencies, large tracts of the Third World are facing starvation under the relentless pressures of exploitation, political instability, environmental degradation and population increase. Although immunisation programmes are one of the most successful elements in the primary health-care

initiative, they will constitute no more than a minor palliative unless basic problems of poverty are addressed. Otherwise there will be an escalation of the health crisis already existing in large parts of Africa, which is already desperate and which has grown steadily worse since 1980.

Health care: in whose service?

Finally, although health services have been provided on a massive scale until they now absorb a significant slice of national wealth, this book has demonstrated that these resources have not been utilised to the maximum beneficial effect. To some extent erroneous judgements were made in full sincerity; they seemed like effective policy at the time. Nevertheless, it is important to realise the extent to which trends within the health services, from 1500 to the present day, have reflected the dominant ideology of the ruling elite, or self-interest of the medical profession, rather than the real needs of the people.

It is difficult to excuse the huge programme of building of workhouses, asylums, mental deficiency institutions, sanatoria, or infectious diseases hospitals in the nineteenth and early twentieth century on grounds of real need. More appropriate, humane and cheaper would have been relief within the community or more prompt use of vaccination and immunisation. Yet incarceration and building of vast hospital networks was favoured by the elite and it advanced the status of the medical profession. Several chapters in this book demonstrate that from the outset the NHS has been dominated by the needs of the acute hospital sector, to the extent that unkind critics have called it the National Hospital Service. In the 1960s the Hospital Plan was pursued at the expense of the parallel and now forgotten Community Care Plan. The opening stages of the 1990s reforms have demonstrated the lesser status of primary care and community care, and they perhaps suggest that the events of the 1960s are likely to be repeated.

This problem reminds us of the real difficulty of introducing drastic change into a system formed by a process of accretion over a long period. Traditions formed decades or even centuries before the NHS was established are likely to influence the course of decision-making. Consequently the objective merits of a case cannot be assessed without attention to limitations imposed by deeply rooted historical determinants. This problem was illustrated in Chapter 7 with reference to the proposals for a radical restructuring of London's health services. With only minor exaggeration, *The Times* health services correspondent claimed that the 1992 Tomlinson plan represented 'the twentieth report in the past 100 years to make this point. The difference this time is that the teaching hospitals face bankruptcy unless they comply' (*The Times*, 6 December 1992). You will of course realise from the above chapters that the problem of incipient bankruptcy is as old as the hospital system itself. Chapters 8 and 9 alert us to the parallel difficulty experienced in the Third World in deflecting resources into primary care.

Although, both in the Western World more generally and in the Third World, changes in direction of policy are being undertaken in the name of the *consumer*, local communities in reality are not adequately informed or consulted, and they possess little control over events. This historical review therefore suggests that the deep-seated tendency to make inappropriate use of the scarce material and human resources available for health care has not been fully corrected. Achievement of the WHO goal for the year 2000 of reaching a level of health that will permit the peoples of the world to lead a socially and economically productive life is likely to remain resolutely beyond our reach. For the attainment of these goals and the creation of appropriate systems of health care the WHO rightly appreciates the need for a much greater exercise of 'national will' for health, which in the more graphic language of earlier decades was called by Sigerist the 'people's war' for health (Sigerist, 1952, p. 362).

The above conclusions may seem unduly pessimistic, yet they draw attention to the very real difficulties involved in translating the product of the modern world economy into real gains for the population as a whole. Nevertheless, it cannot be doubted that the intellectual and material resources exist to devise systems capable of bringing vastly more beneficial results than have so far been available. The discussions in the previous chapters draw attention to the historical determination of the gulf which exists between potentiality and practice. Without taking account of such lessons of history we are unlikely to correct the accumulated errors of the past.

Appendix

Table of abbreviations used in this book

Abbreviation	What it stands for
AA	Alcoholics Anonymous
AHA	Area Health Authority
AIDS	acquired immune deficiency syndrome
ASH	Action for Smoking and Health
ASTMS	Association of Scientific, Technical and Managerial Staffs
BMA	British Medical Association
CHC	Community Health Council
CHW	community health worker
COHSE	Confederation of Health Service Employees
DGH	District General Hospital
DH	Department of Health
DHA	District Health Authority
DHSS	Department of Health and Social Security
DMT	District Management Team
DRG	diagnosis-related group
EC	European Community
EIC	East India Company
EOC	Equal Opportunities Commission
FHSA	Family Health Services Authority
FPC	Family Practitioner Committee
GDP	Gross Domestic Product
GMC	General Medical Council
GNP	Gross National Product
GOBI	growth monitoring, oral rehydration, breast-feeding and immunisation
GP	General (medical) Practitioner
HEA	Health Education Authority
HEC	Health Education Council

Abbreviation	What it stands for
HIV	human immunodeficiency virus
HMO	Health Maintenance Organisation
ICI	Imperial Chemical Industries
ILO	International Labour Office
IMF	International Monetary Fund
IMR	infant mortality rate
LSA	Licence of the (London) Society of Apothecaries
MOH	Medical Officer of Health
MRCS	Member of the Royal College of Surgeons
NHI	National Health Insurance
NHS	National Health Service
NUPE	National Union of Public Employees
OECD	Organisation for Economic Cooperation and Development
PEP	Political and Economic Planning
PHC	primary health care
PPP	purchasing power parity
RAWP	Resource Allocation Working Party
RHA	Regional Health Authority
SGT	self-governing trust
STDs	sexually transmitted diseases
TASO	(translated as) Ugandan AIDS Support Organisation
TB	tuberculosis
UN	United Nations
UNICEF	United Nations Children's Fund
VADs	Voluntary Aid Detachments
VD	venereal disease
WHO	World Health Organisation

References and further reading

References

Abel-Smith, B. (1964) *The Hospitals, 1800–1948*, Heinemann, London.

Age Exchange (1985) *Can we Afford the Doctor? Memories of Health Care* (ed. Schweitzer, P.), Age Exchange Publications, London.

Allsop, J. (1984) *Health Policy and the National Health Service*, Longman, London.

Armstrong, D. (1983) *Political Anatomy of the Body: Medical Knowledge in Britain in the Twentieth Century*, Cambridge University Press, Cambridge.

Arnold, D. (1985) Medical priorities and practice in nineteenth century British India, *South Asia Research*, **5**, pp. 167–83.

Arnold, D. (1987) Touching the body: perspectives on the Indian plague, 1896–1900, in Guha, R. (ed.) *Subaltern Studies V*, Oxford University Press, Oxford, pp. 55–90.

Arnold, D. (1988) Smallpox and colonial medicine in nineteenth century India, in Arnold, D. (ed.) *Imperial Medicine and Indigenous Societies*, Manchester University Press, Manchester, pp. 45–65.

Baggott, R. (1990) *Alcohol, Politics and Social Policy*, Gower/Avebury, Aldershot, Hants.

Baker, N. and Urquhart, J. (1987) *The Balance of Care for Adults with a Mental Handicap in Scotland*, Scottish Health Service Information Services Division, Edinburgh.

Balfour, A. and Scott, H. H. (1924) *Health Problems of the Empire*, Collins, Glasgow.

Ballance, R., Pogany, J. and Forstner, H. (1992) *The World's Pharmaceutical Industries: An International Perspective on Innovation, Competition and Policy*, Edward Elgar for the United Nations Industrial Development Organization, Aldershot.

Bannington, B. G. (1929) *English Public Health Administration*, 2nd edn, P. S. King & Son Ltd, London.

Bayly, C. A. (1988) *Indian Society and the Making of the British Empire*, Cambridge University Press, Cambridge.

Berridge, V. (1979) Opium and oral history, *Oral History*, **7**(2), pp. 48–58.

Berridge, V. (1990) Health and Medicine, 1750–1950, in Thompson, F. M. L. (ed.)*The Cambridge Social History of Britain, 1750–1950*, Vol. 3, Cambridge University Press, Cambridge.

Berridge, V. and Edwards, G. (1987) *Opium and the People: Opiate Use in Nineteenth-Century England*, Yale University Press, New Haven.

Beveridge, W. (1942) *Report on Social Insurance and Allied Services*, Cmd. 6404, HMSO, London (the 'Beveridge Report').

Blyth, M. (1986) A century of health education, *Health and Hygiene*, **7**(3), pp. 105–15.

Bowling, A. (1984) Caring for the elderly widowed—the burden on their supporters, *British Journal of Social Work*, **14**, pp. 435–55.

Bowling, A. and Cartwright, A.(1982) *Life After a Death: A Study of the Elderly Widowed*, Associated Book Publishers, London.

British Medical Association (1938) *A General Medical Service for the Nation*, BMA, London.

British Medical Association (1986) *Alternative Therapy*, BMA, London.

British Medical Association (1993) *Complementary Medicine: New Approaches to Good Practice*, Oxford University Press, Oxford.

Brockington, C. F. (1965) *Public Health in the Nineteenth Century*, Livingstone, Edinburgh.

Brook, C. (1945) *Battling Surgeon*, The Strickland Press, Glasgow.

Brookes, B. (1988) *Abortion in England, 1900–1967*, Croom Helm, Beckenham.

Burgess, M. (1990) Milk shake-up, *The Guardian*, 20 November.

Burstall, M. and Senior, I. (1985) *The Community's Pharmaceutical Industry*, Commission of the European Community, Brussels.

Caldwell, J. C. (1986) Routes to low mortality in poor countries, *Population and Development Review*, **12**(2), pp. 171–220.

Chowdhury, M. and Vaughan, J. P. (1988) Perception of diarrhoea and the use of a homemade oral rehydration solution in rural Bangladesh, *Journal of Diarrhoeal Diseases Research*, **6**(1), pp. 6–14.

CIPFA (Chartered Institute of Public Finance and Accountancy) (1984) *Health Care UK 1984: An Economic, Social and Policy Audit*, CIPFA, London.

Cipolla, C. M. (1976) *Public Health and the Medical Profession in the Renaissance*, Cambridge University Press, Cambridge.

Constantine, S. (1983) *Social Conditions in Britain, 1918–1939*, Methuen, London.

Consultative Council on Medical and Allied Services (1920) *Interim Report on the Future Provision of Medical and Allied Services*, Cmd.693, HMSO, London (the 'Dawson Report').

Corfield, P. J. (1982) *The Impact of English Towns 1700–1800*, Oxford University Press, Oxford; paperback edn reprinted 1989.

Crosby, A. W. (1974) *The Columbian Exchange: The Biological and Cultural Consequences of 1492*, Greenwood, Westport, Connecticut.

Crosby, A. W. (1986) *Ecological Imperialism: The Biological Expansion of Europe, 900–1900*, Cambridge University Press, Cambridge.

Culyer, A. J. (1990) Cost containment in Europe, in OECD, *Health Care Systems in Transition: The Search for Efficiency*, OECD, Paris, pp. 29–40.

Daedalus (1977) *Doing Better and Feeling Worse: Health in the United States* (Winter).

Davies, C. (1988) The health visitor as mother's friend: a woman's place in public health, 1900–14, *Social History of Medicine*, **1**, pp. 39–59.

Day, P. and Klein, R. (1991) Britain's Health Care Experiment, *Health Affairs*, (Fall), pp. 39–59.

Denoon, D. (1989) *Public Health in Papua New Guinea: Medical Possibility and Social Constraints, 1884–1984*, Cambridge University Press, Cambridge.

Department of Health and Social Security (1980) *Inequalities in Health*, Report of a Working Group, DHSS, London (the 'Black Report').

Digby, A. (1989) *British Welfare Policy: Workhouse to Workfare*, Faber, London.

Digby, A. and Bosanquet, N. (1988) Doctors and patients in an era of national health insurance and private practice, 1913–38, *Economic History Review*, **41**(1), pp. 74–94.

Dingwall, R., Rafferty, A. M. and Webster, C. (1988) *An Introduction to the Social History of Nursing*, Routledge, London.

Djukanovic, V. and Mach, E. P. (1975) *Alternative Approaches to Meeting Basic Health Needs*, UNICEF/WHO, Geneva.

Doyal, L. and Pennell, I. (1979) *The Political Economy of Health*, Pluto Press, London.

Draper, P. (ed.) (1991) *Health Through Public Policy: The Greening of Public Health*, Greenprint, London.

Dunnell, K. and Cartwright, A. (1972) *Medicine Takers, Prescribers and Hoarders*, Routledge, London.

Dutt, R. P. (1940) *India Today*, Victor Gollancz, London.

Eckstein, H. (1958) *The English Health Service*, Harvard University Press, Cambridge, Mass.

Edelstein, L. (1967) *Ancient Medicine*, Temkin, O. and Temkin, C. L. (eds) Johns Hopkins University Press, Baltimore.

Elias, N. (1978) *The Civilising Process. I: The History of Manners*, translated by Jephcott, E., Basil Blackwell, Oxford.

Elliott-Binns, C. P. (1973) An analysis of lay medicine, *Journal of the Royal College of General Practitioners*, **23**, pp. 255–64.

Elliott-Binns, C. P. (1986) An analysis of lay medicine: 15 years later, *Journal of the Royal College of General Practitioners*, **36**, pp. 542–4.

Engels, F. (1844) *The Condition of the Working Class in England*; reprinted in 1969 with introduction by E. Hobsbawm, Panther, London.

Enthoven, A. (1991) Internal market reform of the British National Health Service, *Health Affairs*, (Fall), pp. 60–70.

Eyler, J. M. (1979) *Victorian Social Medicine: The Ideas and Methods of William Farr*, Johns Hopkins University Press, Baltimore.

Finch, J. and Groves, D. (eds) (1983) *A Labour of Love: Women, Work and Caring*, Routledge, London.

Flinn, M. W. (ed.) (1965) *Report on the Sanitary Condition of the Labouring Population of Great Britain, by Edwin Chadwick, 1842*, Edinburgh University Press, Edinburgh.

Forsyth, G. (1963) *Doctors and State Medicine*, Pitman, London.

Foster, W. D. (1978) *Sir Albert Cook: A Missionary Doctor in Uganda*, Newhaven Press, Newhaven, Sussex.

Fraser, D. (1973) *The Evolution of the British Welfare State*, Macmillan, London.

French, R. D. (1975) *Antivivisection and Victorian Society*, Princeton University Press, Princeton and London.

Fulder, S. and Monro, R. (1981) *The Status of Complementary Medicine in the United Kingdom*, Threshold Foundation, London.

Gilbert, B. B. (1966) *The Evolution of National Insurance in Great Britain*, Michael Joseph, London.

Godber, G. (1975) *The Health Service: Past, Present and Future*, Athlone, London.

Godber, G. (1983) The Doomsday Book of British Hospitals, *Bulletin of the Society for the Social History of Medicine*, **42**, pp. 4–13.

Graham, H. (1979) Prevention and health: every mother's business; a comment on child health policies in the 1970s, in Harris, C. (ed.) *The Sociology of the Family*, New Directions for Britain, Keele, pp. 160–85.

Gray, N. (1986) *The Worst of Times: An Oral History of the Great Depression in Britain*, Wildwood House, London.

Green, H. (1988) *Informal Carers*, OPCS Social Survey Division, Series GH5, No. 15, Supplement A, HMSO, London.

Haffenden, S. (1991) *Getting It Right for Carers*, Department of Health, Social Services Inspectorate, HMSO, London.

Hardoy, J., Cairncross, S. and Satterthwaite, D. (1990) *The Poor Die Young*, Earthscan Publications Ltd, London.

Harrison, S., Hunter, D. J., Johnston, I. and Wiston, G. (1989) *Competing for Health: A Commentary on the NHS Review*, Nuffield Institute for Health Service Studies, Leeds.

Haynes, B. (1991) *Working-class Life in Victorian Leicester: The Joseph Dare Reports*, Leicestershire County Council, Leicester.

Headrick, D. R. (1988) *The Tentacles of Progress: Technology Transfer in the Age of Imperialism, 1850–1940*, Oxford University Press, Oxford.

Heggenhoughen, K., Vaughan, P., Muhondwa, E. and Rutabanzibwa-Ngaiza, J. (1987) *Community Health Workers: The Tanzanian Experience*, Oxford University Press, Oxford.

Helman, C. (1990) *Culture, Health and Illness*, 2nd edn, Butterworth–Heinemann, Oxford.

Holland, H. (1958) *Frontier Doctor*, Hodder & Stoughton, London.

Honigsbaum, F. (1979) *The Division in British Medicine. A History of the Separation of General Practice from Hospital Care, 1911–68*, Kogan Page, London.

Hunter, D. (1991) Managing medicine: a response to the 'crisis', *Social Science and Medicine*, **32**(4), pp. 441–9.

Hunter, D. and Wistow, G. (1987) *Community Care in Britain: Variations on a Theme*, King Edward's Hospital Fund for London, London.

Hurst, J (1985) *Financing Health Services in the United States, Canada and Britain*, King Edward's Hospital Fund for London, London.

Jeffery, P. *et al.* (1989) *Labour Pains and Labour Power: Women and Childbearing in India*, Zed Press, London.

Jeffery, R. (1988) *The Politics of Health in India*, University of California Press, Berkeley.

Jefferys, M. and Lashof, J. (1991) Preparation for public health practice: into the 21st century, in Fee, E. and Acheson, R. M. (eds) *A History of Public Health Education*, Oxford University Press, Oxford, pp. 314–36.

Jefferys, M. and Sachs, H. (1983) *Rethinking General Practice. Dilemmas in Primary Medical Care*, Tavistock, London.

Jenner, M. (1991) *Early Modern English Conceptions of 'Cleanliness' and 'Dirt' as Reflected in the Environmental Regulation of London c. 1530–c. 1700*, D. Phil. dissertation, University of Oxford.

Jiminez, E. (1986) The public subsidisation of education and health in developing countries: a review of equity and efficiency, *World Bank Research Observer*, **1**, pp. 111–29.

Johnson, J. (1812) *The Influence of Tropical Climates, More Especially the Climate of India on European Constitutions; the Principal Effects and Diseases thereby Induced; and the Means of Preserving Health in Hot Climates*, J. Callow, London.

Jordan, B. (1989) Cosmopolitical obstetrics: some insights from the training of traditional midwives, *Social Science and Medicine*, **28**(9), pp. 925–37.

Kaleeba, N., Ray, S. and Willmore, B. (1991) *We Miss You All*, Women and AIDS Support Network (WASN), Zimbabwe.

Kee, H. C. (1986) *Medicine, Miracle & Magic in New Testament Times*, Cambridge University Press, Cambridge.

King, M. (1966) *Medical Care in Developing Countries*, Oxford University Press, Oxford.

Klein, R. (1983) *The Politics of the National Health Service*, Longman, London.

Lancet (1990) Noticeboard: Marketing of breast milk substitutes, 12 May, pp. 1151–2.

Land, H. (1978) Who cares for the family? *Journal of Social Policy*, **7**(3), pp. 357–84.

Larkin, G. (1987) The licensing of health professions: medical or ministry control? *Bulletin of the Society for the Social History of Medicine*, **40**, pp. 51–3.

Lawrence, C. J. (1975) William Buchan: medicine laid open, *Medical History*, **19**, pp. 20–35.

le Grand, J., Winter, D. and Woodley, F. (1990) The National Health Service: safe in whose hands?, in Hills, J. (ed.) *The State of Welfare. The Welfare State in Britain since 1974*, Clarendon Press, Oxford.

Lean, D. (1992) 'Green thunder' will be aimed at Bush, *The Observer*, 3 May, p. 20.

Lewis, J. (1980) *The Politics of Motherhood*, Croom Helm, Beckenham.

Lewis, J. (1986) *What Price Community Medicine? The Philosophy and Practice of Public Health 1918–1980*, Wheatsheaf, Brighton.

Liddell, A. (1989) Working for patients: a blue-print for the 1990's?, *Public Money and Management* (Summer), pp. 51–4.

Llewellyn Davies, M. (ed.) (1915) *Maternity: Letters from Working Women collected by the Women's Co-operative Guild*, G. Bell & Sons, London; reprinted in 1978 by Virago, London.

Loudon, I. S. L. (1986) *Medical Care and the General Practitioner 1750–1850*, Clarendon Press, Oxford.

Loudon, I. S. L. (1991) On maternal and infant mortality, 1900–1960, *Social History of Medicine*, **4**(1), pp. 29–73.

Lyons, M. (1988) Sleeping sickness, colonial medicine and imperialism: some connections in the Belgian Congo, in MacLeod, R. and Lewis, M. (eds) *Disease, Medicine and Empire: Perspectives on Western Medicine and the Experience of European Expansion*, Routledge, London, pp. 242–56.

MacFarlane, A. and Mugford, M. (1984) *Birth Counts: Statistics of Pregnancy and Childbirth*, HMSO, London.

M'Gonigle, G. and Kirby, J. (1936) *Poverty and Public Health*, Victor Gollancz, London.

Maggs, C. J. (1983) *The Origins of General Nursing*, Croom Helm, Beckenham.

Mahler, H. (1975) Health for all by the year 2000, *WHO Chronicle*, **29**, pp. 457–61.

Mahler, H. (1983) Address to the Thirty-Sixth World Health Assembly, 3 May 1983, unpublished paper, WHA36/DIV/4, WHO, Geneva.

Marks, S. (1988) The historical origins of National Health Services, in *Towards a National Health Service: Proceedings of the 1987 Namda Annual Conference*, Cape Town, South Africa.

Marland, H. (1987) *Medicine and Society in Wakefield and Huddersfield 1780–1870*, Cambridge University Press, Cambridge.

Martin, J. R. (1837) *The Medical Topography of Calcutta*, G. H. Huttman, Calcutta.

Maxwell, R. (1981) *Health and Wealth: An International Study of Health-care Spending*, Lexington Books, Mass., USA.

Maynard, A. and Ludbrook, A. (1981) Thirty years of fruitless endeavour? An analysis of government intervention in the health care market, in Van der Gaag, J. and Perlman, M. (eds) *Health, Economics and Health Economics*, North-Holland, Amsterdam.

Ministry of Health (1944) *A National Health Service*, Cmd. 6502, HMSO, London.

Ministry of Health (1956) *Report of the Committee of Enquiry into the Cost of the National Health Service*, Cmd. 9663, HMSO, London (the 'Guillebaud Report').

Ministry of National Service (1919) *Report upon the Physical Examination of Men of Military Age by National Service Medical Boards from 1st November 1917 to 31st October 1918*, Cmd. 504, HMSO, London.

Morley, D., Rohde, J. and Williams, G. (1983) *Practising Health for All*, Oxford University Press, Oxford; reprinted 1989.

Muraleedharan, V. R. (1987) Rural health care in the Madras Presidency: 1919–39, *Indian Economic and Social History Review*, **24**(3), pp. 323–34.

Newell, K. (1975) *Health by the People*, WHO, Geneva.

Newell, K. (1988) Selective primary health care: the counter revolution, *Social Science and Medicine*, **26**(9), pp. 903–6.

Newman, G. (1939) *The Building of a Nation's Health*, Macmillan, London.

OECD (1991) *OECD Health Data*, Version 1.01, CREDOC/OECD, Paris.

Patterson, T. (1983) Science and medicine in India, in Corsi, P. and Weindling, P. (eds) *Information Sources in the History of Science and Medicine*, Butterworth, London, pp. 457–75.

Pickstone, J. V. (1985) *Medicine and Industrial Society: A History of Hospital Development in Manchester and its Region, 1752–1946*, Manchester University Press, Manchester.

Political and Economic Planning (1939) *Britain's Health*, Pelican Special.

Potter, A. R. (1991) Dealing with two Africas, *British Medical Journal*, **303**, p. 1558.

Pound, J. F. (1971) *The Norwich Census of the Poor 1570*, Norfolk Record Society, Volume XL [Norwich].

Prochaska, F. K. (1980) *Women and Philanthropy in 19th-Century England*, Oxford University Press, Oxford.

Rather, L. J. (ed.) (1985) *Collected Essays on Public Health and Epidemiology of Rudolph Virchow*, Science-History Publications, New York.

Redwood, H. (1987) *The Pharmaceutical Industry: Trends, Problems and Achievements*, Oldwicks Press, Felixstowe, Sussex.

Reidy, A. and Kitching, G. (1986) Primary health care: our sacred cow, their white elephant? *Public Administration and Development*, **6**, pp. 425–33.

Roberts, E. (1980) Oral history investigations of disease and its management by the Lancashire working class, 1890–1939, in Pickstone, J. (ed.) *Health, Disease and Medicine in Lancashire, 1750–1950*, UMIST Occasional Publications, no. 2, Manchester.

Roberts, E. (1984) The working class extended family: functions and attitudes, 1890–1940, *Oral History*, **12**(1), pp. 48–55.

Roberts, F. (1952) *The Cost of Health*, Turnstile, London.

Roberts, R. (1971) *The Classic Slum*, Penguin, Harmondsworth.

Ross, R. (1923) *Memoirs*, John Murray, London.

Rowse, A. L. (1974) *The Casebooks of Simon Forman*, Picador, London.

Royal Commission on Medical Education (1968) *Royal Commission on Medical Education Report 1965–68*, Cmnd.3569, HMSO, London (the 'Todd Report').

Scharlieb, M. (1907–8) Alcohol and the children of the nation, *British Journal of Inebriety*, **5**, pp. 59–82.

Scull, A. (1979) *Museums of Madness: The Social Organisation of Insanity in 19th Century England*, Allen Lane, London.

Seale, C. (1990) Caring for people who die: the experience of family and friends, *Ageing and Society*, **10**, pp. 413–28.

Secretary of State for Health (1989) *Working for Patients*, Cm.555, HMSO, London.

Sheridan, R. B. (1985) *Doctors and Slaves: A Medical and Demographic History of Slavery in the British West Indies 1680–1834*, Cambridge University Press, Cambridge.

Sigerist, H. (1943) *Civilization and Disease*, Chicago University Press, Chicago.

Sigerist, H. (1952) Remarks on social medicine in medical education, in Roemer, M. L. (ed.) *On the Sociology of Medicine*, MD Publications, New York.

Simon, J. (1897) *English Sanitary Institutions*, 2nd edn, Smith, Elder & Co., London.

Slack, P. (1988) *Poverty and Policy in Tudor and Stuart England*, Longman, London.

Snell, K. D. M. (1987) *Annals of the Labouring Poor: Social Change and Agrarian England 1660–1900*, Cambridge University Press, Cambridge.

Stacey, M. (1988) *The Sociology of Health and Healing*, Unwin Hyman, London.

Starr, P. (1982) *The Social Transformation of American Medicine*, Basic Books, New York.

Stevens, R. (1966) *Medical Practice in Modern England: The Impact of Specialization and State Medicine*, Yale University Press, New Haven and London.

Summers, A. (1988) *Angels and Citizens: British Women as Military Nurses 1854–1914*, Routledge, London.

Summers, A. (1989) The mysterious demise of Sarah Gamp: the domiciliary nurse and her detractors, c. 1830–1860, *Victorian Studies*, **32**, pp. 365–86.

Swaan, A. de (1988) *In Care of the State: Health Care, Education and Welfare in Europe and the USA in the Modern Era*, Polity Press, Cambridge.

Taylor, D. (1986) *A Tale of Two Villages*, New Internationalist Publications, Oxford.

Television History Centre (1988) *Making History 5, Birth Control*, Television History Centre, London.

Thompson, E. P. (1975) *The Making of the English Working Class*, Penguin, Harmondsworth.

Thompson, P. (1975) *The Edwardians: The Remaking of British Society*, Weidenfeld & Nicolson, London.

Titmuss, R. (1938) *Poverty and Population*, Macmillan, London.

Townsend, P. (1962) *The Last Refuge*, Routledge, London.

Townsend, P. and Bosanquet, N. (1972) *Labour and Inequality*, Fabian Society, London.

Tudor Hart, J. (1988) *A New Kind of Doctor. The General Practitioner's Part in the Health of the Community*, Merlin Press, London.

Turner, B. (1987) *Medical Power and Social Knowledge*, Sage Publications, London.

Turshen, M. (1989) *The Politics of Public Health*, Zed Press, London.

Ungerson, C. (1983) Why do women care? in Finch, J. and Groves, D. (eds), *A Labour of Love: Women, Work and Caring*, Routledge, London, pp. 31–49.

UNICEF (1990) *The State of the World's Children*, Oxford University Press, Oxford.

United Nations Development Programme (1991) *Human Development Report 1991*, Oxford, Oxford University Press.

Vaughan, M. (1991) *Curing Their Ills: Colonial Power and African Illness*, Polity Press, Cambridge.

Vincent, D. (1991) *Poor Citizens. The State and the Poor in Twentieth Century Britain*, Longman, London.

Vincent-Priya, J. (1991) *Birth Without Doctors*, Earthscan, London.

Vogel, R. (1990) Trends in health expenditures and revenue sources in sub-Saharan Africa. Background paper prepared for *African Health Policy*, World Bank, Washington, DC.

Waddington, C. and Enyimayew, K. (1989) A price to pay: the impact of user charges in Ashanti-Akim District, Ghana, *International Journal of Health Planning and Management*, **4**(11), pp. 17–48.

Walker, A. (ed.) (1982) *Community Care: The Family, the State and Social Policy*, Basil Blackwell and Martin Robertson, Oxford.

Walsh, J. and Warren, K. (1979) Selective primary health care, *New England Journal of Medicine*, **301**(18), pp. 967–74.

Walt, G. (ed.) (1990) *Community Health Workers in National Programmes: Just Another Pair of Hands?* The Open University Press, Milton Keynes.

Webster, C. (1982) Healthy or hungry thirties? *History Workshop*, No. 13, pp. 110–29.

Webster, C. (1991) *Aneurin Bevan on the National Health Service*, Wellcome Unit for the History of Medicine, Oxford.

Weindling, P. J. (1980) Science and sedition: how effective were the Acts licensing lectures and meetings, 1795–1819?, *British Journal for the History of Science*, **13**, pp. 139–53.

Weindling, P. (1989) Population policies under fascism: Germany, Italy and Spain compared, in Teitelbaum, M. S. and Winter, J. (eds) *Population and Resources in Western Intellectual Traditions*, Cambridge University Press, Cambridge.

Winter, J. (1986) *The Great War and the British People*, Macmillan, London.

Wohl, A. S (1983) *Endangered Lives: Public Health in Victorian Britain*, Harvard University Press, Cambridge, Mass.

Woodward, J. (1974) *To Do the Sick no Harm: A Study of the British Voluntary Hospital System to 1875*, Routledge, London.

Worboys, M. (1988a) The discovery of colonial malnutrition between the wars, in Arnold, D. (ed.) *Imperial Medicine and Indigenous Societies*, Manchester University Press, Manchester.

Worboys, M. (1988b) Manson, Ross and colonial medical policy: tropical medicine in London and Liverpool, 1899–1914, in MacLeod, R. and Lewis, M. (eds), *Disease, Medicine, and Empire: Perspectives on Western Medicine and the Experience of European Expansion*, Routledge, London, pp. 21–37.

World Bank (various years) *World Development Report*, Oxford University Press, Oxford and New York.

World Bank (1987) *Financing Health Services in Developing Countries: An Agenda for Reform*, a World Bank policy study, World Bank, Washington, D.C.

World Bank (1992) *Zimbabwe: Financing Health Services: A World Bank Country Study*, World Bank, Washington, DC.

World Health Organisation (1973) *Organizational Study on Methods of Promoting the Development of Basic Health Services*, Annex II, Official Records of the WHO, No. 206, WHO, Geneva.

World Health Organisation–UNICEF (1978) *Alma Ata 1978*, Primary Health Care Health for All Series, No. 1, WHO, Geneva.

World Health Organisation (1984) *The supervision of traditional birth attendants*, Unpublished paper HMD/NUR/84.1, Division of Health Manpower Development, WHO, Geneva.

Wyman, A. L. (1984) The surgeoness: the female practitioner of surgery 1400–1800, *Medical History*, **28**, pp. 22–41.

Yoder, R. A. (1989) Are people willing and able to pay for health services? *Social Science and Medicine*, **29**(1), pp. 35–42.

Young, M. and Willmott, P. (1957) *Family and Kinship in East London*, Routledge, London; paperback edition, Pelican, 1962.

Zwi, A. and Ugalde, A. (1991) Political violence in the Third World: a public health issue, *Health Policy and Planning*, **6**(3), pp. 203–17.

Further reading

The following lists are designed to supplement the information contained in the References. We have confined this additional guidance largely to books, most of which are recent and reasonably accessible. The further reading is organised under the five recurrent themes specified in Chapter 1, preceded by items of a more general nature. Within each list, you will notice that the sources are given in the order of their approximate chronological coverage rather than in alphabetical order.

As you will notice from the References, we have utilised an extremely wide range of sources. Consequently it is not possible to refer you to any book conveniently covering the entire, or even a major, part of our subject matter. For introductory purposes you might like to read D. E. Nagy, *Popular Medicine in Seventeenth-Century England* from section 2 of the following list (difficult to obtain, but a short, inexpensive paperback), and R. Klein, *The Politics of the National Health Service*, given in the References. An important (but difficult) recent book relating to various sections of our survey is A. de Swaan, *In Care of the State*, given in the References; this book should only be attempted at the end of your studies.

1   General

Corsi, P. and Weindling, P. (eds) (1983) *Information Sources in the History of Science and Medicine*, Butterworth, London.

Shryock, R. H. (1979) *The Development of Modern Medicine*, University of Wisconsin Press, Bloomington, Indiana.

Pelling, M. and Smith, R. M. (eds) (1991) *Life, Death and the Elderly: Historical Perspectives*, Routledge, London.

Wear, A. (ed.) (1992) *Medicine in Society*, Cambridge University Press, Cambridge.

Wrigley, E. A. and Schofield, R. S. (1981) *The Population History of England 1541–1871*, Edward Arnold, London.

Laslett, P. (1979) *The World We Have Lost*, Methuen, London (and later editions).

Thomas, K. (1980) *Religion and the Decline of Magic*, Penguin, Harmondsworth.

Wrigley, E. A. (1983) The growth of population in eighteenth-century England: a conundrum resolved, *Past and Present*, No. 98, pp. 121–50.

2 Lay care/formal care

Drummond, J. C. and Wilbraham, A. (1991) *The Englishman's Food: Five Centuries of English Diet*, Pimlico, London.

Webster, C. (ed.) (1979) *Health, Medicine and Mortality in the Sixteenth Century*, Cambridge University Press, Cambridge.

MacDonald, M. (1981) *Mystical Bedlam: Madness, Anxiety and Healing in Seventeenth-Century England*, Cambridge University Press, Cambridge.

Nagy, D. E. (1988) *Popular Medicine in Seventeenth-Century England*, Bowling Green State University Popular Press, Bowling Green, Ohio.

Fissell, M. E. (1991) *Patients, Power, and the Poor in Eighteenth-Century Bristol*, Cambridge University Press, Cambridge.

Porter, R. and Porter, D. (1988) *In Sickness and in Health: the British Experience 1650–1850*, Fourth Estate, London.

Smith, F. B. (1979) *The People's Health 1830–1910*, Croom Helm, London.

3 Environment/public health

Slack, P. (1985) *The Impact of Plague in Tudor and Stuart England*, Routledge, London.

Rosen, G. (1958) *A History of Public Health*, MD Publications, New York.

Rosen, G. (1974) *From Medical Police to Social Medicine: Essays on the History of Health Care*, Science History Publications, New York.

Longmate, N. (1966) *King Cholera: The Biography of a Disease*, Hamish Hamilton, London.

Pelling, M. (1978) *Cholera, Fever and English Medicine 1825–1865*, Oxford University Press, Oxford.

Finer, S. E. (1952) *The Life and Times of Edwin Chadwick*, Methuen, London.

Lambert, R. (1963) *Sir John Simon 1816–1904 and English Social Administration*, MacGibbon & Kee, London.

Rosner, D. and Markowitz, G. (eds) (1987) *Dying for Work: Workers Safety and Health in Twentieth-Century America*, Indiana University Press, Bloomington, Indiana.

Weindling, P. J. (ed.) (1985) *The Social History of Occupational Health*, Croom Helm, Beckenham.

4 Professionalisation

Pelling, M. (1987) Medical practice in early modern England: trade or profession? in Prest, W. (ed.) *The Professions in Early Modern England*, Croom Helm, Beckenham, pp. 90–128.

Cook, H. J. (1986) *The Decline of the Old Medical Regime in Stuart London*, Cornell University Press, Ithaca and London.

Donnison, J. (1977) *Midwives and Medical Men: A History of Interprofessional Rivalries and Women's Rights*, Heinemann, London.

Freidson, E. (1975) *Profession of Medicine: A Study of the Sociology of Applied Knowledge*, Dodd, Mead & Co., New York.

Stacey, M., Reid, M., Heath, C. and Dingwall, R. (eds) (1977) *Health and the Division of Labour*, Croom Helm, London.

Davies, C. (ed.) (1980) *Rewriting Nursing History*, Croom Helm, London.

Larkin, G. V. (1983) *Occupational Monopoly and Modern Medicine*, Tavistock, London.

Dingwall, R. and Lewis, P. (eds) (1983) *The Sociology of Professions: Lawyers, Doctors and Others*, Macmillan, London.

5 Health-care systems

Busfield, J. (1986) *Managing Madness. Changing Ideas and Practice*, Hutchinson, London.

Esping-Andersen, G. (1990) *The Three Worlds of Welfare Capitalism*, Polity Press, Cambridge.

Hennock, E. P. (1987) *British Social Reform and German Precedents: The Case of Social Insurance 1880–1914*, Oxford University Press, Oxford.

Crowther, A. (1988) *British Social Policy 1914–39*, Macmillan, London.

Gough, I. (1979) *The Political Economy of the Welfare State*, Macmillan, London.

6 Europe and the rest of the world

Hartwig, G. W., and Patterson, K. D. (eds) (1978) *Disease in African History: An Introductory Survey and Case Studies*, Duke University, Durham, North Carolina.

McNeill, W. H. (1976) *Plagues and Peoples*, Basil Blackwell, Oxford.

Harrison, G. (1978) *Mosquitoes, Malaria and Man: A History of the Hostilities since 1880*, John Murray, London.

Weindling, P. (1989) *Health, Race and German Politics between National Unification and Nazism, 1870–1945*, Cambridge University Press, Cambridge.

Sand, R. (1952) *The Advance to Social Medicine*, Staples Press, London.

Flora, P. and Heidenheimer, A. J. (eds) (1981) *The Development of Welfare States in Europe and America*, Transaction, New Brunswick and London.

Evans, P., Rueschemeyer, D. and Skocpol, T. (eds) (1988) *Bringing the State Back In*, Cambridge University Press, Cambridge.

Answers to self-assessment questions

Chapter 1

1 The imposing scale of the Great Hospital and the Norfolk and Norwich Hospital, and the unusual example of the Bethel Hospital (endowed by a woman for patients with mental illness), indicate the high status of philanthropy directed at caring for the sick. The Great Hospital (a monastic institution) also emphasises the capacity and willingness of the medieval church to engage in medical philanthropy, and the importance it attached to this work. Notice also that the Lazar House was endowed by a Bishop of Norwich. The remote situations of the Lazar House, the Workhouse Infirmary, the Victorian County Lunatic Asylum and the Isolation Hospital indicate the extent of fear of infection and the stigmatisation of the insane. The dismal appearance of publicly funded institutions such as the Workhouse Infirmary also reveals the prevailing view that the poor were deviant rather than unfortunate. These buildings often survived as geriatric or mental hospitals in the twentieth century, which perhaps indicates that discrimination against vulnerable groups survives to a greater degree than we generally appreciate.

2 Turshen is not calling for the idea of modernisation to be abandoned. But this author warns against simplistic interpretation which imposes a simple linear, evolutionary pattern on economic and social change, under which Europe advances first, and then is followed by the Third World after a considerable delay. Our example of the links between Africa, the West Indies and Lancashire shows that economic integration between Europe and the wider world was well established by the mid-eighteenth century. Other countries, e.g. Papua New Guinea, escaped Western influence for longer but, as Denoon points out, in the twentieth century this remote culture became exposed to infectious diseases imported from the West.

Diseases associated with urbanisation and industrialisation are prevalent in any part of the world where high population density and particular industries occur. The quotation from Chadwick underlined the similarity of health conditions in Mexico and Britain. From about 1750 to the present day, all societies have experienced a process of modernisation, although the pace of change has not been uniform, for instance in the speed of industrialisation, or in the growth of urban populations.

3 The profound impact of poverty demonstrates the scale of avoidable disease. Adequate and secure household income is therefore the essential basis for maintenance of health. From this source follows improved security of nutrition, housing, education, and self-respect, all necessary components of health protection.

At the other end of the social scale, the affluent can adjust their lifestyle to attain better health without direct medical intervention. But even if these social measures are optimised, there remains a substantial residue of unavoidable problems which necessitate medical intervention. With growing expectations, increasing life expectancy, emergence of fresh threats to health, and the increasing capacities of medical science, direct medical intervention of all kinds, involving lay, alternative, public health and high technology aspects, will continue to be essential and will absorb a substantial share of national resources.

4 Medical sociology has tended to adopt terminology evolved for consideration of other departures from the normal, especially the control of criminality by policing agencies. Thus the sick may be described as deviants. The professionals involved in dealing with the sick are said to be engaged in surveillance and control. At an extreme, medical 'police' initiate a process which ends with 'incarcerating' the sick in institutions. By the use of this terminology, hospitals are equated with prisons. This terminology is obviously of limited value in the case of acute hospitals (involving emergency medical intervention), but it is not entirely inappropriate in the case of mental hospitals, or other long-stay hospitals where patients are detained, sometimes without active treatment and rehabilitation.

The term *medicalisation* suggests the intrusion of medical values into increasing areas of life, possibly to the detriment of the groups affected. Such terminology relates sickness to other forms of deviance, and medical occupations to other means of preserving social norms.

Chapter 2

1 Women were involved in medical practice at many levels (though they were excluded from most formal systems of education). The example of Lady Margaret Hoby shows how a local gentlewoman could build up a reputation involving even serious surgical intervention, at least in desperate cases and in more remote areas. Figure 2.2 shows the role of more humble women, and in particular the midwife. Although men are shown in the background, casting the horoscope of the child about to be born, childbirth, even in a textbook, is still being shown as managed by women. We can also infer that Lady Margaret Hoby's patient was an infant, although it would be wrong to infer that she would never be asked to treat adults. Her case also shows the role of community sanction in the activities of lay practitioners. This can also be said of English midwives, because we know that the ecclesiastical system of regulation of midwives was very imperfect. (Formal training for midwives did exist in towns elsewhere in northern Europe.)

2 The quotation shows: lay people taking responsibility for potential threats to the public health; that conditions could be imposed on the use of buildings; that some control was exerted in cities on noxious trades; and that lay administrators were afraid of the concentration of infection from plague and venereal disease in particular. In addition, the quotation illustrates how many sick people could be accommodated outside hospitals; and how attempts were made during epidemics to restrict this common practice.

3 The poem implies (and other evidence confirms) that during epidemics the formally qualified physicians followed the example of their elite patrons by fleeing for safety into the country, leaving the less well-off to fend for themselves. (This was defended at the time in terms of the need for the elite to be able to call on medical advice, and the public value of physicians—and, by implication, their scarcity value.) Forman expresses the contemporary loss of faith in physicians and their search for status, as compared with the usefulness of the lower levels of practitioner, who were more prepared to treat the poor.

4 The quotation gives examples of the gradual discovery by the authorities of pre-industrial towns of the extent and causes of poverty among the 'respectable', resident poor. The reference to the 'storm of…sickness' shows an appreciation of how easily ill-health could lead to poverty, with the implication that timely assistance during sickness could prevent beggary and long-term dependence. The Cambridge authorities, like those of Sheffield, were driven to 'number the poor' in their community, but in their case the administrative response was caused by a crisis of epidemic disease. Few societies would think it appropriate or possible to provide institutional support for 36 per cent of their populations. Cambridge's experience suggests that epidemics underlined the need for flexible systems of out-door relief.

5 Like the epidemiological exchange described by Crosby and others, the exchange of medical knowledge was a very unequal one. Europeans in the tropics were confronted with diseases like yellow fever which they had never encountered before, and which took a heavy toll among them. Lacking knowledge of how to treat these diseases effectively, European practitioners initially became dependent on local medicinal plants (many of which were very effective) and, in many cases, on local medical practitioners. Medical knowledge and medicinal substances from Asia and the New World also found their way back to Europe, where they transformed the treatment and prevention of certain diseases. By contrast, Europeans were able to offer indigenous peoples little in return, and, in the case of slaves, only the most rudimentary health care was provided, in order to increase the profitability of the trade and of plantations.

Chapter 3

1 Both quotations illustrate the growth of class divisions during industrialisation, with the burden of the effects of industrialisation falling on the working class. You may feel that Johnson was not entirely serious, and you may suspect that some of the older towns, like Lichfield, were in some senses being 'left behind' by the industrial boom towns like Birmingham, 15 miles away. Nonetheless, Johnson betrays the gap already existing between the middle classes and the labouring poor. The second quotation shows how the situation had worsened in the intervening decades—and how necessary was the process of 'revelation' of which the Commission was itself part. The physical proximity is greater—Brook and Holroyd 'live within a few miles'—and they belong to professions which might be expected to be well informed about social conditions, yet they have to confess to not knowing what conditions in the mines were like. Their ignorance is also a measure of the lack of supervision or regulation of conditions at work, which of course affected men and women as well as children. (It may also strike you that poor working conditions made it possible for industrialists to produce coal and iron at the low cost essential for rapid economic growth.)

2 One aspect of urbanisation was the attempt by the middle classes in smaller centres to imitate the

sophisticated amenities of larger towns—or even of the resorts of continental Europe. The search for health was a sufficiently strong motive for a health-related amenity to be a good commercial speculation, likely to improve local prosperity. At the same time, such resorts provided opportunities for social display and social contacts, which required agreeable surroundings. (For the middle classes, industrialisation may have sharpened enjoyment of such pastoral features as the rustic bridge—to which the 'rustics' themselves would not have had access.) It is possible, too, that the Lockwood entrepreneurs were hoping to capitalise on the sulphur well's local reputation for curative qualities.

3   The 'General Practitioner' label was relatively new in 1827, which was also a time of increased competition among practitioners for 'respectable' practice. 'General Practitioner' would have hoped to improve his clientele by acquiring 'College and Hall' qualifications—the MRCS of the Royal College of Surgeons and the LSA of the Society of Apothecaries. However, this was well before the Medical Act of 1858 which, though limited, did offer some advantage to the formally qualified. In 1827, the MRCS and LSA would have improved 'General Practitioner''s status, but would have had little effect on his unqualified competitors—who were very much in the majority. (Provisions in the Apothecaries' Act of 1815 against unqualified practice had had no effect.) 'General Practitioner''s grievance is clearly also directed against the elites of the London medical organisations who put up barriers for rank-and-file practitioners to climb, without controlling unqualified practice or helping to guarantee an adequate return for the time and money involved in pursuing qualifications.

4   In political terms, environmental conditions were at this time 'no one's responsibility'. In better-off areas, the inhabitants could raise the funds and promote the legislation necessary for improving their surroundings. These were essentially local (or commercial) initiatives. By contrast, it was not possible for the poor to help themselves, and it was not yet perceived as in anyone else's interests to improve slum housing. The role of central government in health matters was extremely limited. Southwood Smith also makes the important point that the poor were obliged to live near their work—and were therefore most exposed to the effects of industrial pollution. You may also note, however, that Smith's account places the blame not on the workplaces of the poor, but on their living conditions—illustrating the Benthamites' limited willingness to interfere directly with the economy.

5   The quotation shows that the attitude of the poor to hospitals was not necessarily positive; that attendance as outpatients was often better suited to their circumstances; that it could be assumed that the living conditions of the poor did not include 'free air, wholesome…diet, and clean…attendance'; and that the medical and surgical procedures conducted in the voluntary hospitals could be relatively limited (partly to avoid deterring prospective patients). You may also have noticed that, at this time, the hospitals were still functioning more like the pre-Reformation monastic foundations, rather than as acute hospitals in the modern sense (i.e. short-stay and emergency admissions); it was realised that good nutrition could do as much as medical intervention to improve the state of health among the poor. You might also have speculated that the poor's fear of hospitals could in part be based on experience of compulsory removal to pesthouses and mass burial during the plague epidemics of the previous century—and perhaps also on an increasing sense of social isolation.

6   These extracts signify two important developments which took place in colonial medicine in India in the 1820s and 1830s, both of which were associated with the growing influence of Benthamite principles. Indian medicine, along with Indian culture, morals and political institutions, were compared unfavourably with their Western counterparts, the latter supposedly being more rational, efficient, and enlightened. Whereas Europeans had once learned from indigenous medicine and hygienic practices, the Indian people and their customs were now identified as part of the sanitary problem confronting the British in India. But, like many of his contemporaries, Martin reserved a certain amount of admiration for the 'martial races' of northern India, whose physical appearance and culture were closer to those of the British.

Chapter 4

1   The quotation signals the change from thinking in terms of environmental causes, which were largely out of the poor's control, to a view focusing upon personal responsibility. In particular, we see the start of concern about the effects of the employment of mothers on the health of infants and children—'maternal inefficiency' was stressed to explain why, at the end of the century (and in spite of sanitary reform), infant mortality had failed to fall as had adult mortality.

2   Although traditions of lay care remained strong, this quotation shows how homes were increasingly being invaded by outside help and advice. This advice also shows clearly the dual function of outside intervention: to help and advise, but also to provide moral leadership and

to inculcate habits of thrift, cleanliness, and morality which were norms in middle-class society. The health visitor was also expected to emphasise the individual aspects of health. There is no appreciation in this advice that 'bad smells' and 'feeding and clothing' might also be dependent upon influences (such as drainage, and employment) outside the family's control.

3   Miss Phipps was, as a middle- to upper-class amateur nurse, in the *minority* at this time. Her practice among her 'farm people' links her with the gentlewoman practitioners we have seen in earlier chapters. Her background experience shows her connections with philanthropic outlets for women. She was writing during the 'thirty-year nursing war' which began around 1880. She may later have joined those pressing for professional status for nurses.

4   The British scheme had a number of advantages for insured people, compared with its German predecessor:

    (a)   Contributions were not graduated, but paid at a flat rate.

    (b)   Worker and employer contributed equal amounts, whereas German workers contributed twice as much as their employer.

    (c)   Maternity benefits were paid to all working women in the scheme, whereas in Germany they were discretionary.

    (d)   The scheme was open to all workers from the outset, whereas in Germany the scheme at first covered only certain categories of urban worker (but was extended to all later).

    (e)   Sexually transmitted diseases were not excluded in Britain, as they were in Germany before 1911.

    However, the British scheme had certain significant limitations, which it shared with the German scheme:

    (i)   Dependants of the insured worker were excluded (although both schemes were modified at a later date to include them in limited ways).

    (ii)   Treatment options were limited; for example in Britain, hospital treatment was covered only for people with tuberculosis.

    (iii)   Cash benefits were a fixed amount regardless of the severity of an illness, accident or disability.

5   Colonial medical practitioners often claimed that it was the duty of Europeans to 'civilise' indigenous peoples by inducing them, through the provision of health care, to accept Christianity and other 'Western' values. The rhetoric of colonial medicine cast European civilisation in a superior light and portrayed indigenous peoples as morally as well as physically diseased. But, by 1918, colonial medicine had bestowed few medical benefits upon indigenous peoples, since, with the exception of medical missions, it continued to concentrate on the health of Europeans and on improving economic efficiency. Colonial medicine also expressed European fears of the indigenous population, with medicine providing a justification for racial segregation, which left indigenous Africans in settlements with inferior housing and poor sanitation.

Chapter 5

1   Health-care provision remained geographically patchy and uncoordinated. The location of voluntary hospitals was often unrelated to need and their work was totally separate from that of the workhouse infirmaries and local authority hospitals. Local authorities provided an increasing range of services, from ante-natal clinics to STD clinics. But there was no coordination with GP 'panel' services provided under the NHI scheme. There was no universal right of access to services (women and children were particularly poorly served) and to specialist hospital services in particular. Attempts to reform and rationalise the funding of services were prevented by economy measures taken by government and by the attitude of the approved societies, which administered the NHI scheme.

2   This quotation indicates the continuing vitality of lay care and advice and the access to non-commercial means of self-medication. It also underlines the importance of the pharmacist in working-class health care. But the boundaries were beginning to shift towards a greater reliance on formal health-care provision. This tendency was most apparent in the area of childbirth and child care; hospital-based childbirth and the advice and assistance of outside 'experts' such as trained midwives and health visitors (including advice on birth control) became more common.

3   Nineteenth-century public health had seen its remit as covering environmental questions—housing, sanitation, and their effect on disease as well as matters of individual hygiene. In the twentieth century this focus narrowed to one on questions of individual ill-health and the prevention of ill-health. In addition, in the inter-war years, MOHs in the local authorities took on a considerable range of administrative responsibilities, running local hospitals and a battery of local-authority services. Historians have argued that MOHs were simply taking on

whatever activities offered themselves without thinking of what was distinctive about the public-health approach. There has also been criticism of the narrower focus on individual rather than environmental causes of ill-health.

4 In theory, the nurses achieved partial professional status in 1919. But many practising nurses did not meet the registration requirements and still wanted to continue nursing. The state and the voluntary hospital sector also had an interest in diluting professionalisation, since this kept nursing numbers up and costs therefore down. Trades-union activism spread among the unregistered nurses. A new and lower grade of nurse, the enrolled nurse, was recommended just before the outbreak of World War II. The move towards professionalisation was thus beset by internal and external difficulties—internally by different conceptions of nursing's role, and externally by the intervention of the Ministry of Health and the demands of government economic policy.

5 Dutt was undoubtedly correct in stating that the needs of the working population of India, as in other colonies, had not been adequately addressed by systems of health care which privileged white interests above those of the indigenous population. The colonial powers did practically nothing in this period to alleviate the widespread poverty and malnutrition which were the underlying causes of ill-health among indigenous peoples. Equally, the problem of chronic disease, as opposed to epidemic and infectious disease, was largely ignored. Yet Dutt fails to take account of the many genuine attempts that were made to improve the health of Indians and other colonial peoples in the inter-war period: attempts that constituted a significant shift from the limited interventionism of the nineteenth century.

Chapter 6

1 The acute hospital services were given priority when resources were scarce for a number of reasons:

(a) The under-resourced hospitals inherited from the pre-NHS system were in urgent need of bringing up to the standard elsewhere in Europe and the USA.

(b) The revolution in high-technology medicine created a demand for surgery, X-rays, pathology laboratories and blood transfusion services, all of which could only be supplied by hospitals. There was also increasing demand for childbirth in hospitals.

(c) It was politically easier to focus resources on hospitals because they were under state control.

However, prioritising the acute hospitals meant that the bias in health care shifted towards the curative services. The preventive and primary health-care services became Cinderellas, starved of resources and attention. Only after a long delay, with rising demand for community care and avoidance of unnecessary institutionalisation, was the concept of a first-class service altered to involve better balance between services.

2 As indicated in Chapter 5, Bevan inherited the wartime faith in rational and integrated planning with a view to securing the most economical and effective use of scarce human and material resources. This ideally involved administration of all local health services by local government, which was also responsible for other personal services such as housing and education.

However, the government was forced into making concessions to medical vested interests. Unification of health services under local government was unacceptable to the medical profession. Because of opposition to integration by the BMA, primary care was administered by Executive Councils, which were merely updated National Insurance Committees. Also, to meet the demands of the powerful organisations representing consultants, each teaching hospital was given complete independence, while individual hospitals were granted a high degree of autonomy, under committees upon which consultants and former trustees of voluntary hospitals were dominant. Finally, the pattern of expenditure of the new health services replicated most of the inequalities of the pre-war system.

3 Community care in the immediate post-war period meant care at home supported by a wide range of local-authority, voluntary and health-authority-provided services. In the 1950s and 1960s, it also came to mean residential care in the community in residential homes, for elderly people in particular, and domiciliary care was downgraded. In practice, because of the poor coordination between different services providing domiciliary care and the patchy provision of residential accommodation, the role of lay care, i.e. care by family and friends, remained considerable.

4 The status of the GP in the immediate post-war period was low. The GP's rise in status between 1948 and 1974 involved: the establishment of a new image and 'function' for the GP; a new professional body, the College of General Practitioners; government support for general practice and primary health care, and GP management of other health-care occupations, e.g. health visitors.

5 Public-health doctors lost their hospital 'empires'. Many health campaigns were run by single-issue pressure groups rather than involving MOHs. Examples you

could cite are campaigns on air pollution; birth control; abortion; and housing.

6   Your answer should include some of the following points:

(a)   Strong confidence in, and the prestige associated with, Western medical and pharmaceutical technology led to the importation of expensive drugs and therapeutic and diagnostic equipment for referral hospitals. This skewed the health budget towards hospitals in capital cities.

(b)   Indigenous systems of medicine were undermined and devalued by the emphasis on the perceived scientific superiority of Western medicine.

(c)   The establishment of research bodies and medical schools run on European lines, with comparability of standards, led to the teaching of irrelevant curricula, and the perception that the best training could only be obtained 'abroad'. Third World professionals often left their own countries to specialise in industrialised countries, and were not encouraged to return because they could not practise medicine under the same conditions, or earn as much.

(d)   Social reform of the type that occurred in some European countries (e.g. West Germany and France) after World War II was discussed but not, on the whole, implemented in Third World countries for a number of complex reasons, e.g. opposition from within the political and administrative structures, resistance of the medical profession to change, and Cold War ideology.

Chapter 7

1   The changes of 1974 were detrimental to local accountability by:

(a)   eliminating the direct local-authority stake in the health services, which was the only part of the health service directly accountable to local electorates;

(b)   increasing the managerial bias of the three-tier structure of health authority administration; and

(c)   placing greater authority with consensus management teams representing the professions.

The changes of the 1980s reinforced the effect of (a) and (b) by progressively reducing local-authority and trades-union membership of health authorities and increasing management control. The restructuring of 1991 formally ratified these changes. Representation of consumer interests has increasingly depended on the effectiveness of Community Health Councils, which themselves are not formally accountable to the public. The 1991 structure relies on GP fund-holders and District Health Authority purchasing policies to represent the interests of the consumer.

2   There is much to say for the hypothesis of continuity between 1948 and 1988. The Conservative Party perhaps favoured modifying the NHS, but in practice, there was considerable continuity of policy between Labour and Conservative administrations. The only shifts in policy before 1988 which were alien to the Labour Party were limited experiments in privatisation, the escalation of direct charges on prescriptions, erosion of the teeth and eye services, and the Griffiths management changes. The Labour Party's main complaint related to the level of funding for the NHS.

Since 1988 the purchaser–provider split, and the ongoing fragmentation of the service into competing units marks a fundamental break with the principles of the wartime planners and the 1948 system, and in some respects it is a reversion to the pre-war system in which local authorities purchased services from a variety of independent and competing agencies, especially the voluntary hospitals, which have clear similarities with the new hospital Trusts. The fund-holder scheme for general practice, introduced in 1991, is without historical precedent in British health care.

3   The concept of community care was redefined to mean not just care *in* the community, but also care *by* the community. The assumption was that female labour in the family would supply the deficiencies of statutory services. Many women did try to fulfil this role, although demographic changes made it harder. More women lived at a distance from elderly relatives, and more worked full- or part-time. Little financial help was available for women who stayed at home to care. Many studies show that much of lay care in the community was provided by elderly people for other elderly people; this was again a relationship where women, rather than men, did most of the caring.

4   This case illustrates what might be the logical outcome of the emphasis on managerialism and the importance of general managers as opposed to the traditional power of the medical profession. The quotation illustrates a significant change in the balance of power between non-medical and medical in health services. But, as the discussion in Chapter 7 indicates, these changes have not yet been overwhelming. The power of the medical profession has not yet been significantly eroded. Managerialism has had an impact on nursing, where it exacerbated tensions between different conceptions of nursing. It should not be forgotten that managerialism was not the only tendency at this period. Unionisation

was also a strong force among nurses as it was among hospital ancillary workers and among doctors through the BMA and the hospital doctors' unions.

5   The consensus around health education as a tool of health policy established itself through the relatively non-controversial nature of such education. Health education did not overtly attack vested interests—it was attractive to politicians for giving the appearance of concern without demanding substantive action against economic interests (for instance the alcohol, tobacco and food industries). The focus on health education suited the 'single issue' focus of public health in the 1970s and 1980s and it fitted the model of health problems as the result of individual behavioural defects. Health education thus had a moral as well as a health dimension.

Chapter 8

1   Your answer should include some of the following points:

(a)   The Chinese barefoot doctor was a stimulus for thinking about the mutually beneficial relationship between community and health worker.

(b)   Social research encouraged ideas that lay people were already, and could be more, involved in health care, providing a link between formal health services and communities.

(c)   Concern about consumer dissatisfaction within international organisations such as the WHO led to active searching for ways in which communities could be involved in health and health care.

2   Your answer should include some of the following points:

(a)   Third World countries cannot afford to train doctors and nurses in the necessary numbers to ensure that the whole population has access to a health professional. Many community health workers (or traditional midwives) can be trained for the price of training one nurse or doctor. Because their training is shorter, they can be paid much lower salaries than professionals, and some work unpaid.

(b)   Many health professionals dislike living and working in rural areas, and refuse to spend any length of time in the countryside.

(c)   People in small communities feel more comfortable with someone from their own area, and prefer taking health problems to them than to a professionally trained health worker who may not speak the same language, or know that part of the country, or the habits and customs of the community.

3   *Selective* programmes tend to be vertically organised, and not integrated with other health services; they focus on one health problem, diverting attention and resources away from other, equally or more important, problems; they are often based on simplistic assumptions about people's behaviour, and do not take into sufficient account the various socio-economic and cultural factors affecting behaviour; they may not be sustainable over the long run; they focus on outputs (numbers of immunisations undertaken, numbers of oral rehydration packets sold) but often cannot say what the impact of the programme has been on the particular problem.

Comprehensive PHC, on the other hand, is based on a broad philosophy about health and disease, which is difficult to put into operation without clear overall government policy. It demands a redistribution of resources across a number of sectors including the environment, education and employment—not only health. Within the health sector, it means building up health services in general, and not focusing only on one or two diseases, although any comprehensive PHC programme will also have a programme of priorities.

4   Lack of resources because of continuing debt and economic constraints; ecological deterioration through overgrazing, destruction of forests, desertification, loss of topsoil, and chemicals that are damaging to the ozone layer or water-polluting; in urban areas, overcrowding, lack of resources for infrastructure, e.g. provision of adequate housing, clean water, drainage (especially where flooding is likely), sewage and garbage disposal, etc.

Chapter 9

1   There is a broad association between national income and health spending, as shown for example in Figure 9.1. However, there are many instances of countries spending more or less than might be predicted on the basis of their national income, as Figure 9.1 makes clear. In addition, the chapter suggested (Figure 9.2) that as national income increases countries tend to devote a higher *proportion* of it to health care.

2   The United Kingdom is unusually reliant on general taxation to fund health care, and out-of-pocket expenses form a relatively small part of health-care funding in the United Kingdom. More generally, the public-sector share of health spending in the United Kingdom is quite high in comparison to that of the OECD countries as a whole. However, the broad trends in Britain seem to have been in line with other countries in recent decades: a slow growth in public-sector financing until the mid-1970s, followed

by a decline in the late 1970s and 1980s as the policy emphasis shifted towards the private sector and direct charges.

3   Researchers have suggested the existence of a phenomenon known as supplier-induced demand: doctors can in effect decide how much of their own services to 'demand'. If financial incentives exist to increase the amount of care provided, as where fee-for-service payment operates, the phenomenon may be reinforced. Thus attempts to overcome a 'shortage' of doctors by increasing their numbers could result in even more demand being generated for their services, and the 'shortage' continuing.

4   It is broadly true that pharmaceutical companies concentrate on areas where a market exists. Unfortunately many of the commonest diseases, especially infectious and parasitic diseases, are found in the Third World, where markets are small because incomes are low. This leads to a lower research priority in these areas, which in turn reduces the likelihood that appropriate drugs will be developed for particular health problems in the Third World.

Index